Endoscopy in the Diagnosis of Small Intestine Diseases

Toshiyuki Matsui • Takayuki Matsumoto
Kunihiko Aoyagi
Editors

Endoscopy in the Diagnosis of Small Intestine Diseases

Springer

Editors
Toshiyuki Matsui
Department of Gastroenterology
Fukuoka University Chikushi Hospital
Chikushino, Japan

Kunihiko Aoyagi
Department of Gastroenterology and Medicine
Fukuoka University Faculty of Medicine
Fukuoka, Japan

Takayuki Matsumoto
Department of Medicine and Clinical Science
Graduate School of Medicine
Kyushu University
Fukuoka, Japan

ISBN 978-4-431-54351-0 ISBN 978-4-431-54352-7 (eBook)
DOI 10.1007/978-4-431-54352-7
Springer Tokyo Heidelberg New York Dordrecht London

Library of Congress Control Number: 2013956236

Printed on acid-free paper

Springer is part of Springer Science+Business Media (www.springer.com)

Preface

This volume was about one year in the planning, and was inspired by the realization that capsule endoscopy and double-balloon endoscopy frequently reveal findings that nevertheless do not result in diagnosis. Another reason was our recognition of the difficulty in distinguishing findings of ulcerative colitis from those of Crohn's disease and other disorders in small intestinal endoscopy. Of course, we have seen numerous case presentations at academic conferences and have also read several books on small intestinal endoscopy. However, these frequently do nothing more than list a large number of disorders without providing a detailed analysis of findings. European and American reference works also seem to fail to address issues such as radiographic comparisons. When endoscopic findings were discussed at an international conference on double-balloon endoscopy held in Japan a few years ago, a leading Western researcher was unaware of such basic observations as the fact that ulcers of the small intestine present on the side of mesenteric attachment in Crohn's disease and on the opposite side in tuberculosis. Probably this lack of awareness was mainly because the researcher had never seen an accurate macroscopic depiction of a resected specimen. Although the United States and European nations are advanced in terms of capsule endoscopy, Americans and Europeans still face many problems in diagnostic imaging for this very reason. We therefore decided to put together a large number of carefully selected Japanese examples of small intestinal lesions, in an effort to compare and contrast small intestinal lesions that exhibit consistent findings and morphologies.

The basic premise of this book is differential diagnosis on the basis of endoscopic findings, and readers should start by taking a close look at the individual endoscopic findings illustrated on the left side of each full-page spread. We have then added an explanation of each finding on the right side, together with radiographic images and macroscopic depictions of resected specimens for comparison. This layout was designed with everyday clinical practice in mind, and we hope that readers will interpret the elements that compose each of these endoscopic findings with the aim of understanding the pathology and distinguishing features of each condition. Radiographic comparisons comprise another important element of the findings. There are limitations to endoscopic observations when it comes to long or large lesions of the small intestine, with its many curves. Therefore, we have also emphasized radiographic findings in this volume. In Japan, many institutions still practice double-contrast imaging, providing beautiful results, and we believe this point will resonate with many readers. Since a single disorder may exhibit great variety, this volume includes multiple depictions of the same disorders. We have also included lesions in both active and inactive phases. This is because both appearances are highly likely to be encountered simultaneously in actual clinical practice. Presenting a good overall balance of these cases would require a huge page area. We therefore decided to limit the number of findings depicted and to put together only carefully selected cases. In producing a work such as this, we thought it important to reflect the underlying concept in the title. After consulting among all the editors, we decided on *Endoscopy in the Diagnosis of Small Intestine Diseases*.

Because we wanted this book to be published before the Japan Digestive Disease Week (JDDW) held in Fukuoka in the fall of 2011, we had only about six months to spend on production. The editors were in communication with one another on a daily basis and brought in colleagues to share diagnostic knowledge. The cases presented in this volume were assembled jointly from three institutions: the Department of Gastroenterology at Kyushu University, the Department of Gastroenterology at Fukuoka University, and the Department of Gastroenterology at Fukuoka University Chikushi Hospital. A number of cases were requested from leading researchers at external institutions in the event that no suitable case was available from any of these three institutions. Within our group, we regularly hold joint seminars and undertake joint clinical trials. As we were already using the same methods for diagnosing small intestinal disease and applying radiographic procedures and treatment methods, we could assemble cases at the same pace. This meant that each institution ultimately held responsibility for a very similar number of cases.

As members of our group have some predecessors in common, we have a long history of joint research into disorders of the small intestine, such as Crohn's disease. We have also treated and accumulated a large number of cases. *Shōchō shikkan no rinshō* (Clinical Treatment of Small Intestinal Disease), edited by Tsuneyoshi Yao and Mitsuo Iida, was a major compilation of a large number of disorders published by Igaku Shoin in 2004. Since then, dramatic advances have been made in the field of small intestinal endoscopy. The simplicity of diagnostic operations has also meant that an increased number of images are now shared among multiple institutions. However, the inadequacy of a number of aspects has also become evident, including comparisons with radiography, pathological diagnosis, and handling of cases. We therefore regarded as a matter of great importance the publication of this volume focusing on accurate diagnosis and procedures for differentiating between conditions on the basis of endoscopic findings.

We are grateful for the assistance of Mr. Shingo Ano from the Medical Publications Department of Igaku Shoin in the production of this book. He established the original plan, provided swift editing, and overcame numerous problems in assembling the manuscript. We would also like to express our warm thanks to the pathologists who provide everyday diagnostic support for our clinical work. We are profoundly grateful to Dr. Akinori Iwashita (Department of Pathology, Fukuoka University Chikushi Hospital), Dr. Minako Hirahashi (Department of Anatomic Pathology, Graduate School of Medical Sciences, Kyushu University), Dr. Satoshi Nimura (Department of Pathology, Fukuoka University Faculty of Medicine), and Dr. Takashi Yao (Department of Human Pathology, Juntendo University School of Medicine; formerly of the Department of Anatomic Pathology, Graduate School of Medical Sciences, Kyushu University), who not only were involved in diagnosing the cases presented in this volume, but also have been passionately dedicated to the macroscopic and histological diagnosis of small intestinal disease for many years. It is thanks to their efforts that we were able to compile this volume. If our purpose in proposing this book is widely understood and arouses interest in the interpretation of findings rather than being viewed solely as a collection of rare cases, we will have succeeded beyond our expectations.

Chikushino, Japan

Toshiyuki Matsui
On behalf of the editors

Preface to the English Edition

The original Japanese edition of this book was prepared in October 2011. It has subsequently been published as an English atlas, and its content remains extremely valuable. In this preface to the English edition, we would like to emphasize several points.

We are currently in the era of small intestinal diagnostic endoscopy. Since 2000, the advent of double-balloon endoscopy and capsule endoscopy has shed new light on small intestine diseases. Thanks to the results of substantial research, a large number of small intestine diseases can now be diagnosed. In particular, the pathology of obscure gastrointestinal bleeding (OGIB) has now been almost completely explained. However, for many small intestine diseases, the diagnostic sensitivity and specificity of endoscopy remains low. This may be due to the poor resolution of the endoscopic images obtained, or the inability, for a variety of reasons, to depict small intestinal lesions accurately. The small intestine is extremely long; therefore, inserting the endoscope and completing the examination can be difficult. Both skill and creativity are required to overcome these problems. In addition, although small intestine diseases themselves are relatively few in number, they may display wide variations in morphology, which may also contribute to the difficulty of endoscopic diagnosis. For this reason, it is important to study in advance endoscopic images of key diseases in an atlas. Here, we should learn from the study of diagnostics in other fields. Endoscopic diagnosis of the severity of ulcerative colitis is surprisingly difficult, and determinations of the Mayo score frequently differ greatly between observers. This is because the definitions in the documents are inconsistent with the decisions made during actual diagnostic endoscopy. Production of an endoscopy atlas with an emphasis on severity has been shown to improve inter-observer consistency. Such subtle inter-observer variability also occurs in diagnostic image-enhanced endoscopy (IEE). This is because completely new diagnostic imaging criteria are used, and shared awareness of how to use them is currently lacking. In this situation, too, the production of an atlas is regarded as useful for establishing common perspectives. Atlases are thus used in many new fields of diagnostics.

Diseases of the small intestine may display many morphological variations, even if they share the same diagnosis. Simply providing a catalog of numerous endoscopic images for each diagnosis is not an efficient method to facilitate learning. Therefore, this atlas has adopted the format of categorizing lesions by morphology and providing a catalog of the corresponding diseases, both for the reason mentioned above and for consistency with the actual diagnostic process. Although this is a novel format, we consider it a highly effective approach to learning. This atlas has also been designed with problems set out on the left-hand page and their answers and explanations on the right, in the hope of cultivating an inquiring mind on the part of readers. Several major problems with the diagnosis of small intestine disease remain, and it is not a perfect form of diagnostics. If this book eventually becomes known as a milestone on the journey toward effective diagnostics, it would far exceed even the greatest hopes of the editors.

Here we would like to give a simple description of the characteristics of diagnostic endoscopy in Japan. The Japanese tend to emphasize comparisons either with macroscopic images or with macroscopic and histological images of resected specimens as the basis of diagnostic endoscopy. They are thus constantly aware of the rationalization and interpretation of endoscopic images, and for this reason, they pay special attention to resected materials. They also frequently bear the findings of endoscopic observation in mind when immobilizing or resecting specimens. Their detailed expertise in the endoscopic diagnosis of both early gastric cancer and early colorectal cancer has been cultivated in this way. We believe it is appropriate to apply this concept to small intestine diseases. Therefore, macroscopic images of resected specimens also appear in this atlas for comparison, as the morphological characteristics should help improve the interpretation of endoscopic images. Comparisons of radiographic and endoscopic images are also fundamental to Japanese diagnostics, for the same reason. Here we would like to mention some examples from other fields. For example, colitis-associated cancer is difficult to diagnose. It has been previously regarded as beyond the diagnostic capability of modern endoscopy, with diagnosis possible only by means of blind biopsy. If it had not been for the Japanese style of diagnostics, which involves painstakingly cutting out resected colorectal materials and comparing them with findings from diagnostic endoscopy (such as the extent of redness, as well as detailed patterns and differences in level), endoscopic diagnosis of this condition would have remained a pipe dream. However, endoscopic diagnosis of various small intestine diseases, driven by improvements to procedures and the development of new devices, is gradually becoming a reality.

The morphology of small intestine diseases may be difficult to accurately imagine in two dimensions for many reasons, including whether a lesion is in the active phase, whether it is hemorrhaging, its orientation, and its relationship with the long axis. Observations may often be inadequate due to the lumen being immobilized by adhesions, fistula formation, and so on. Of course, endoscopic observation is often impossible if stenosis is present. To overcome these problems, it may be necessary to combine endoscopy with procedures such as barium contrast, computed tomography, and magnetic resonance imaging. We regard diagnostic radiography of the small intestine as preferable from the perspectives of panoramic imaging of small intestinal disease and visualization of the mucosal surface, and have endeavored to master diagnostic radiography for many years. However, the impact of diagnostic endoscopy normally far outweighs diagnostic radiography, and endoscopy is gradually becoming the main method of diagnosis.

Histopathological diagnosis also had limitations in the small intestine. Little biopsy material is typically available, and histological diagnosis may end unsatisfactorily for reasons such as unresectability. When producing this atlas, we requested numerous diagnoses from pathologists. From among those diagnoses, we have concentrated on cases with adequate diagnostic results. For rare diseases, this frequently involved a large amount of work from the diagnostic perspective. Therefore, we would like to express our profound gratitude to those pathologists here. Of course, we requested individuals with ideas similar to our own to author the clinical side. Due to the large number of items, we asked young doctors from the departments of gastroenterology at Kyushu University, Fukuoka University, and Fukuoka University Chikushi Hospital to provide case descriptions. These three universities have grown from a shared foundation and are constantly holding joint case conferences and study groups. On this point, a shared perspective on endoscopy has already been established. The pathologists of these universities have also developed from a shared foundation, meaning that differing viewpoints are not an issue.

Some of the problems we encountered in the production of this atlas were that images were somewhat small and their resolution was not fully utilized, and it was not possible to provide adequate space to other images. However, the compact design of the atlas was chosen because our priority was to include as many images as possible. We hope that readers will understand the purpose of this atlas and will utilize it to train young endoscopy practitioners.

Chikushino, Japan
Fukuoka, Japan

Toshiyuki Matsui
Kunihiko Aoyagi
Takayuki Matsumoto

Contents

Part III Basic Knowledge and Classification

Contributors

Koichi Abe (Chapter 18.11, Chapter 27) Department of Gastroenterology and Medicine, Fukuoka University Faculty of Medicine, Fukuoka, Japan

Kunihiko Aoyagi (Chapter 7, Chapter 12, Chapter 13, Chapter 18.2, 7, Chapter 23.7, Chapter 26.2) Department of Gastroenterology and Medicine, Fukuoka University Faculty of Medicine, Fukuoka, Japan

Kouichi Asano (Chapter 23.5) Department of Medicine and Clinical Science, Graduate School of Medical Sciences, Kyushu University, Fukuoka, Japan

Takahiro Beppu (Chapter 4, Chapter 9, Chapter 19.1, Chapter 22.3, Chapter 23.14) Department of Gastroenterology, Fukuoka University Chikushi Hospital, Chikushino, Japan

Issei Egashira (Chapter 16.11, Chapter 24.1) Department of Medicine and Clinical Science, Graduate School of Medical Sciences, Kyushu University, Fukuoka, Japan

Koichi Eguchi (Chapter 18.4, Chapter 23.13, Chapter 26.1) Department of Gastroenterology and Medicine, Fukuoka University Faculty of Medicine, Fukuoka, Japan

Motohiro Esaki (Chapter 3, Chapter 19.10, Chapter 23.12, Chapter 24.5) Department of Medicine and Clinical Science, Graduate School of Medical Sciences, Kyushu University, Fukuoka, Japan

Shin Fujioka (Chapter 18.1, Chapter 24.2) Department of Medicine and Clinical Science, Graduate School of Medical Sciences, Kyushu University, Fukuoka, Japan

Ritsuko Fujisawa (Chapter 18.10) Department of Medicine and Clinical Science, Graduate School of Medical Sciences, Kyushu University, Fukuoka, Japan

Kohei Fujita (Chapter 17.10) Department of Gastroenterology, Fukuoka Red Cross Hospital, Fukuoka, Japan

Sadahiro Funakoshi (Chapter 16.3, Chapter 17.1) Department of Gastroenterology and Medicine, Fukuoka University Faculty of Medicine, Fukuoka, Japan

Minako Hirahashi (Chapter 25.4) Department of Medicine and Clinical Science, Graduate School of Medical Sciences, Kyushu University, Fukuoka, Japan

Fumihito Hirai (Chapter 2, Chapter 4, Chapter 8, Chapter 19.12, 13) Department of Gastroenterology, Fukuoka University Chikushi Hospital, Chikushino, Japan

Atsushi Hirano (Chapter 14.2) Department of Medicine and Clinical Science, Graduate School of Medical Sciences, Kyushu University, Fukuoka, Japan

Takashi Hisabe (Chapter 23.9, Chapter 24.4, Chapter 29) Department of Gastroenterology, Fukuoka University Chikushi Hospital, Chikushino, Japan

Hideki Ishibashi (Chapter 16.7, 10, Chapter 19.14) Department of Gastroenterology and Medicine, Fukuoka University Faculty of Medicine, Fukuoka, Japan

Satoshi Ishikawa (Chapter 19.15, Chapter 22.2) Department of Gastroenterology, Fukuoka University Chikushi Hospital, Chikushino, Japan

Takao Kanemitsu (Chapter 17.2) Department of Gastroenterology, Fukuoka University Chikushi Hospital, Chikushino, Japan

Yoshihiko Karashima (Chapter 16.2) Department of Gastroenterology, Fukuoka University Chikushi Hospital, Chikushino, Japan

Hiroshi Kawano (Chapter 14.4, Chapter 18.8) Division of Gastroenterology, Department of Medicine, Kurume University School of Medicine, Kurume, Japan

Fukunori Kaneshiro (Chapter 23.8) Department of Endoscopy, Faculty of Medicine, University of the Ryukyus, Okinawa, Japan

Ken Kinjo (Chapter 21.7, Chapter 22.1) Department of Gastroenterology, Fukuoka University Chikushi Hospital, Chikushino, Japan

Masahiro Kishi (Chapter 25.6) Department of Gastroenterology, Fukuoka University Chikushi Hospital, Chikushino, Japan

Kazuto Kishimoto (Chapter 23.8) Department of Endoscopy, Faculty of Medicine, University of the Ryukyus, Okinawa, Japan

Mayumi Kodama (Chapter 21.5) Center for Digestive and Liver Diseases, Miyazaki Medical Center Hospital, Miyazaki, Japan

Naoya Kubokura (Chapter 19.11, Chapter 20.5) Department of Medicine and Clinical Science, Graduate School of Medical Sciences, Kyushu University, Fukuoka, Japan

Yuji Maehata (Chapter 14.1, Chapter 18.3) Department of Medicine and Clinical Science, Graduate School of Medical Sciences, Kyushu University, Fukuoka, Japan

Takayuki Matsumoto (Chapter 1, Chapter 3, Chapter 11, Chapter 15, Chapter 17.8, Chapter 20.7, 8, 9, Chapter 23.1) Department of Medicine and Clinical Science, Graduate School of Medicine, Kyushu University, Fukuoka, Japan

Tomohiko Moriyama (Chapter 21.6, Chapter 25.3) Department of Medicine and Clinical Science, Graduate School of Medical Sciences, Kyushu University, Fukuoka, Japan

Takashi Nagahama (Chapter 25.7) Department of Gastroenterology, Fukuoka University Chikushi Hospital, Chikushino, Japan

Shotaro Nakamura (Chapter 6, Chapter 17.5, 6, Chapter 18.6, Chapter 19.3, Chapter 20.3, Chapter 25.1, Chapter 28) Department of Medicine and Clinical Science, Graduate School of Medical Sciences, Kyushu University, Fukuoka, Japan

Tomoko Nawata (Chapter 19.16) Department of Gastroenterology and Medicine, Fukuoka University Faculty of Medicine, Fukuoka, Japan

Kazeo Ninomiya (Chapter 16.5, 9) Department of Gastroenterology, Fukuoka University Chikushi Hospital, Chikushino, Japan

Naoki Ohmiya (Chapter 5, Chapter 23.3, Chapter 25.5) Department of Gastroenterology, Nagoya University Graduate School of Medicine, Nagoya, Japan

Kensei Ohtsu (Chapter 20.6, Chapter 23.2, 4) Department of Gastroenterology, Fukuoka University Chikushi Hospital, Chikushino, Japan

Yoichiro Ono (Chapter 19.6, 7, Chapter 24.3) Department of Gastroenterology, Fukuoka University Chikushi Hospital, Chikushino, Japan

Yuho Sato (Chapter 16.1) Department of Gastroenterology, Fukuoka University Chikushi Hospital, Chikushino, Japan

Mitsue Sogawa (Chapter 19.8, 17, Chapter 22.4) Department of Gastroenterology, Osaka City University Graduate School of Medicine, Osaka, Japan

Haruhiko Takahashi (Chapter 17.9) Department of Gastroenterology, Fukuoka University Chikushi Hospital, Chikushino, Japan

Yasuhiro Takaki (Chapter 23.6) Department of Gastroenterology, Fukuoka University Chikushi Hospital, Chikushino, Japan

Noritaka Takatsu (Chapter 17.3, 7) Department of Gastroenterology, Fukuoka University Chikushi Hospital, Chikushino, Japan

Yoshitaka Tomioka (Chapter 18.9, Chapter 19.18. Chapter 20.10) Department of Gastroenterology and Medicine, Fukuoka University Faculty of Medicine, Fukuoka, Japan

Shinji Tsukamoto (Chapter 20.1) Department of Gastroenterology and Medicine, Fukuoka University Faculty of Medicine, Fukuoka, Japan

Kozue Tsurumi (Chapter 19.4, 5) Department of Gastroenterology, Fukuoka University Chikushi Hospital, Chikushino, Japan

Kenji Watanabe (Chapter 19.8, 17, Chapter 22.4) Department of Gastroenterology, Osaka City University Graduate School of Medicine, Osaka, Japan

Takashi Watanabe (Chapter 19.9, Chapter 20.4) Department of Gastroenterology and Medicine, Fukuoka University Faculty of Medicine, Fukuoka, Japan

Masashi Yamaguchi (Chapter 17.4, Chapter 19.2, Chapter 20.2) Department of Gastroenterology and Medicine, Fukuoka University Faculty of Medicine, Fukuoka, Japan

Shunichi Yanai (Chapter 14.3, Chapter 25.2) Japan Seamen's Relief Association Moji Hospital, Kitakyushu, Japan

Tomonori Yano (Chapter 10, Chapter 16.6, 8, Chapter 21.1, 2, 3, 4) Department of Internal Medicine, Division of Gastroenterology, Jichi Medical University, Shimotsuke, Japan

Yutaka Yano (Chapter 18.5) Department of Gastroenterology, Fukuoka University Chikushi Hospital, Chikushino, Japan

Part I

General Considerations

1 Diagnostic Process for Small Intestinal Disease

Takayuki Matsumoto

1.1 Symptomatology of Small Intestinal Disease

The small intestine is the longest organ of the digestive tract, with main functions of digestion, absorption, and maintenance of innate immunity. Accordingly, symptoms of small intestinal disease comprise impaired digestion and absorption due to widespread damage to the intestinal mucosa, as well as diarrhea, abdominal pain, and malnutrition caused by immune abnormalities. The development and widespread adoption of small intestinal endoscopic techniques has increased the frequency with which small intestinal lesions are diagnosed following hemorrhage from a small lesion. Symptoms of small intestinal disease must therefore be categorized into two types: gastrointestinal hemorrhage; and other symptoms. The latter are suggestive of more widespread small intestinal disease.

1.1.1 Gastrointestinal Hemorrhage

Hemorrhagic lesions may occur at any point along the gastrointestinal tract, from the oral cavity to the anus. If the apparent source of bleeding cannot be identified on upper gastrointestinal endoscopy or colonoscopy, this is known as "obscure gastrointestinal bleeding" (OGIB). OGIB is categorized as overt OGIB, in which red blood or black excretions comprising the metabolic products of hemoglobin are visible, or occult OGIB, which can only be confirmed by recurrent or persistent iron-deficiency anemia or a positive result on testing for fecal occult blood [1].

T. Matsumoto (✉)
Department of Medicine and Clinical Science, Graduate School of Medicine, Kyushu University, 3-1-1 Maidashi, Higashi-ku, Fukuoka, 812-8582, Japan
e-mail: matane@intmed2.med.kyushu-u.ac.jp

With overt OGIB in small intestinal disease, blood is excreted via the anus. The color of this blood is affected by the location and amount of hemorrhage, with stool being black or tarry for a small hemorrhage occurring *on the proximal side of GI tract*, and tinged with red in the case of a large hemorrhage or one occurring on the distal side.

1.1.2 Other Symptoms

1.1.2.1 Diarrhea

In healthy adults, around 9 L of orally ingested liquid and intestinal fluid flow into the small intestine each day, but the majority is reabsorbed, with only around 100–200 mL of liquid excreted in feces. Diarrhea is a condition comprising the repeated excretion of feces with increased liquid content, although there is no clear definition of the frequency or amount of liquid involved. The mechanisms whereby diarrhea occurs can be categorized as hyperosmosis of intestinal contents, increased exudation and hypersecretion by the intestinal mucosa due to small intestinal disease, and intestinal dysmotility (Table 1.1).

1.1.2.2 Edema, Pleural Effusion, and Ascites

Malabsorption syndrome or protein-losing enteropathy due to widespread damage to the small intestinal mucosa can cause hypoproteinemia. As a result, the colloidal osmotic pressure of serum drops, and edema, pleural effusion, and ascites occur. Normally, edema appears systemically and symmetrically as pitting edema. Improvement and exacerbation appear in accordance with changes in total serum protein levels. Serum protein levels are low, but serum lipid levels are normal. In many cases, the condition is accompanied by other signs of malnutrition, including weight loss, weakness, diarrhea, tetany, and osteomalacia. If lymphangiectasis is present, pleural effusion and ascites are milky.

T. Matsui et al. (eds.), *Endoscopy in the Diagnosis of Small Intestine Diseases*,
DOI 10.1007/978-4-431-54352-7_1, © Springer Japan 2014

Table 1.1 Mechanisms of diarrhea and associated disorders

	Osmotic diarrhea	Exudative diarrhea	Secretory diarrhea	Intestinal dysmotility
Mechanism	Increased liquid content due to rise in osmotic pressure within the intestine	Increased exudation by inflammatory lesions	Hypersecretion by the intestinal mucosa	Reduced transit time due to hyperperistalsis Intestinal bacterial proliferation due to hypoperistalsis
Features	Worsens with eating, improves with fasting	Worsens with eating, does not resolve completely even after fasting	Does not improve with fasting	Infrequently woken at night by diarrhea
	Steatorrhea, watery diarrhea	Bloody diarrhea, mucous and bloody stool present	Watery diarrhea, sometimes steatorrhea	Watery diarrhea
Main underlying disorders: acute	Oral saline laxatives	Infectious enteritis (infectious type)	Infectious enteritis (toxin production type)	
	Ingestion of non-absorbable sugars	Drug-induced enteropathy	Abuse of laxatives	
	Overeating	Ischemic enteritis		
Main underlying disorders: chronic	Malabsorption syndrome Short bowel syndrome	Chronic inflammatory bowel disease	Zollinger-Ellison syndrome WDHA syndrome	Irritable bowel syndrome Hyperthyroidism Scleroderma Amyloidosis Neurological disorders

1.1.2.3 Abdominal Distension and Flatulence

These are symptoms caused by the accumulation of excess gas or liquid in the small intestinal lumen or abdominal cavity, or the development of a massive tumor, with gas frequently accumulating due to intestinal stenosis. Under physiological conditions, the volume of gas in the intestines is maintained at around 100 mL. This volume increases, however, as a result of stenotic lesions of the intestinal tract or reduced intestinal motility, leading to abdominal distension and flatulence. In particular, nausea and vomiting are evident in cases of gastrointestinal stenosis, and may lead to alkalosis or hypochloremia if severe.

1.1.2.4 Abdominal Pain

This is the most common symptom of gastrointestinal disorders, and is non-specific. Depending on the mechanism involved, abdominal pain may be visceral, somatic or referred.

Visceral abdominal pain occurs when a stimulus to the intraluminal sensory nerve is transmitted through the intraluminal nerve plexus via sympathetic nerve afferent fibers to the brain. Transmission speed is slow, and an aching pain is felt that is not clearly localized. Somatic abdominal pain is a sharp, localized pain transmitted from receptors located in the peritoneum and mesenterium via the encephalomyeloneuropathic sensory conduction route, and is associated with symptoms of peritoneal irritation. Referred pain occurs when a strong stimulus from visceral abdominal pain spills over into somatic afferent nerves that run through the dorsal spinal root, resulting in the pain being perceived as somatic abdominal pain. The majority of abdominal pain in small intestinal disease is visceral abdominal pain in the periumbilical area. If caused by severe transmural inflammation and perforation, somatic abdominal pain becomes pronounced. Symptoms of peritoneal irritation may not be present during the acute phase of widespread ischemic small intestinal lesions, however, and caution is therefore required.

1.2 Diagnostic Procedure for Small Intestinal Disease

1.2.1 Patient Interview and Current Symptoms

As for other conditions, conducting the patient interview is often central to the diagnosis of small intestinal disease. This applies not just at the point when a lesion is suspected; reconfirmation of clinical information after a lesion has been confirmed must never be neglected. The small intestine is a common site for the occurrence of lesions as localized symptoms of systemic disorders, and it is important to ask about family history, including place of birth, and previous medical history (particularly tuberculosis infection, previous oral medication, foreign travel, autoimmune disorders, allergic disorders, radiation exposure, inflammatory bowel disease, and polyposis of the digestive tract). In terms of current symptoms, particular attention should be paid to the presence and nature of lesions of the skin, lips and oral cavity, and anal area, and a specialist should be consulted proactively for cases in which such findings are present.

1.2.2 Clinical Test Results

In addition to general testing such as blood and biochemical tests, Sudan III should be used to test for steatorrhea, and blood vitamin levels (vitamin K, vitamin B_{12}, and folic acid) can be measured using simple absorption tests. The α-1 antitrypsin clearance test is an appropriate technique for quantifying small intestinal protein exudate, and offers a valuable objective testing method if protein-losing enteropathy is strongly suspected or when strict indications such as response evaluation apply.

A wide range of testing methods have been developed for testing the absorption of sugars, protein, and lipids, but from the perspectives of reliability and clinical necessity, there is little opportunity to utilize these at present. Tests such as intestinal mucosa permeability tests using orally administered sugars as markers and fecal calprotectin can also be used as indirect indicators of small intestine inflammatory cell infiltration, but are not yet in wide use.

1.2.3 Imaging Techniques Other Than Small Intestinal Radiography and Endoscopy

The least invasive of these is abdominal ultrasonography, which can also be used to screen for a thickened bowel wall. In recent years, visualization of the small intestine by multidetector row computed tomography (MDCT) and magnetic resonance imaging (MRI) has improved, and in the United States and Europe the use of CT-enterography and MR-enterography is becoming more widespread. These techniques can also be expected to replace small intestinal radiography in Japan in the future. Nuclear medical techniques such as hemorrhagic scintigraphy and protein-losing scintigraphy have already been in use for some time, and today offer comparatively good diagnostic performance.

1.3 Diagnostic Algorithm for Small Intestinal Disease

1.3.1 OGIB

Small intestinal endoscopy has been shown in prospective studies to have a high rate of positive findings in OGIB compared with other diagnostic methods. This fact means that two approaches incorporating either capsule endoscopy or balloon endoscopy are recommended for OGIB [2, 3].

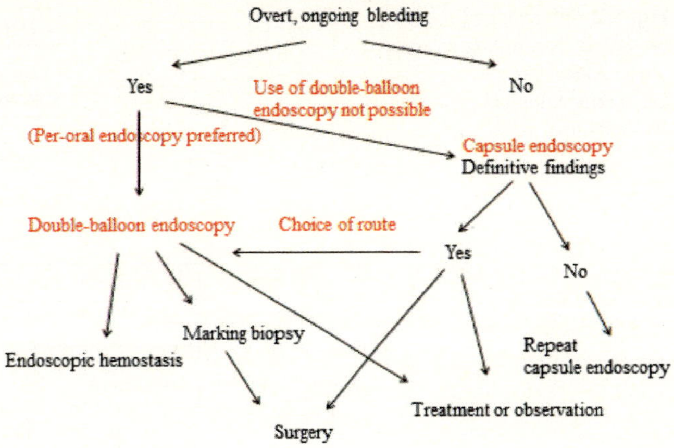

Fig. 1.1 Diagnostic process for OGIB (recommendations of the first international workshop on double-balloon endoscopy consensus meeting)

Figure 1.1 shows an algorithm centering on double-balloon endoscopy that was devised with the participation of Japanese small intestinal endoscopists [3]. Per-oral double-balloon endoscopy, which does not require any pretreatment, is used for overt OGIB, whereas capsule endoscopy is the first choice in cases of occult OGIB or when double-balloon endoscopy is difficult to perform. When using either of these diagnostic methods, the performance of endoscopic hemostasis and histological diagnosis by double-balloon endoscopy in cases with positive findings is assumed. This approach thus takes efficient treatment into account.

Figure 1.2 shows the algorithm proposed by the American Gastroenterology Association, which focuses on capsule endoscopy as the diagnostic method [2]. Capsule endoscopy is the first choice in cases of both overt and occult OGIB, and angiography is given as an option in cases of overt OGIB. Dealing with cases in which results of capsule endoscopy are negative is also referred to, with laparoscopic investigation and intraoperative endoscopy given as options.

In Japan, balloon endoscopy is widely used, and the diagnostic and treatment frameworks in use emphasize the first approach. Diagnosis and treatment of cases of overt OGIB are also performed with contrast CT as the first choice and interventional radiography as an additional treatment option. Given the fact that hemorrhagic lesions may have been missed by previous upper and lower gastrointestinal endoscopy, however, there should be no hesitation in performing repeated tests. If capsule endoscopy is preferred, the possibility of retention due to unexpected stenosis must be kept in mind.

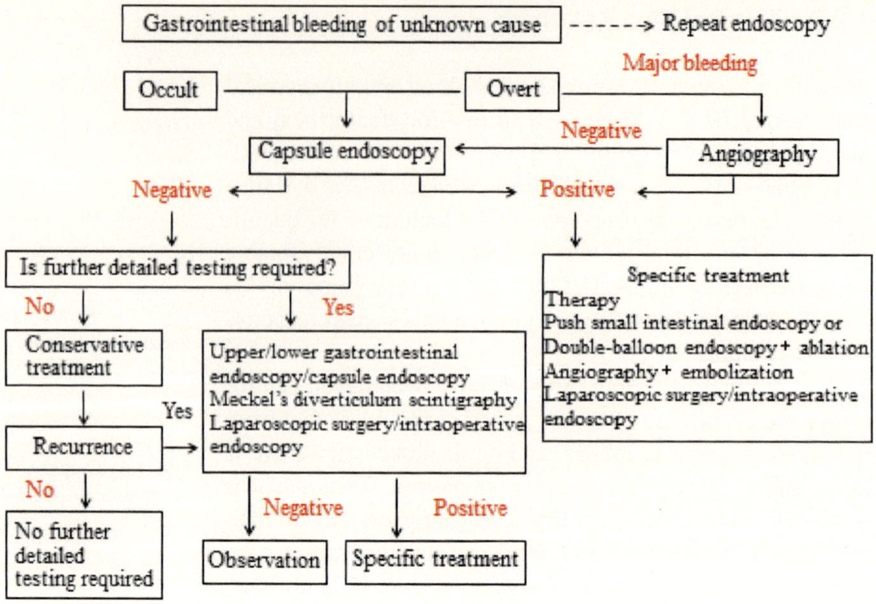

Fig. 1.2 Diagnostic process for OGIB (recommendations of the American Gastroenterological Association)

1.3.2 Small Intestinal Disease Other Than OGIB (Fig. 1.3)

For conditions other than OGIB, it is important to suspect small intestinal disease on the basis of the patient interview, physical findings, and general test results. In this process, it should be remembered that diffuse lesions and multisystem disorders are common. This means that information that is conclusive for diagnosis can frequently be obtained from diagnostic imaging, such as upper and lower gastrointestinal endoscopy, abdominal ultrasonography, and abdominal CT.

Decisions on whether to use radiography or endoscopy should also be made with care. Endoscopy is better suited to the diagnosis of small lesions and localized disease, whereas radiography is more useful for evaluating the extent of the affected area and the distribution of lesions. Radiography is particularly valuable for stenotic lesions and lesions located principally within the intestinal wall [4].

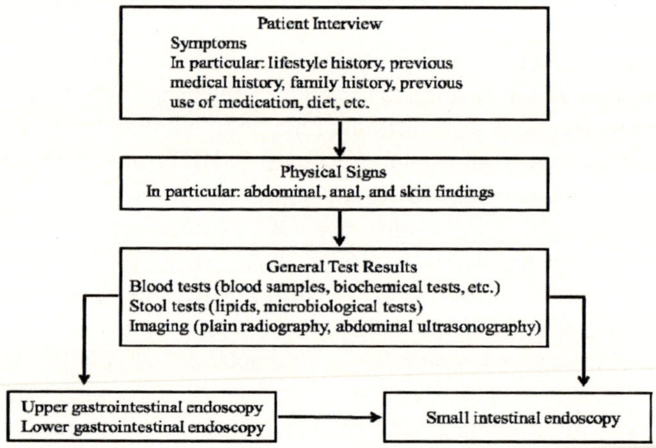

Fig. 1.3 Diagnostic process for small intestinal disease other than OGIB

References

1. Zuckerman GR et al. AGA technical review on the evaluation and management of occult and obscure gastrointestinal bleeding. Gastroenterology. 2000;118:201–21.
2. Raju GS et al. American Gastroenterological Association (AGA) institute technical review on obscure gastrointestinal bleeding. Gastroenterology. 2007;133:1697–717.
3. Sugano K, Marcon N. The first international workshop on double balloon endoscopy: a consensus meeting report. Gastrointest Endosc. 2007;66(3 Suppl):S7–11.
4. Matsumoto T et al. Is small-bowel radiography necessary before double-balloon endoscopy? AJR Am J Roentgenol. 2008;191:175–81.

2 Small Intestinal Radiography

Fumihito Hirai

2.1 Practical Importance of Radiographic Diagnosis

The advent of capsule endoscopy (CE) and balloon-assisted endoscopy (BAE) is revolutionizing the diagnosis of small intestinal disease, which has hitherto relied on radiographic methods. Endoscopic examination offers a range of advantages, and its future development and widespread adoption are expected. Conversely, the use of radiography can be anticipated to decline still further. However, it is unlikely that it will ever be possible to diagnose small intestinal disease using endoscopy alone, without any need for radiography. The small intestine is bordered on the proximal end by the esophagus, stomach, and duodenum, and on the distal end by the large intestine, and is the longest organ in the human body. These anatomical characteristics mean that it is no easy task to observe the small intestine in its entirety, even with the help of capsule and balloon endoscopy. Endoscopy may also encounter problems due to stenosis, adhesions, or unusual dispositions following surgery. From the disease perspective, although malignant conditions are less frequent compared with other parts of the gastrointestinal tract, chronic inflammatory disorders such as Crohn's disease and lesions associated with systemic disorders are common. In such disorders, grasping the entire picture and describing responses to treatment and the natural course objectively is more important than observing localized areas in detail. Radiography is clearly superior to endoscopy in terms of grasping the entire picture and objectively describing areas or lesions. If imaging is performed properly and interpreted by a competent practitioner, radiography will still have an important role to play in the diagnosis of small intestinal disease. Mechanical advances have also improved visualization by CT and MRI, and these modalities have recently been used for procedures such as enterography and enteroclysis. Unlike regular radiography, these methods also provide information external to the lumen, and have the advantages of being performable even if intestinal tract obstruction is present as well as minimal invasiveness, meaning they will continue to hold important places in diagnostic imaging of the small intestine.

2.2 Radiography of the Small Intestine [1–3]

Small intestinal radiography may be broadly divided into the per-oral method, in which contrast agent is administered by mouth, and the per-tube method, in which it is administered via a probe placed deep into the duodenum (in the neighborhood of the ligament of Treitz) or otherwise injected. Another special method is selective contrast administration following endoscopy of the large or small intestine. In actual clinical practice, the condition of the patient, suspected disease, and pathology of existing disorders are taken into account, and a method is selected in accordance with the objectives of radiography. Table 2.1 shows the contrast agents used in different methods, and the associated advantages and disadvantages [1–3]. Radiography is indicated in most types of small intestinal disease, but the use of barium in radiography is contraindicated in patients with obvious intestinal obstruction or generalized peritonitis.

2.2.1 Per-Oral Method

This can be performed simply to look for small intestinal lesions following gastric fluoroscopy, or with the small intestine as the sole target. In the former case, the objective of radiography is to identify gastric lesions and undertake detailed investigation, with the small intestine as the subject

F. Hirai (✉)
Department of Gastroenterology, Fukuoka University Chikushi Hospital, 1-1-1 Zokumyoin, Chikushino, Fukuoka 818-8502, Japan
e-mail: fuhirai@cis.fukuoka-u.ac.jp

T. Matsui et al. (eds.), *Endoscopy in the Diagnosis of Small Intestine Diseases*,
DOI 10.1007/978-4-431-54352-7_2, © Springer Japan 2014

Table 2.1 Comparison of methods of small intestinal radiography

	Contrast agent, etc.	Advantages	Disadvantages
1. Per-oral method	50–100 w/v %	Simple, minimally invasive	Poor visualization of small lesions
	200–300 mL	Can be used for screening	Easily affected by conditions
2. Per-tube method	50–100 w/v %	Capable of visualizing extensive lesions	Invasive (probe insertion)
(a) Double-contrast method (b) Herlinger's method	250–400 mL + 600–800 mL air	Good visualization of small lesions	Accuracy depends on operator
	70–90 w/v %	Short radiography time	Poor visualization of small lesions
	250–300 mL + 1.5-2.0 L 0.5 % methyl cellulose	Easy separation of loops of small intestine	Inferior visualization of lower ileum
3. Retrograde ileography	50–100 w/v % 100–250 mL +	Capable of visualizing intrapelvic lesions	Pain (due to insertion of endoscope into small intestine or large intestine), invasiveness
	200–500 mL air	Enables evaluation of proximal side of stenoses through which an endoscope is unable to pass	Complex procedure

Modified from Nakamura et al. [1], Yao [2]

of secondary observation. This discussion focuses on the latter case.

For barium, 200–250 mL of a 50–100 w/v % suspension is used. In our department, we normally administer 250 mL of 100 w/v % barium by mouth. Because of individual differences in transit time through the small intestine and the area to be investigated, however, this must be adjusted for each patient. A basic principle common to all small intestinal radiography is to separate the loops of small intestine as far as possible and eliminate overlap, to improve radiographic accuracy. In particular, as barium-filled and compression images are the main types of image with this technique, it is important for the small intestine to be completely filled with barium and for the loops of small intestine to be carefully compressed when searching. Different procedures are required for different areas to avoid overlapping of the small intestine. For the upper small intestine, a shallow left anterior oblique position is adopted, and observation and imaging are performed while the patient takes a deep breath. For the central small intestine, frontal imaging and a right anterior oblique position are adopted, and imaging is normally performed while the patient breathes in. In both cases, a small quilt may be used as necessary to apply an appropriate level of compression. The ileum within the small pelvic cavity and the terminal ileum are frequent sites of lesions, but are often difficult to separate. The use of sedatives and compression with a quilt are both effective, and clear separation can be achieved in many cases by putting the patient in the prone position and placing the quilt over the lower abdomen (Fig. 2.1a–c). Transanal air insufflation may also prove effective.

During fluoroscopy, or when interpreting images, it is important to focus on whether abnormal disposition edema, deformity, or stenosis is present. In particular, deformity is an important key to the identification of small intestinal disease. If a deformity is observed under fluoroscopy, applying pressure may permit some type of cause to be recognized in the surrounding area (Fig. 2.2a, b). It is vital to be well acquainted with the characteristic images seen in each different disorder in order to interpret radiographic images. For example, the presence of the widespread spoke-like lesions seen in systemic lupus erythematosus (SLE) (Fig. 2.3), or the longitudinal aphthae evident in Crohn's disease (Fig. 2.4) in themselves comes close to a confirmed diagnosis. Detailed descriptions of the various disorders are given in Part II, "Specific Findings of Small Intestinal Lesions," and are therefore omitted here, but it is important to carry out any additional tests required for diagnosis in an efficient manner based on the results obtained by this method.

2.2.2 Per-Tube Method

Two different methods are used: the double-contrast method [1, 2] utilizing air; and Herlinger's method [3] in which barium transit is enhanced by the use of methyl cellulose. In both cases, a 12- to 16-Fr probe is used, which is normally inserted per-nasally as far as the neighborhood of the ligament of Treitz under fluoroscopy. This technique is unaffected by gastric juices or transit time through stomach, unlike the per-oral method, and has the advantage that the

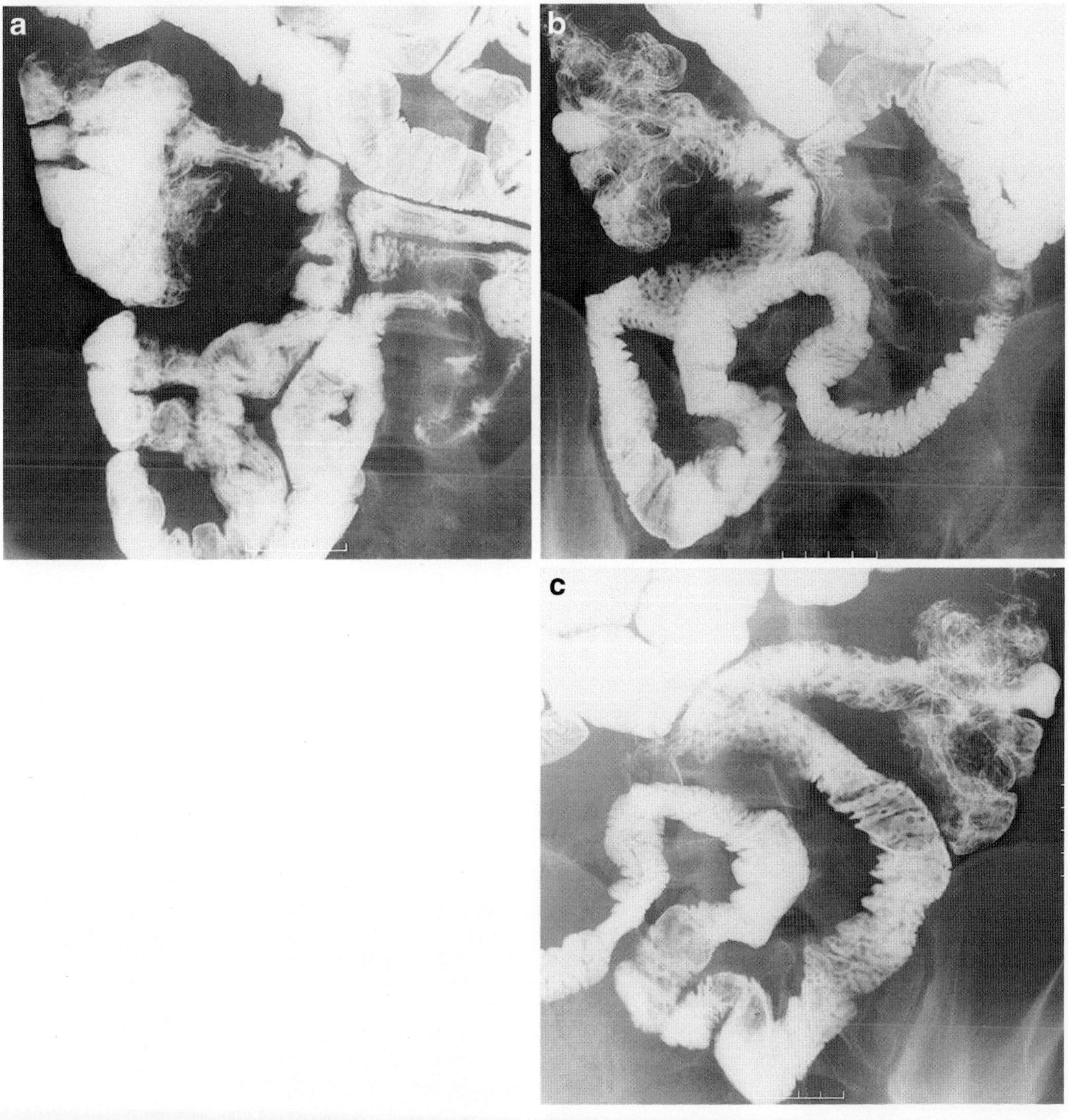

Fig. 2.1 Performance of per-oral small intestine contrast imaging. (**a**) X-ray image focusing on the lower ileum once the contrast agent has reached the terminal ileum. The intrapelvic small intestine is not separated. Peristalsis is present, making evaluation of the mucosal surface difficult. (**b**) Image obtained after intramuscular sedative injection and application of pressure with a quilt. The small intestine within the pelvis is almost completely separated, and lymph follicles are visualized in the terminal ileum. (**c**) When imaging is performed with the patient in the prone position and a quilt placed on the abdomen, the small intestine within the pelvis is completely separated. This image can be interpreted as showing the presence of multiple lymph follicles, restricted to the terminal ileum

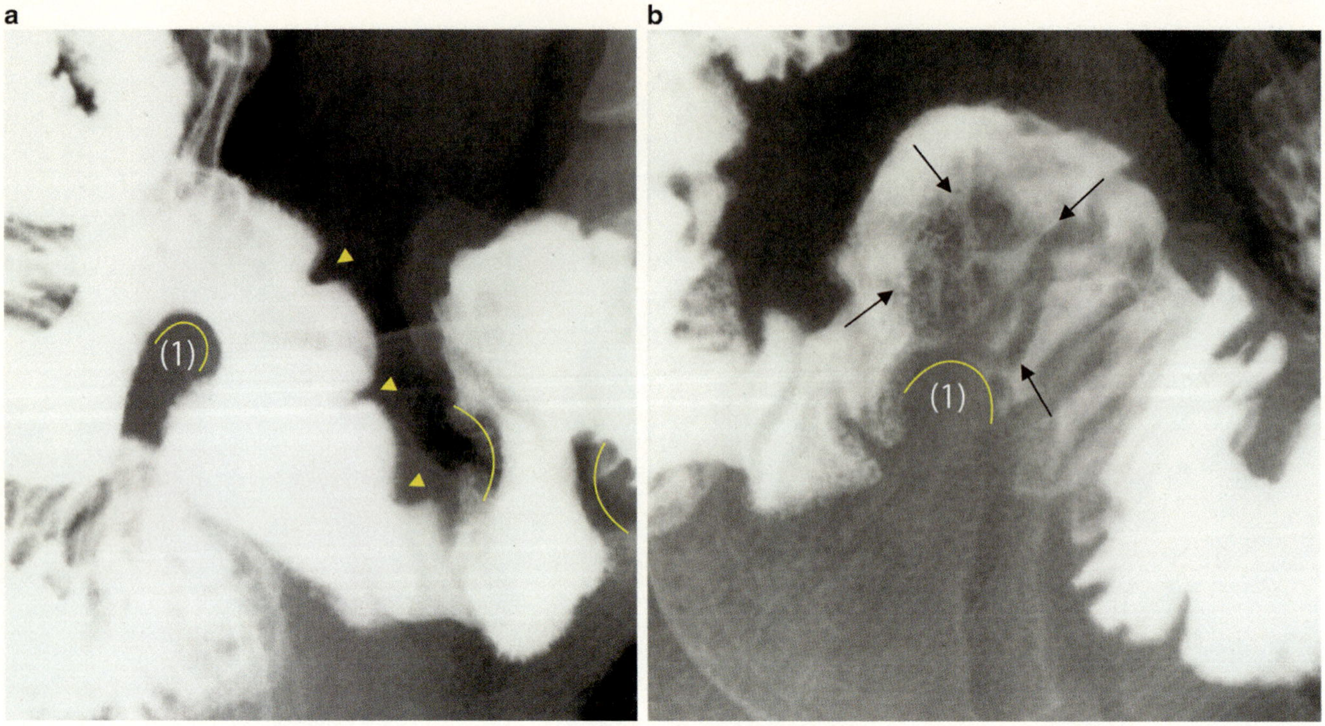

Fig. 2.2 Use of compression to visualize findings of deformity. (**a**) Multiple deformities of the ileum seen in chronic non-specific multiple ulcers of the small intestine (CNSU). The barium-filled image shows indentations of different sizes within a small area of the ileum (the area marked (*1*) is a comparatively severe indentation). (**b**) When the severe indentation marked (*1*) on the barium-filled image was carefully compressed, ulcerative lesions with mild activity and slight protrusion were visualized in the surrounding area (*arrows*)

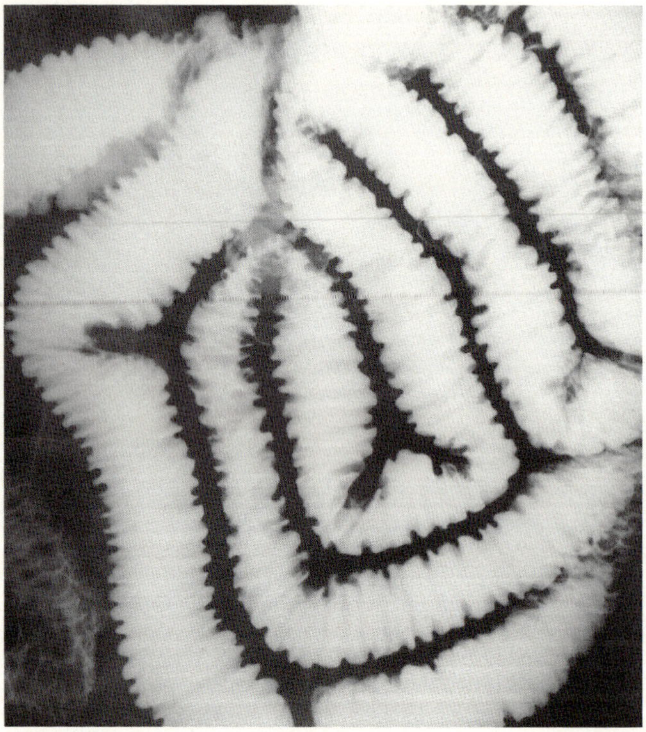

Fig. 2.3 Small intestinal lesions in SLE. Diffuse, spoke-shaped lesions are evident across a wide area from the jejunum to the ileum. This finding is characteristic of the enteritis seen in SLE

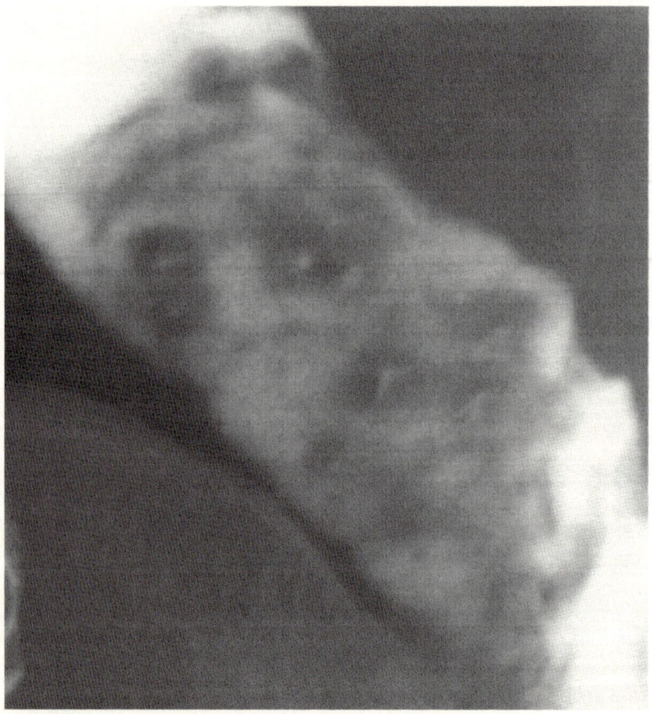

Fig. 2.4 Visualization of small aphthae by compression. Multiple aphthae of the ileum seen in Crohn's disease. Aphthae with a prominent pattern of protrusions are visualized in this compression image

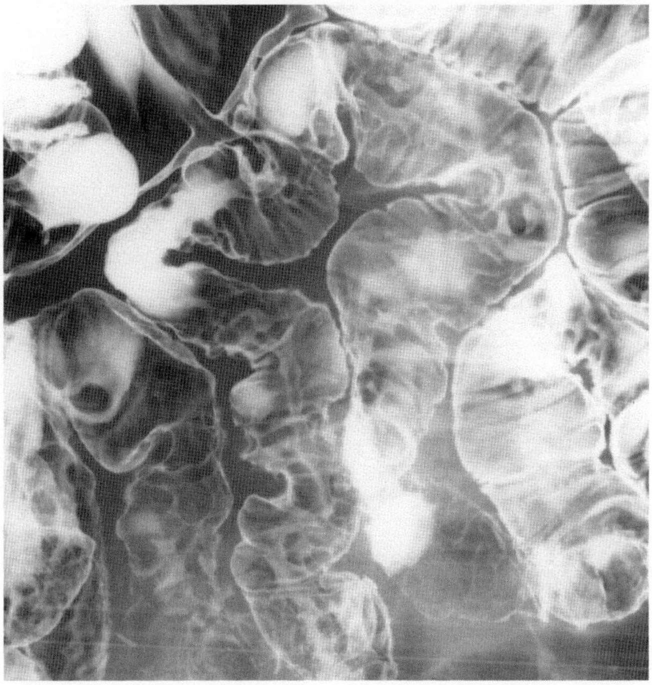

Fig. 2.5 Double-contrast image of longitudinal ulceration. Longitudinal ulceration of the ileum seen in Crohn's disease. Double-contrast images have been obtained over a wide area from the lower ileum to the terminus of the ileum, and the lesions are clearly visualized

volume of barium can be adjusted while its passage through the small intestine is observed.

2.2.2.1 Double-Contrast Method

The double-contrast method is capable of visualizing tiny lesions in the small intestinal mucosa over a wide area, and is therefore suited to detailed investigations (Fig. 2.5). The barium concentration is varied as appropriate, but in general is around 50–100 wv %, with 250–300 mL often used. In our department, we place the patient in the left lateral decubitus position or a steep right anterior oblique position, and normally start with an initial introduction of 100–150 mL of 80 wv % barium. We then move the patient to a position from supine to left anterior oblique and observe the passage of the barium, adding a further 100–200 mL. As increasing the amount of barium makes it more difficult to obtain double-contrast images over a wide area, it is preferable that the terminus of ileum be reached with a volume of around 300 mL if possible. We perform the procedure while massaging the barium manually toward the distal end, but as barium degrades if this takes too long, we also administer water or inject metoclopramide (Primperan®) if necessary to speed the process along. Air insufflation is initiated after barium has reached the terminal ileum. To start with, 200–300 mL is injected, and movement of the air toward the distal end is monitored. A further 100–200 mL is then injected while the position of the patient is repeatedly varied, until the air reaches the terminal ileum. Under favorable conditions, double-contrast images can be obtained across a wide area of the small intestine, but there are always at least a few points at which the barium pools and continues to fill the intestine, or where it has been preceded by air and barium adhesion is insufficient. It is therefore necessary to adjust the procedure to enable clear visualization by double-contrast imaging of the location where visualization is most desired (Fig. 2.6a, b). Once the air has reached the terminal ileum and the target location contains sufficient air, a sedative is administered (normally an intravenous injection of 1-2A hyoscine butylbromide (Buscopan®) and imaging is performed. It is no exaggeration to state that the quality of radiographic films is determined by the timing of sedation, and this therefore requires care.

Interpretation of double-contrast images is basically the same as for the per-oral method, but there is a greater possibility of obtaining information on matters such as tiny bumps and patterns on the mucosal surface (Fig. 2.7), abnormal disposition of Kerckring's folds (Fig. 2.8), and the degree of deformity (when extended). Because lesions that go unnoticed during screening may be picked up during image interpretation, imaging should be performed for areas in which lesions frequently occur for the suspected disease while varying body positions and angles.

2.2.2.2 Herlinger's Method [3]

The greatest advantage of this method is that radiography can be completed during a short space of time. Methyl cellulose is used to speed up passage of the barium, which is effective in reducing the time required and preventing loops of small intestine from overlapping. Around 250–300 mL of barium of around 50–100 wv % concentration is used. When 1.5–2.0 L of 0.5 % methyl cellulose is introduced immediately after barium introduction, sequential double-contrast images can be obtained from the proximal end of the small intestine. Visualization of lesions, however, is poor compared with both good compression images obtained by the per-oral method and double-contrast images obtained by utilization of air (Fig. 2.9). The barium also degrades the closer it approaches the distal end of the ileum, and this method is therefore not generally used.

2.2.3 Retrograde Ileography

One disadvantage of double-contrast imaging is the difficulty of visualizing the intrapelvic small intestine and the terminal ileum. Barium frequently fails to reach these locations even after some time has passed, or becomes denatured, reducing the quality of radiography. Barium may also fail to flow smoothly, making double-contrast images difficult to

a b

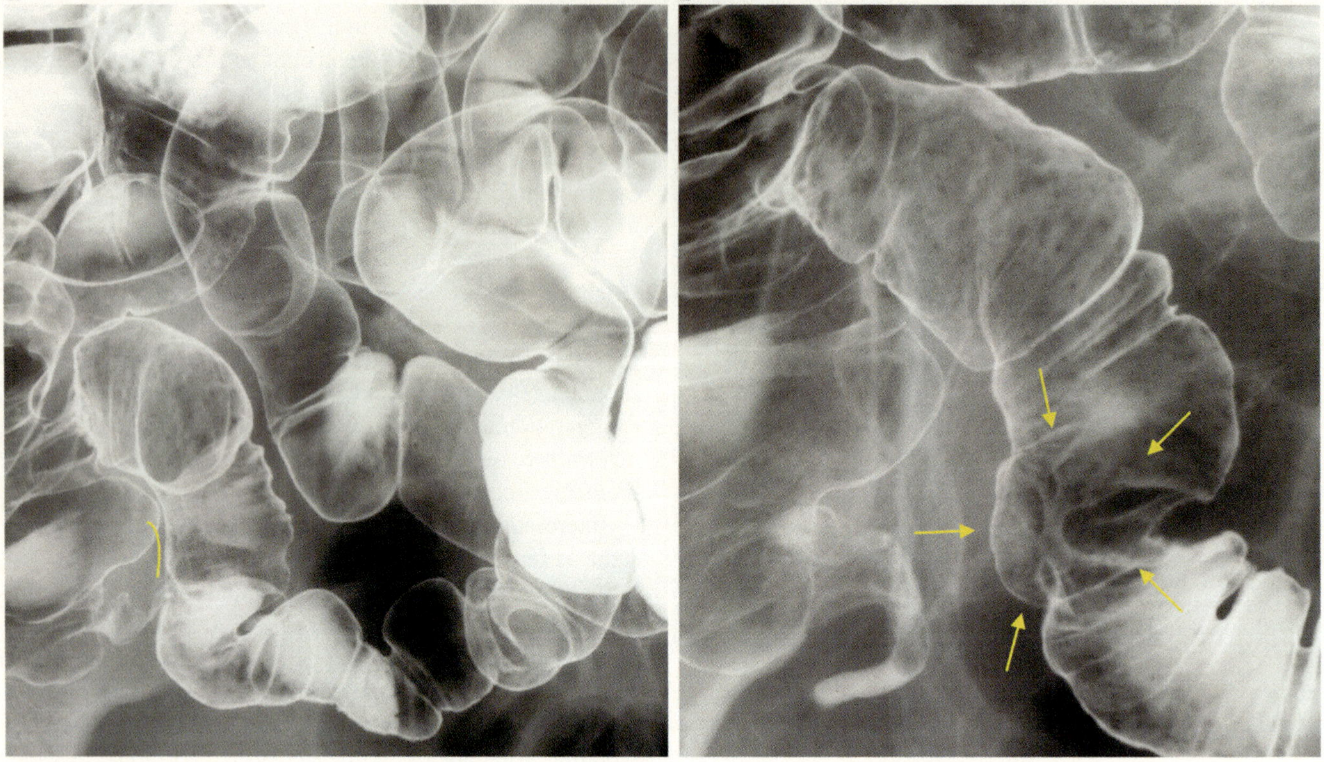

Fig. 2.6 Double-contrast imaging in practice. (**a**) Double-contrast imaging focusing on the lower ileum. Barium is pooled in some areas, and there are overlapping loops of bowel. A lesion of the terminus of the ileum was originally suspected in this case, so radiography focused on that area, and a sclerotic area was noticed during scanning. (**b**) When imaging was performed from a different angle, a somewhat bumpy concave lesion was visualized (*arrows*). Non-steroidal anti-inflammatory drug (NSAID)-induced enteropathy was diagnosed on the basis of the patient's history of NSAID use, biopsy results, and the fact that improvement was observed after medication was discontinued

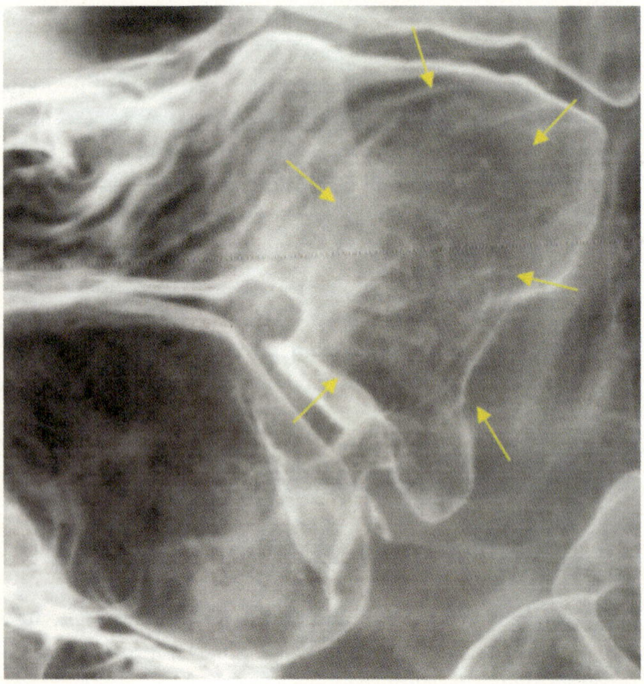

Fig. 2.7 Double-contrast image of small intestinal tuberculosis. Ileal stenosis seen in intestinal tuberculosis. Kerckring's folds have disappeared on the proximal side of the stenotic area, and the mucosal surface is roughened (areas of atrophic scarring). Shallow depressions can be seen in the same area (*arrows*)

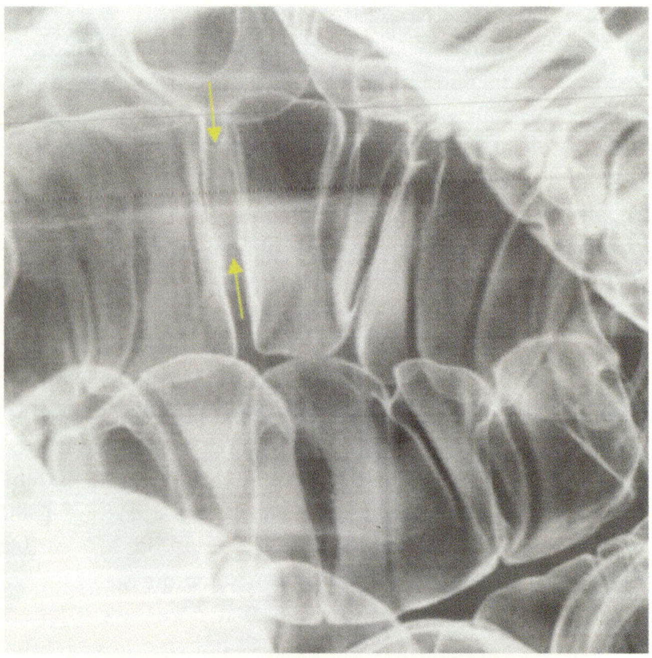

Fig. 2.8 Annular stenosis seen in NSAID-induced enteropathy. Abnormal Kerckring's folds seen in NSAID-induced enteropathy. The disposition of folds is inconsistent, with uneven spacing and width. Mild membranoid stenosis is also evident (*arrows*)

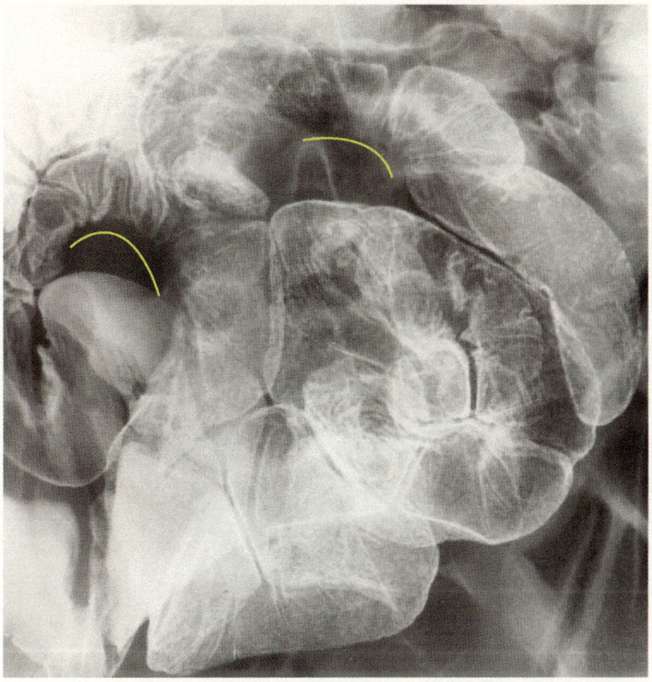

Fig. 2.9 Herlinger's method. Small intestine contrast image obtained by using Herlinger's method from a patient with Crohn's disease during remission (after total parenteral nutrition therapy). Longitudinal ulcerative scarring and lateral deformity can be seen, but dilution and degradation of the barium mean that the properties of the mucosal surface cannot be determined

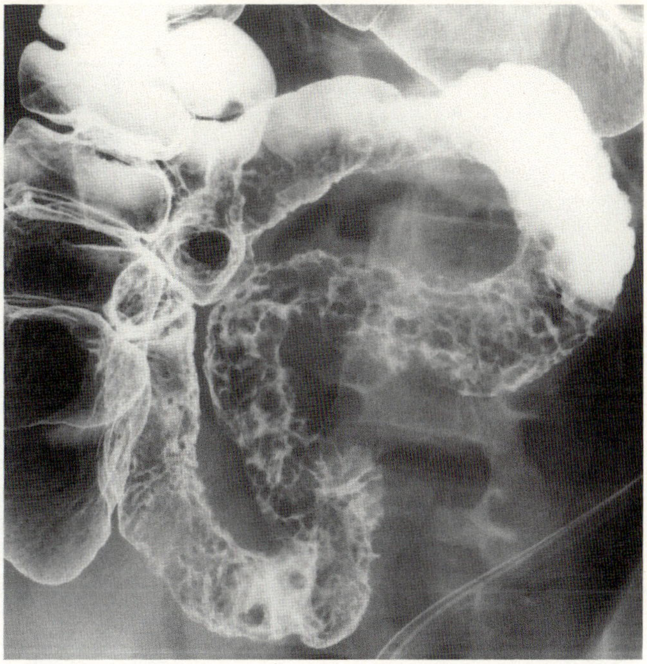

Fig. 2.10 Cobblestone appearance of the ileum visualized by retrograde ileography. Retrograde ileography image taken following on from colonoscopy. The typical cobblestone appearance of Crohn's disease is evident mainly from the terminal ileum to the intrapelvic ileum, together with lateral deformity

obtain, and an inability to separate loops of small intestine despite changing positions, applying pressure, and taking other measures is also common. Retrograde ileography has been devised as a selective contrast method to compensate for these disadvantages of double-contrast imaging. The method was formerly performed following colonoscopy [4], and involved: (1) inserting a lower gastrointestinal endoscopy scope as far as the terminus of the ileum via a sliding tube, and placing a guidewire via the forceps port; (2) withdrawing the scope, and inserting a contrast tube along the guidewire left inside the sliding tube; (3) after the contrast tube had been placed in the terminus of the ileum, inflating the balloon at its tip; and (4) using barium and air from the tip of the tube for selective contrast of the ileum. This method enables high-quality double-contrast images to be obtained using comparatively small volumes of barium and air even for the intrapelvic small intestine, which is difficult to separate (Fig. 2.10). The complexity of using a sliding tube, however, as well as the difficulty of inserting and placing the contrast tube, mean that this method frequently ends unsatisfactorily. In recent years, the use of balloon-assisted endoscopy (BAE) has become widespread, facilitating endoscopic observation of the small intestine and resulting in something of a decline in the significance of conventional retrograde ileography. BAE, however, is also limited in its range of observation in cases of stenosis or severe adhesions that do not permit passage of the scope, and difficulties in assessing lesions are frequently encountered, particularly in inflammatory disorders such as Crohn's disease. In such cases, many institutions introduce a water-soluble contrast agent (such as diatrizoate meglumine (Gastrografin®)) via the forceps port during BAE as a simple way of performing contrast. Good double-contrast images cannot be obtained, however, and investigation by this method frequently ends unsatisfactorily. The authors have devised a special probe for small intestinal radiography (made of polyvinyl chloride, which slides easily and is strong and flexible), and have reported the value of a new technique of retrograde ileography that improves on the conventional method [4]. This technique utilizes the overtube used in balloon endoscopy to enable safe, more selective contrast, and renders the guidewire unnecessary due to the improved probe, providing major improvements to the disadvantages of the conventional method (Fig. 2.11a–d). This approach can also be used following BAE via the peroral approach, and adapted for the jejunum or upper ileum. It may be necessary in future to develop investigative frameworks that utilize BAE and radiography in a complementary fashion, including this technique.

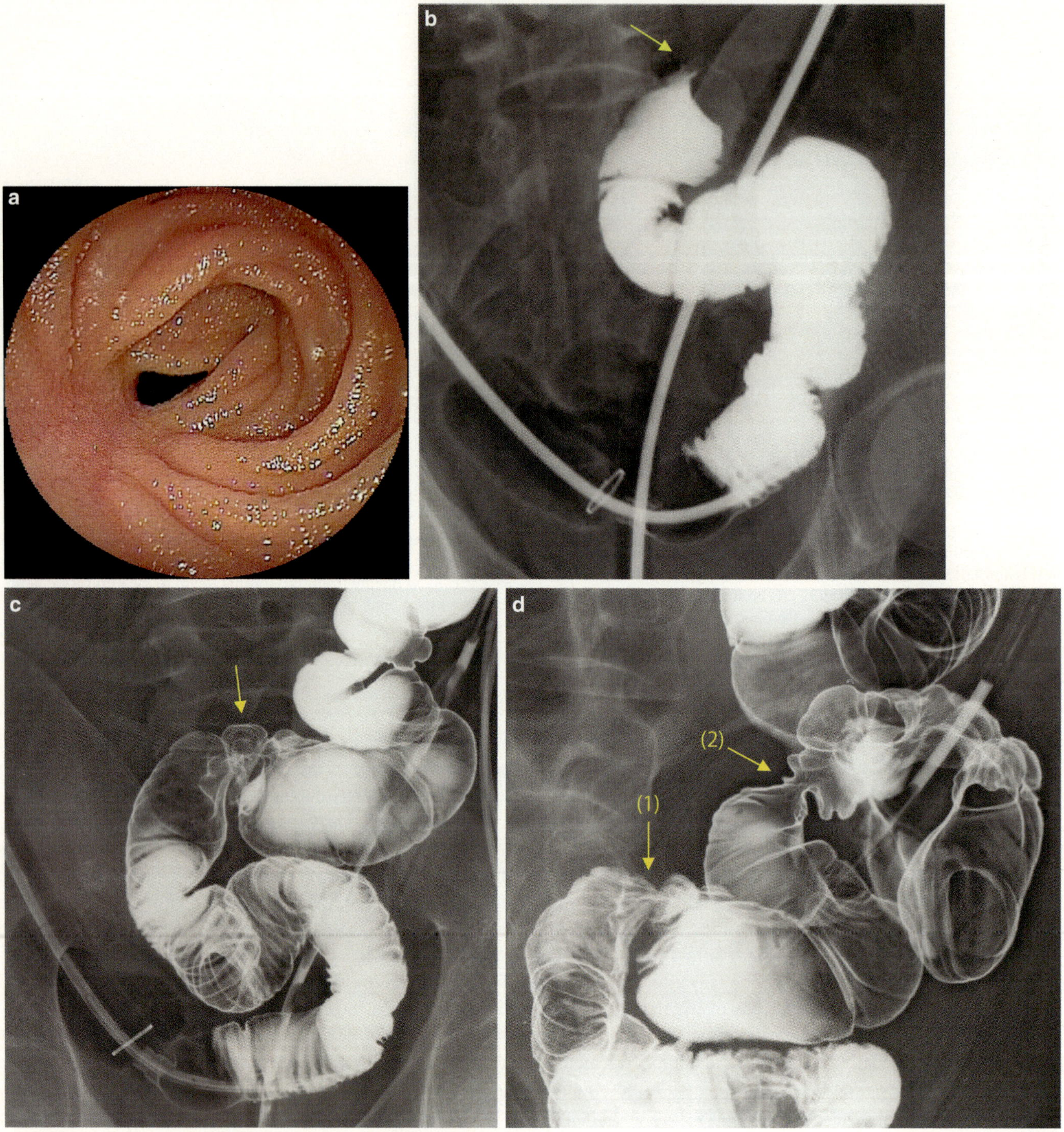

Fig. 2.11 Practice of retrograde ileography using double-balloon endoscopy. (**a**) Double-balloon endoscopy was performed via a peranal approach in a patient with Crohn's disease, but stenosis prevented viewing any further toward the proximal end. (**b**) A contrast tube was placed on the tip of the over-tube, and 100 mL of barium introduced. The site of stenosis (*arrow*) observed endoscopically can be seen. (**c**) After the barium had been observed to flow in retrograde fashion through the site of stenosis (*arrow*), a total of 250 mL of air was slowly introduced. (**d**) Double-contrast observation of the proximal side of the site of stenosis (*1*) showed not only deformation of the intestinal tract, but also a second stenosis (*2*). Endoscopic balloon dilatation was performed the following day, enabling surgery to be avoided

2.3 CT and MRI Diagnostics

In recent years, the development of MDCT has led to dramatic improvements in spatial separability [5, 6]. It is now possible to visualize the gastrointestinal tract clearly by means of CT. Advances in the computers used for data-processing have also enabled detailed multiplanar reconstruction (MPR) based on the information acquired from CT. As CT is minimally invasive, this modality can be applied even when serious conditions such as intestinal obstruction or perforation are suspected (Fig. 2.12). In the field of small intestinal disease, CT is used for a wide range of indications, including obscure gastrointestinal bleeding (OGIB), suspected small intestinal tumor, and inflammatory bowel disease of unknown cause. In some institutions, CT enterography (Fig. 2.13a, b) is performed by filling the small intestinal lumen with a negative contrast agent such as air, water, or polyethylene glycol solution (PEG) or a positive contrast agent (including iodine and barium) to produce three-dimensional images [7–10]. Compared with small intestinal radiography, CT requires less expertise on the part of the practitioner. It can still be performed even if passage is obstructed, and has the advantage of providing information about the intestinal wall and areas outside the digestive tract. However, it is not possible to evaluate tiny bumps and depressions on the mucosal surface. CT also has the disadvantages that visualization of a target location may not be possible, depending on conditions, and that time is required for image production.

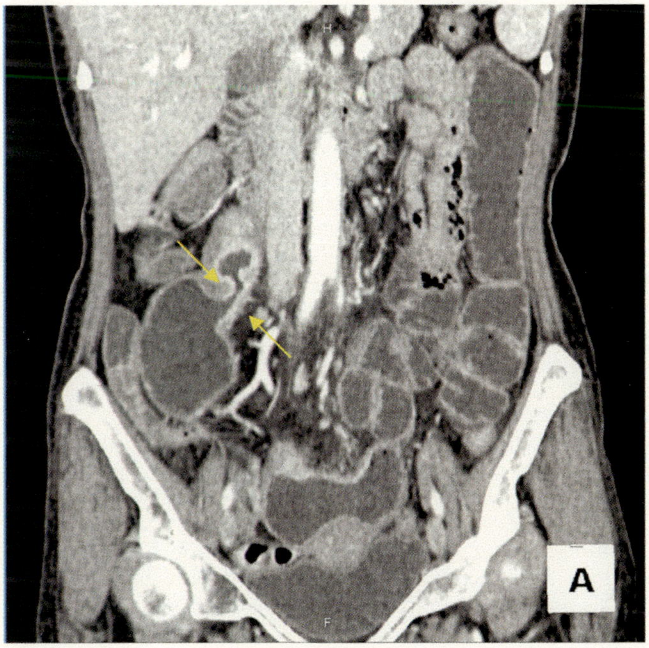

Fig. 2.12 Abdominal CT MPR image. MPR image of a patient with Crohn's disease and intestinal obstruction. The small intestine is visualized to a comparatively wide extent due to the backing up of intestinal fluid. Stenosis of the ileum is evident, with thickening of the intestinal wall, and the intestinal tract is dilated on the proximal side. This was regarded as the culprit lesion

Thanks to advances in MRI equipment that have reduced the time needed for imaging, this modality can now also be applied to small intestinal disease in the same way as CT. Although MRI has many similarities with CT in terms of imaging of the small intestine, its features include superior concentration resolution and the fact that no radiation exposure is involved. In Europe and the United States, there is a tendency to prefer MRI to CT or small intestinal radiography, both of which require radiation exposure, in chronic inflammatory conditions such as Crohn's disease that require repeated scanning. Studies comparing MRI with endoscopy have also been reported [7, 8] and MRI may be used with increasing frequency in future, particularly in Europe and the United States. MR enterography is also regarded as useful [9, 10] as, unlike CT enterography, it offers advantages such as dynamic evaluation, and there are hopes for its future development.

CT and MRI are expected to undergo further advances in engineering in future. At present, MPR imaging, which does not require the introduction of air or liquid, is the main form of imaging in all but a few institutions. There is no sign of the widespread adoption of CT enterography or MR enterography and the methods of dilatation of the small intestine also differ between institutions. Establishment of consistent methods to both enable clear visualization of the small intestine and offer superior simplicity and safety would thus be desirable.

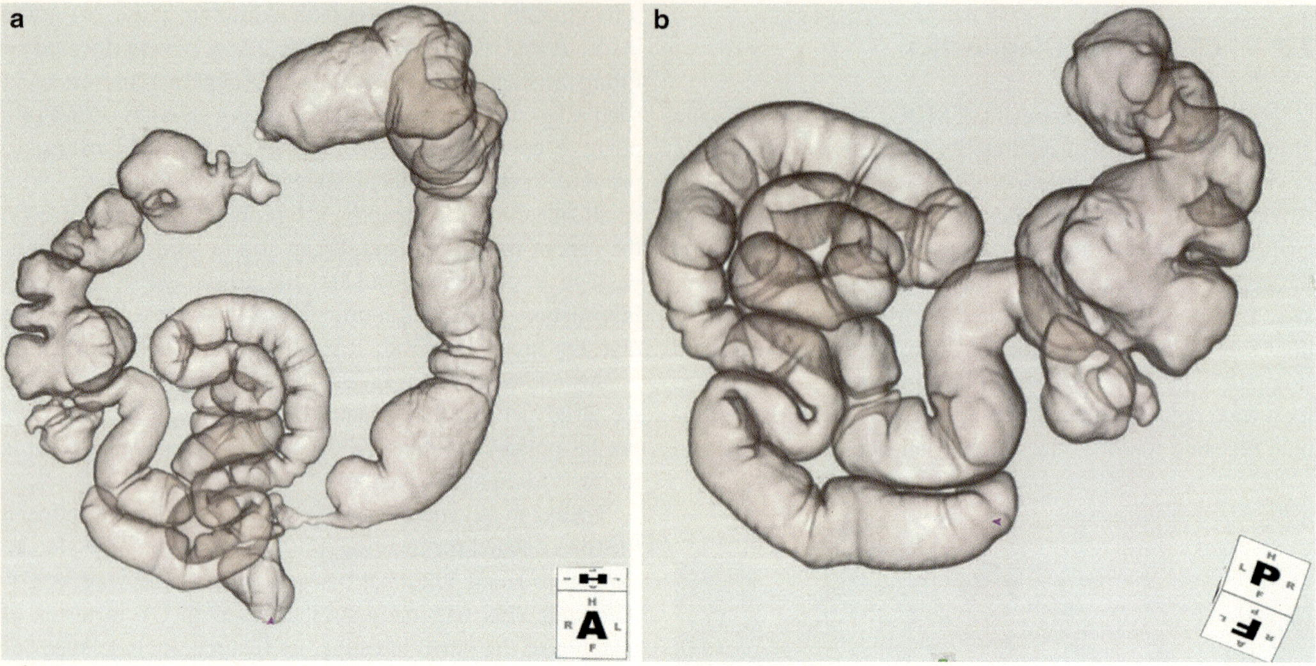

Fig. 2.13 Enterocolonography of large intestine stenosis. (**a**) Enterocolonography image of a patient with Crohn's disease with stenosis of the sigmoid and transverse colon. Air was introduced peranally, and the intestine was observed from the lower ileum to the colon. (**b**) There is clear visualization from the intrapelvic ileum to the terminal ileum, and this can be adjusted to any angle. Active lesions, fistulae, and the like can be ruled out, although it is not possible to evaluate small lesions such as aphthae

References

1. Nakamura U et al. X-ray examination of the small intestine by means of duodenal intubation—double contrast study of the small bowel. Stom Intest. 1974;9:1461–9.
2. Yao T. Double contrast enterolysis with air. In: Freeny PC, Stevenson GW, editors. Malgulis and Burhenne's alimentaly tract radiology. St Louis: Mosby; 1994. p. 548–51.
3. Herlinger H. Enteroclysis technique and variations. In: Herlinger H, Maliglinte DDT, Birnbaum BA, editors. Clinical imaging of small intestine. 2nd ed. New York: Springer; 1999. p. 95–123.
4. Yorioka M et al. Newly devised small bowel sonde for air contrast barium study after enteroscopy. Stom Intest (in Japanese). 2011;46:500–6.
5. Colombel JF et al. Quantitative measurement and visual assessment of ileal Crohn's disease activity by computed tomography enterography. Gut. 2006;55:1561–7.
6. Paulsen SR et al. CT enterography as a diagnostic tool in evaluating small bowel disorders: review of clinical experience with over 700 cases. Radiographics. 2006;26:641–57.
7. Low RN et al. Crohn disease with endoscopic correlation: single-shot fast spin-echo and gadolinium-enhanced fat-suppressed spoiled gradient-echo MR imaging. Radiology. 2002;222: 652–60.
8. Koilakou S et al. Endoscopy and MR enteroclysis: equivalent tools in predicting clinical recurrence in patients with Crohn's disease after ileocolic resection. Inflamm Bowel Dis. 2010;16: 198–203.
9. Umschaden HW et al. Small-bowel disease: comparison of MR enteroclysis images with conventional enteroclysis and surgical findings. Radiology. 2000;215:717–25.
10. Negaard A et al. Magnetic resonance enteroclysis in the diagnosis of small-intestinal Crohn's disease: diagnostic accuracy and inter-and intra-observer agreement. Acta Radiol. 2006;47: 1008–16.

Capsule Endoscopy

3

Motohiro Esaki and Takayuki Matsumoto

3.1 Mechanisms of Capsule Endoscopy Devices

Two types of device for small intestinal capsule endoscopy (CE) are currently available in Japan, manufactured by GIVEN Imaging and Olympus. These devices show few differences in terms of mechanisms and performance, and this chapter will therefore describe the diagnostic imaging system for the capsule endoscope manufactured by GIVEN Imaging.

3.1.1 Capsule Endoscope Main Unit (Fig. 3.1a, b)

Figure 3.1a, b shows an exterior view and the internal configuration of the main unit of the Pillcam® capsule endoscope. A white light-emitting diode (LED), a battery, a transmitter, a turn coil sensor array to transmit image data, and an image sensor are contained within a biocompatible plastic capsule measuring 11 × 26 mm. One *side* of the capsule comprises a clear dome, and endoscopic images are acquired twice a second simultaneously with a flash of the LED light [1]. The improved Pillcam SB2 incorporates both an extended field of view (156°) and a multistratified lens with automatic light-adjustment functionality, providing greatly improved image quality. The operating time has also been extended compared with the previous model, enabling imaging for over 8 h. The image data transmitter uses an application-specific integrated circuit to send ultrahigh frequency-band radio waves (432 MHz) beyond the body at a frequency that does not affect the human body.

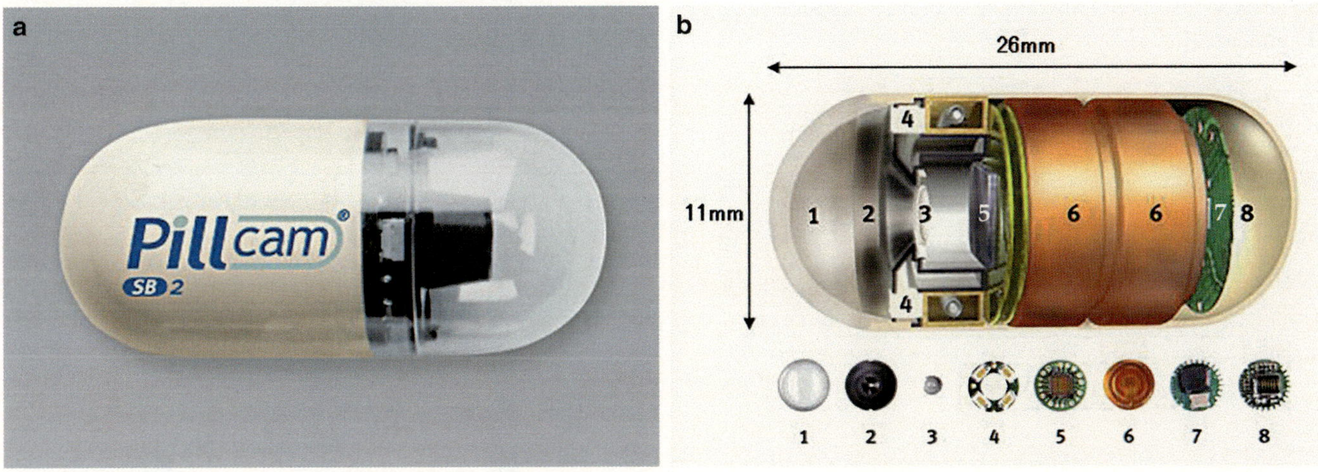

Fig. 3.1 Small intestine capsule endoscope. (**a**) External view of capsule endoscope (Pillcam® SB2). (**b**) Internal configuration of capsule endoscope. (*1*) Clear dome. (*2*) Lens holder. (*3*). Single-focus aspherical lens. (*4*) Light-emitting diode (LED) for illumination. (*5*) Image sensor: complementary metal oxide semiconductor. (*6*) Battery. (*7*) Transmitter: application-specific integrated circuit. (*8*) Turn coil sensor array

M. Esaki (✉) • T. Matsumoto
Department of Medicine and Clinical Science, Graduate School of Medicine, Kyushu University, 3-1-1 Maidashi, Higashi-ku, Fukuoka 812-8582, Japan
e-mail: mesaki@intmed2.med.kyushu-u.ac.jp

T. Matsui et al. (eds.), *Endoscopy in the Diagnosis of Small Intestine Diseases*, DOI 10.1007/978-4-431-54352-7_3, © Springer Japan 2014

3.1.2 Data Recorder Set (Fig. 3.2)

This is a device for receiving and recording image data transmitted from the CE main unit, consisting of a sensor array that receives image data and a data recorder that records it.

The array of eight sensors attached to the patient's abdomen not only receives image data, but also incorporates the capacity to calculate and display the location of the capsule in the body on the basis of signal strength. The main components of the data recorder comprise a radiofrequency module, a microprocessor, a motherboard, and a recording component capable of storing a little under 60,000 images per test. The stored data can be replayed or displayed as images after transfer to a visual display unit. In addition, RAPID® Real Time software can be used to observe images as they are acquired during the examination.

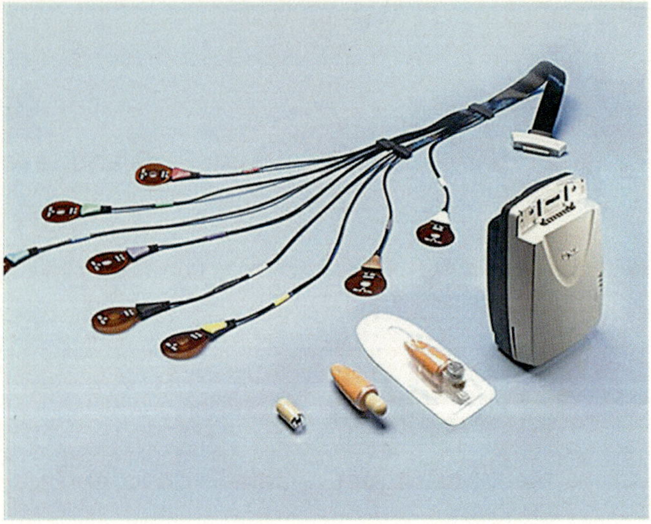

Fig. 3.2 External view of the data recorder set

3.1.3 RAPID® Real Time Workstation (Fig. 3.3)

Image data recorded in the data recorder are downloaded to a RAPID workstation, and video images converted to AVI format and saved can be replayed using image-reading software (RAPID® software) for diagnosis. RAPID®6 software incorporates Fuji film's flexible spectral imaging color enhancement (FICE) function. Image enhancement functionality is also anticipated to be useful for capsule imaging diagnosis [2].

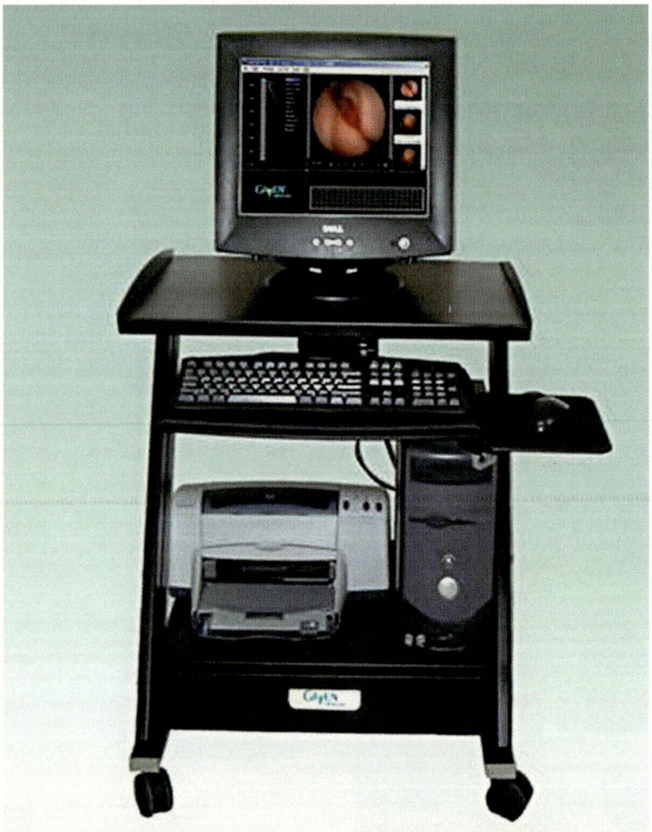

Fig. 3.3 RAPID® workstation

3.2 Practical Points of Capsule Endoscopic Diagnosis

3.2.1 Advanced Explanation

The greatest problem with CE is retention in the intestine. Before the start of the examination, it must be explained to patients that: (1) observation of the entire small intestine may not be possible; (2) if passage of the capsule cannot be confirmed within 2 weeks, plain abdominal radiography will be used to check for the capsule; and (3) if the capsule is retained, surgery may be required to remove it. Magnetic resonance imaging (MRI) is also contraindicated until excretion of the capsule has been confirmed.

3.2.2 Procedure for Examination

1. Input patient information into the data recorder, and charge the battery.
2. Instruct the patient to fast from 12 h before the examination, and administer an oral defoaming agent 30 min before the start of the procedure. Isotonic magnesium citrate solution or polyethylene glycol solution may also be administered several hours before the procedure with the aim of improving imaging conditions [3].
3. Attach the array of eight sensors to the patient's abdomen (Fig. 3.4a), and connect the cable to the data recorder. The patient should put on the vest containing the data recorder (Fig. 3.4b).
4. Remove the capsule from the package. When the magnetic switch is released and the light starts to flash, bring the capsule close to the sensor array and check that the light on the recorder is flashing synchronously with the light on the capsule.
5. Have the patient swallow the capsule with some water (100–200 mL). To encourage early passage into the duodenum within 1–2 h after swallowing, instruct the patient not to adopt a supine or left lateral decubitus position during this time.
6. Allow the patient to drink water from 2 h after swallowing the capsule, and to eat from 4 h after.
7. Remove the data recorder and other devices 8 h after the capsule has been swallowed. If the patient is hospitalized, RAPID® Real Time can be used to confirm in advance that the capsule has reached the large intestine.

3.2.3 Practical Points of Image Analysis

Figure 3.5 shows the RAPID®6 analysis screen. The horizontal bar extending from the center to the right at the bottom of the screen is the temporal axis, with the color reflecting the color inside the gastrointestinal lumen. Immediately above the temporal axis is the suspected blood indicator (SBI), shown as a red line indicating regions of suspected hemorrhage. The interpreter views endoscopic images as video footage in the central video screen. Frame count and playback speed can be adjusted in accordance with experience, and if an abnormality is suspected, stills and frame-by-frame playback can be used to confirm the presence and nature of a

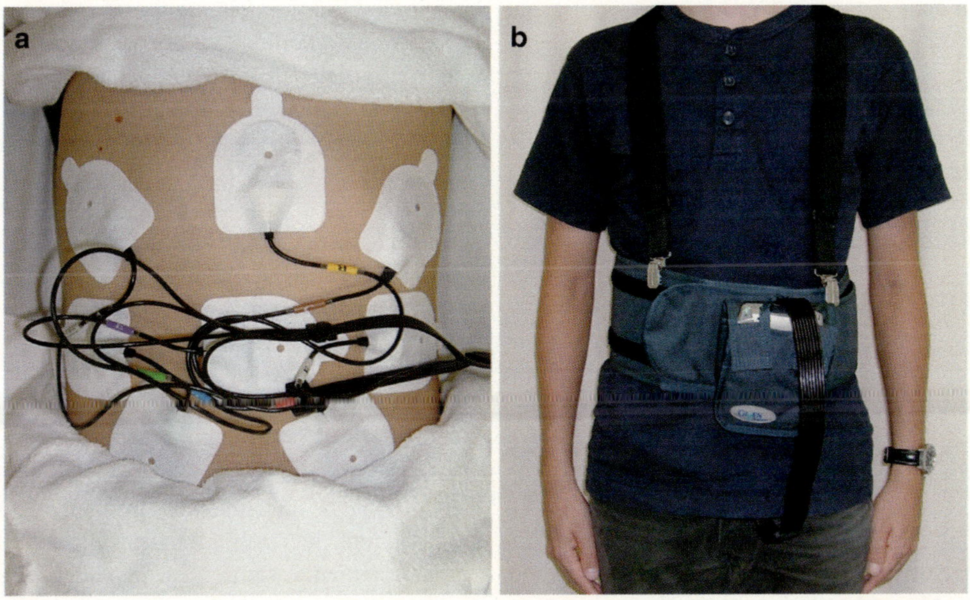

Fig. 3.4 Fitting the digital recorder set. (**a**) Attaching the sensor array to the abdomen. (**b**) Wearing the vest containing the data recorder

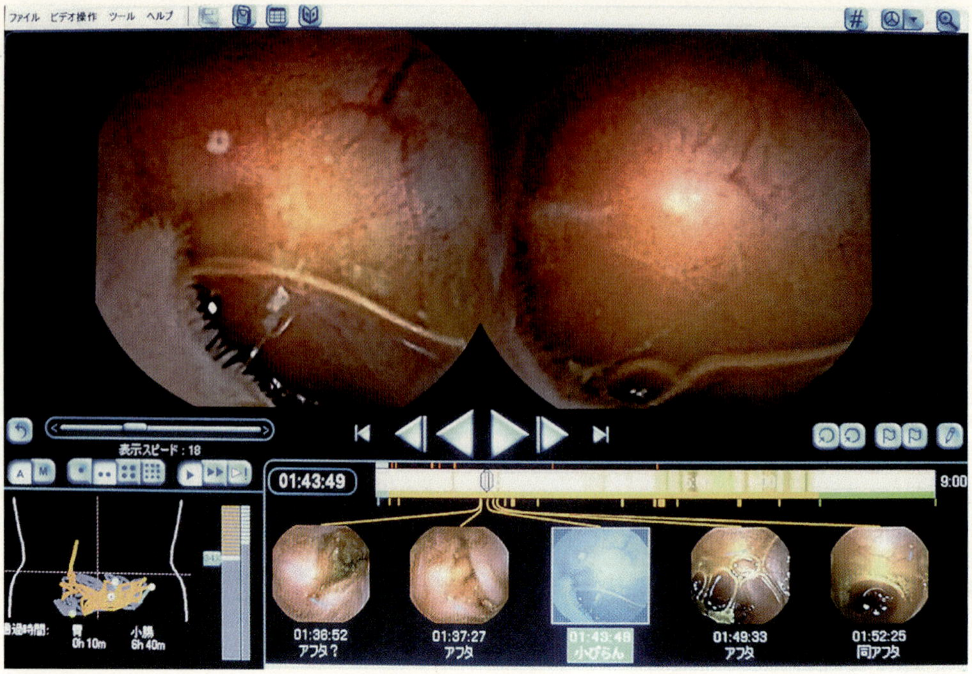

Fig. 3.5 RAPID®6 analysis screen

lesion. Sites of abnormalities can be saved as thumbnail images with findings attached.

This image analysis procedure requires around 30–60 min. Upgrades to image analysis software have incorporated a range of computer-aided diagnosis (CAD) functions into RAPID®6, and these can be utilized to reduce the time needed for interpretation. However, SBI may not necessarily identify sites of bleeding correctly [4, 5] and false-negative results may be generated if only the Quick View function for previewing video images is used. CAD functions must thus be regarded as nothing more than auxiliary functions.

3.3 Indications, Contraindications, and Problems with CE

3.3.1 Indications and Contraindications

CE is indicated mainly for *OGIB* for which a cause cannot be determined by upper gastrointestinal or lower gastrointestinal examination (including endoscopic examination). In practice, however, the value of CE has been demonstrated for numerous small intestinal diseases without overt bleeding, including gastrointestinal polyposis and malabsorption syndrome, as well as inflammatory bowel disease and non-steroidal anti-inflammatory drug (NSAID)-induced enteropathy in the absence of stenosis [6, 7].

The greatest problem with CE is retention in the intestine, and this approach is thus contraindicated in patients with obvious obstruction or stenosis of the gastrointestinal tract or with known or suspected fistula. If stenosis or fistula is suspected, prior evaluation by radiography of the small intestine is important, but in some cases stenosis or fistula may be difficult to rule out. The utility of a dummy capsule of the same shape and size as the main unit of the capsule endoscope (Agile J Patency Capsule) is currently under investigation in Japan. This patency capsule consists of a main component made chiefly of lactose and a timer plug component to control the time required for the capsule to dissolve, and the main component is formulated with 10 % barium sulfate to render it visible under radiographic examination. Use of such a device appears likely to prove useful for advance confirmation in patients for whom retention is a possibility.

CE is not indicated for patients with implanted internal electronic devices such as cardiac pacemakers, but no problems have yet been encountered in practice. The safety of using CE in pregnant women has yet to be established.

3.3.2 Problems

Even in the absence of lesions that might potentially cause retention in the intestine, the capsule may not reach the small or large intestine within the time allocated for examination. In such patients, some form of underlying gastrointestinal dysfunction may be present, and administration of erythromycin [8] or metoclopramide [9] may prove effective. With the Pillcam® SB2, however, the capsule operating time is extended, and RAPID® Real Time can also be used to monitor the state of progress of the capsule, contributing to an improved rate of reaching the cecum.

In the lower small intestine, residual food and bile not uncommonly cause difficulties in observation. The use of dimethicone, which possesses a foaming action, can improve visibility in the upper and middle small intestine, but is ineffective in the lower part [10]. Some studies have reported that pretreatment with enteric lavage can improve visibility in the small intestine, but no consensus has yet been reached [7].

References

1. Iddan G et al. Wireless capsule endoscopy. Nature. 2000;405:417.
2. Imagawa H et al. Improved visibility of lesions of the small intestine via capsule endoscopy with computed virtual chromoendoscopy. Gastrointest Endosc. 2011;73:299–306.
3. Esaki M et al. Bowel preparations for capsule endoscopy:a comparison between simethicone and magnesium citrate. Gastrointest Endosc. 2009;69:94–101.
4. D'Halluin P et al. Does the "Suspected Blood Indicator" improve the detection of bleeding lesions by capsule endoscopy? Gastrointest Endosc. 2005;61:243–9.
5. Buscaglia JM et al. Performance characteristics of the suspected blood indicator feature in capsule endoscopy according to indication for study. Clin Gastroenterol Hepatol. 2008;6:298–301.
6. Lewis BS. Expanding role of capsule endoscopy in inflammatory bowel disease. World J Gastroenterol. 2008;14:4137–41.
7. Ladas SD et al. European Society of Gastrointestinal Endoscopy (ESGE): recommendations (2009) on clinical use video capsule endoscopy to investigate small-bowel, esophageal and colonic diseases. Endoscopy. 2010;42:220–7.
8. Caddy CR et al. The effect of erythromycin on video capsule endoscopy intestinal–transit time. Gastrointest Endosc. 2006;63:262–6.
9. Selby W. Complete small-bowel transit in patients undergoing capsule endoscopy: determining factors and improvement with metoclopramide. Gastrointest Endosc. 2005;61:80–5.
10. Albert J et al. Simethicone for small bowel preparation for capsule endoscopy: a systematic, single-blinded, controlled study. Gastrointest Endosc. 2004;59:487–91.

4 Double-Balloon Endoscopy

Takahiro Beppu and Fumihito Hirai

4.1 Traditional Examinations for Small Intestinal Disease

Double-balloon endoscopy (DBE) constitutes a major advance in endoscopic examination of the small intestine. Traditionally, methods of small intestinal endoscopy have been limited to the tube method, in which the endoscope is advanced by peristalsis, and the push method, whereby the endoscope is pushed in while the stomach and duodenum are straightened. However, both methods are painful for patients and require specialist skills, and observation of a sufficiently wide area and endoscopic treatment can be difficult. In many cases, this meant that radiography was used for detailed investigation of the small intestine, as described in detail in other chapters. As radiography can only provide indirect findings, however, definitive diagnosis of neoplastic or ulcerative lesions is difficult.

This was the context in which Yamamoto et al. first reported the principles and methods of DBE in 2001 [1], after which the technique came into clinical use in 2003 and was rapidly adopted. Today, this approach is regularly used in over 200 institutions in Japan, and is contributing to the elucidation of the pathology of small intestinal diseases.

DBE examination is frequently insufficient in patients with inflammatory bowel disease (IBD) in whom stenosis, adhesions, fistula, or deep ulceration are present, and we have previously reported a comparison between DBE and radiography in terms of detectability and utility for IBD of the small intestine. We found that radiography was valuable for the overall assessment of widespread lesions and observation beyond regions of stenosis, whereas DBE was useful for localized small lesions and areas of overlapping intestine where radiographic depiction was problematic. We concluded that radiography is better in disorders such as Crohn's disease, where stenosis or deformity is present and an overall assessment is important, while DBE is better for diseases with small lesions such as NSAID-induced enteropathy and intestinal tuberculosis.

CE devices, which came on the market at around the same time as DBE, are non-invasive and simple to use, and are therefore extremely useful for diagnosing obscure gastrointestinal bleeding (OGIB) [2]. Using CE and DBE in combination to supplement each other has clearly improved diagnostic performance for small intestinal diseases.

4.2 Principle and Mechanism

The small intestine is an organ 6–7 m long, situated between the stomach and large intestine and consisting of three parts: duodenum; jejunum; and ileum. The jejunum and ileum are not anchored in the peritoneal cavity after passing the ligament of Treitz until the ileocecal region, and form a continuous series of loops within the peritoneal cavity. This anatomical feature is one of the factors preventing insertion of a regular endoscope into the deeper parts of the small intestine. Inserting a conventional push-type endoscope into these loops of intestine results only in stretching them out, without actually advancing the endoscope into the deeper part of the intestine (Fig. 4.1). DBE uses an overtube (OVT) to prevent the intestinal loops from extending, enabling the tip of the endoscope to advance while the insertion distance remains the same (Fig. 4.2).

Two balloons are also used to grasp the intestine and draw it backward to shorten the intestine and simplify the approach as much as possible. This action causes the intestine to shorten in accordion fashion over the OVT, while simultaneously simplifying the shape of the intestine into which the endoscope will be inserted next, thus facilitating insertion (Fig. 4.3). The balloon at the tip of the endoscope is deflated, and the tip is advanced deeper into the small intestine.

T. Beppu (✉) • F. Hirai
Department of Gastroenterology, Fukuoka University Chikushi Hospital, 1-1-1 Zokumyoin, Chikushino, Fukuoka 818-8502, Japan
e-mail: bouzutb@yahoo.co.jp

T. Matsui et al. (eds.), *Endoscopy in the Diagnosis of Small Intestine Diseases*, DOI 10.1007/978-4-431-54352-7_4, © Springer Japan 2014

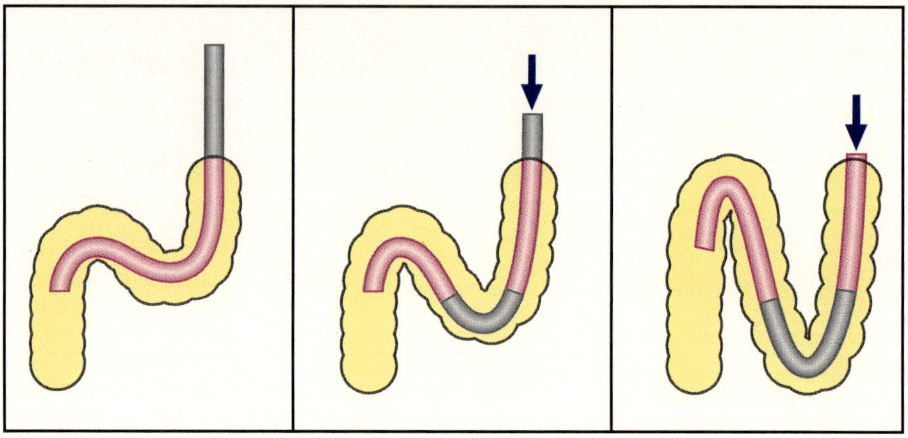

Fig. 4.1 Push-type endoscopy: intestinal loops. Inserting a conventional push-type endoscope into an intestinal loop only stretches the intestine, without the tip of the endoscope actually advancing deeper into the intestine

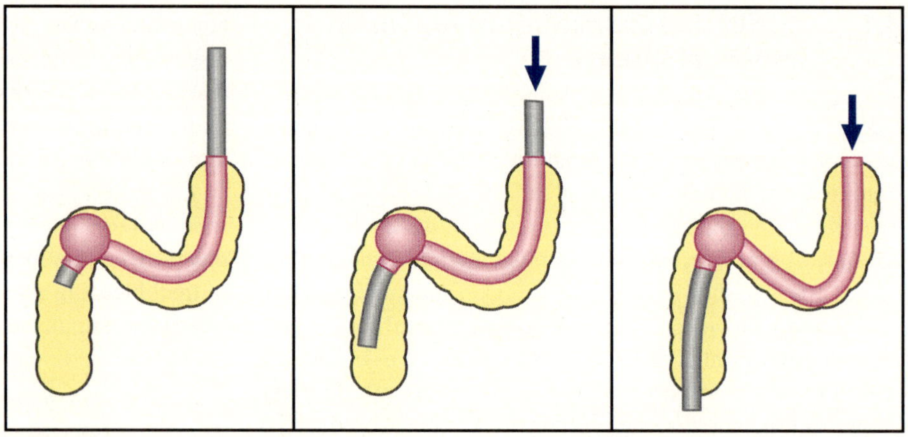

Fig. 4.2 DBE: intestinal loops. Use of an overtube (OVT) prevents the intestinal loop from extending, enabling the tip of the endoscope to advance while the insertion distance remains the same

In patients with no adhesions, the entire small intestine can be observed. As time is required to observe the entirety of the small intestine in a single examination, however, dividing the examination into two parts using antegrade and retrograde approaches is both safer and more efficient.

One feature of DBE is provision of a high degree of operability for the endoscope in deeper parts of the small intestine. As the distance and angle with respect to lesions can be controlled, not only regular biopsy, but also hemostasis, polypectomy, balloon dilation, and other endoscopic treatments can be performed. Inflating the balloon at the tip of the endoscope also prevents the reverse flow of contrast agent, enabling selective enhancement of lesion sites.

DBE systems consist of the system main unit, a balloon controller, an endoscope, and an OVT (Fig. 4.4a, b). The pressure within each balloon is monitored by means of the balloon controller (PB-10 or PB-20), which is set to maintain the pressure automatically at 6.0 kPa (approx. 45 mm Hg) when dilated. An alarm rings in the event of a sudden increase in pressure inside the balloon due to endoscope operation or peristaltic movement, or if the balloon does not reach the required pressure despite continued insufflation for a set period of time.

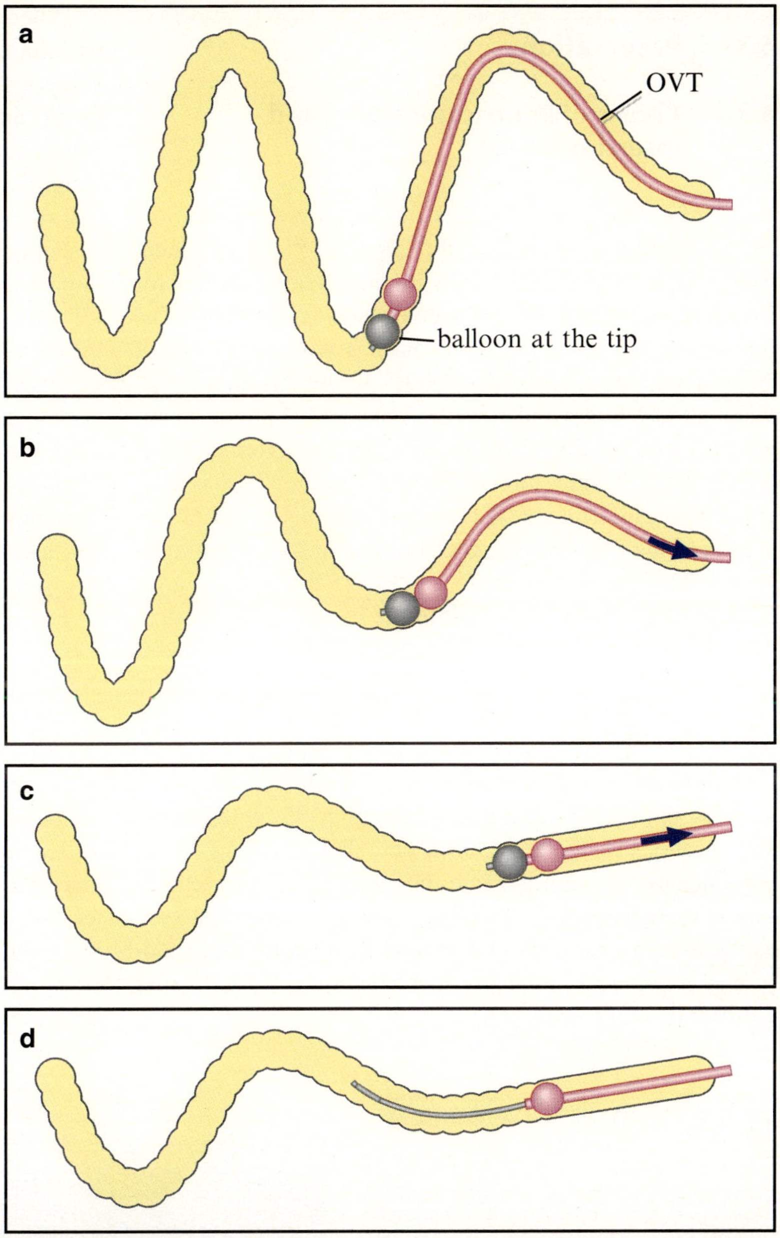

Fig. 4.3 Simplification and shortening. (**a**) The overtube (OVT) is advanced, and the intestine is gripped by two dilated balloons. (**b**) The entire device is pulled back, shortening the intestine above the OVT and simplifying the course of the section of intestine into which the endoscope will be advanced next. (**c**) The intestine is shortened in accordion fashion, facilitating the next insertion of the endoscope. (**d**) The balloon at the tip of the endoscope is deflated, and the tip is advanced deeper into the small intestine

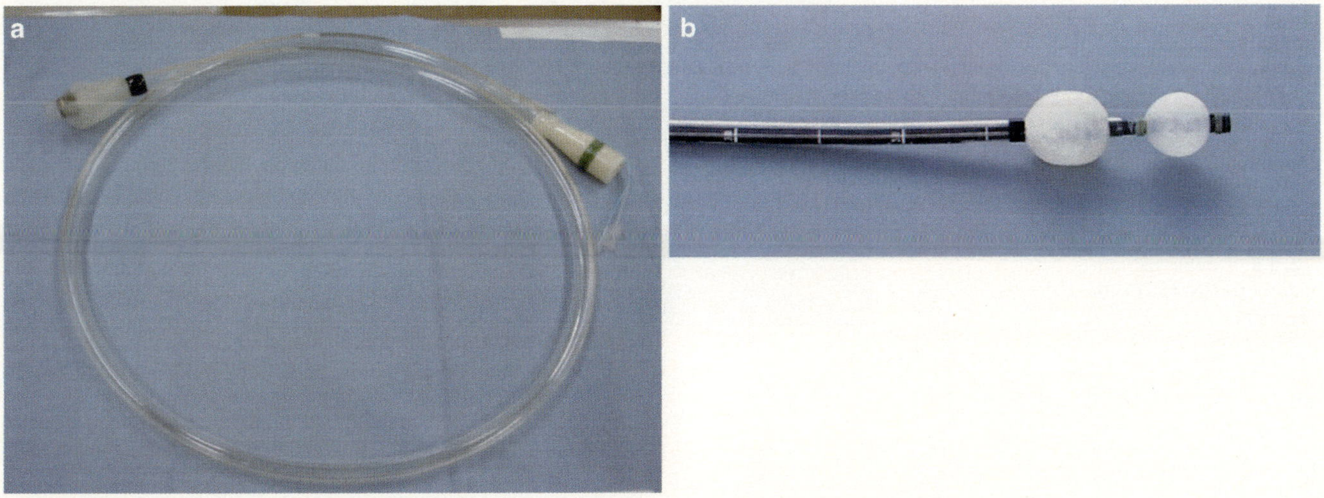

Fig. 4.4 Overtube and balloons. (**a**) Overtube (OVT). (**b**) The OVT is fitted over the endoscope EN-450P5

4.3 Preparation

4.3.1 Choice of Endoscope Model and Insertion Route

As of May 2011, three models of DBE were on sale: the EN-450P5® for examination; the EN-450T5® for treatment (Fig. 4.5); and the EC-450BI5® with short working length for cases showing difficulty with colonoscopic insertion. The EN-450P5 and EN-450T5 both have a working length of 200 cm, with a 145-cm OVT. The EN-450P5 has an external diameter of 8.5 mm and a forceps channel 2.2 mm in diameter, whereas the EN-450T5 is larger with an external diameter of 9.4 mm and a forceps channel 2.98 mm in diameter, enabling the insertion of snares, clips, balloons for dilatation, argon plasma coagulation (APC) probes, and other treatment tools. Although the EN-450T5 and EC-450BI5 are designed for use in treatment and enable the use of a large range of treatment tools, the endoscopes themselves are somewhat stiff due to their thickness, and may be difficult to insert in patients with adhesions affecting the peritoneal cavity. As the EC-450BI5, with its shorter working length, has a more limited range, use is restricted to cases showing difficulty in colonoscopic insertion. However, the EI-530B, with similar specifications to the EC-450BI5 and short working length but capacity for insertion into the small intestine, went on sale in early June 2011, enabling biliary tree treatment such as Roux-en-Y anastomosis after total gastrectomy and endoscopic retrograde cholangiopancreatography (ERCP) after Billroth II surgery.

When selecting the insertion route for DBE, the first important point is to take a medical history. This must cover matters such as medication history (NSAIDs, antiplatelet drugs, etc.), underlying conditions, location of abdominal pain, nature of stools, systemic symptoms such as fever and weight loss, and previous medical history (history of abdominal surgery, trauma).

For neoplastic or inflammatory lesions, contrast radiography of the small intestine or abdominal contrast-enhanced CT may offer clues regarding which approach to use. If the location of the lesion can be estimated by imaging, insertion via the closer approach is chosen. If the location of the lesion cannot be identified, then retrograde insertion should be used, followed by antegrade insertion if no signs are evident. This is because per-oral DBE entails a risk of inducing complications such as acute pancreatitis and aspiration pneumonia, and great care is required when performing antegrade insertion for drawn-out examinations and in elderly patients.

For patients with suspected small intestinal bleeding, the presence of fresh blood in stools may indicate bleeding from the ileum, whereas black to reddish-black stool more frequently indicates bleeding from the jejunum or middle small intestine. In current patients with OGIB, CE is often used to search for the general source of bleeding, after which DBE is performed. As CE is contraindicated for patients with suspected stenosis, however, contrast radiography of the small intestine should first be performed to check for stenotic lesions. If overt bleeding is present, fresh blood or clots flowing from the proximal side may be difficult to see using the retrograde approach, making it difficult to search for the source of bleeding. In principle, antegrade insertion should be attempted in such cases to search for the bleeding site.

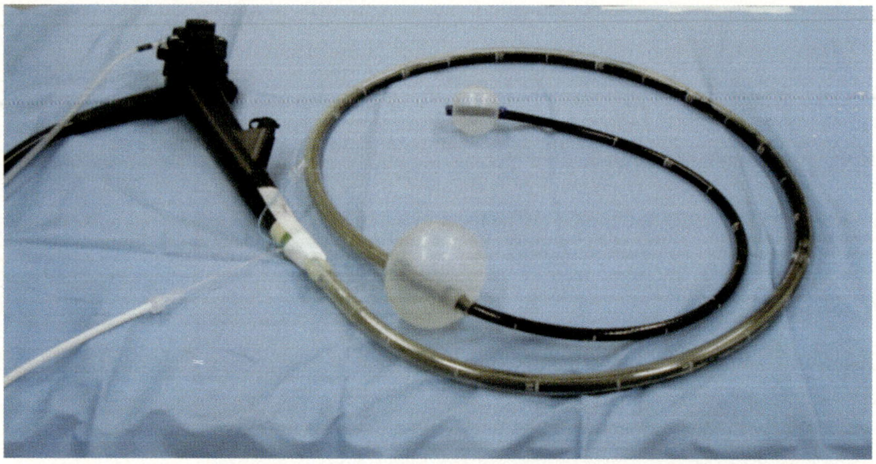

Fig. 4.5 Double-balloon endoscopy EN-450T5 for treatment

4.3.2 Indications and Contraindications (Table 4.1)

DBE is indicated not only for the small intestine, but in other cases when the postoperative intestinal canal or large intestine cannot be reached by conventional endoscopy or the superior operability offers an advantage over conventional endoscopy.

The following is an overview of indications.

In IBD, DBE is used for the diagnosis of Crohn's disease, intestinal tuberculosis, NSAID-induced enteropathy, chronic non-specific multiple ulcers of the small intestine (CNSU), Behçet disease, simple ulcer, and ischemic colitis. Ulcerative lesions in IBD tend to be longitudinal in Crohn's disease, circular or consistent with Peyer's patches in intestinal tuberculosis, and circular in NSAID-induced enteropathy. It should also be kept in mind that lesions are more common on the mesenteric side in Crohn's disease and on the antimesenteric side in intestinal tuberculosis.

Because the introduction of biologic drugs for Crohn's disease in recent years has made mucosal healing an important factor in response evaluation, DBE now plays a major role in monitoring after treatment with infliximab or adalimumab. DBE can also be used to perform endoscopic balloon dilation for benign stenosis in IBD.

In terms of hemorrhagic lesions, DBE is indicated for both OGIB and overt bleeding. In cases of severe anemia or unstable general condition, however, DBE should be performed only after the patient's hemodynamics has been stabilized by blood transfusion or intravenous fluids. Bleeding from small angioectasias or hemangiomas, or ulcers in inflammatory bowel disease such as Crohn's disease, can frequently be treated. The EN-450T5 for treatment use has a forceps channel 2.8 mm in diameter, enabling a wide variety of hemostatic treatments including APC, clipping, and snare-tip high-frequency ablation. The EN-450T5 should therefore be prepared from the start in cases when hemostasis may be required. In patients for whom endoscopic hemostasis may be difficult due to arteriovenous malformation or other causes, a tattoo may be placed near the lesion in preparation for surgical treatment.

In many cases, neoplastic lesions such as cancer, malignant lymphoma, GIST, Peutz-Jegher's syndrome (PJS), and familial adenomatous polyposis can be diagnosed by biopsy. Endoscopic polypectomy, endoscopic mucosal resection (EMR), and intussusception reduction can be performed in cases of polyposis. In the case of neoplastic conditions for which endoscopic treatment is not indicated, examination concludes with biopsy and tattooing alone. Caution is required in cases of neoplastic lesions in which ulceration is also present, as biopsy of the bottom of a particularly deep ulcer carries a risk of perforation.

DBE is also indicated in cases of intestinal obstruction, including post-laparotomic adhesions and ulcers. In cases of chronic intestinal obstruction due to adhesion, diagnosing intestinal adhesions from curving or twisting of the intestine may be possible. A tattoo should be placed at the site of adhesion, and synechiotomy performed laparoscopically at a later date to reduce invasiveness and alleviate the burden on the patient.

DBE is also indicated in cases showing difficulty with colonoscopic insertion, as the balloon endoscope can be inserted deeply in cases of elongated sigmoid or transverse colon or when insertion is difficult due to postoperative adhesions. DBE can also be used to perform colonoscopy treatments (EMR, endoscopic submucosal dissection (ESD)) with the aim of stabilizing the field of view and operability.

Table 4.1 DBE indications and contraindications (P.27)

Diseases for which DBE is indicated	
1. Inflammatory bowel disease	Crohn's disease, intestinal tuberculosis, NSAID-induced enteropathy, chronic non-specific multiple ulcer of the small intestine, Behçet disease, simple ulcer, ischemic colitis
2. Hemorrhagic diseases	Angioectasia, capillary hemangioma, arteriovenous malformation, portal hypertensive enteropathy, small intestinal varices
3. Neoplastic diseases	Small intestinal cancer, malignant lymphoma, GIST, polyposis, metastatic intestinal carcinoma, lipoma
4. Intestinal obstructions	Adhesional ileus, malignant tumor, Meckel's diverticulum
5. Cases showing difficulty with colonoscopic insertion	Patients with elongated sigmoid or transverse colon, patients for whom insertion is difficult due to postoperative adhesions
6. Bile duct and pancreatic diseases	Roux-en-Y anastomosis after total gastrectomy, ERCP after Billroth II surgery following partial gastrectomy, stent placement, lithotomy, etc.
7. Removal of foreign body from the small intestine	
Contraindications for DBE	
1. Patients with suspected perforation 2. Patients with severe inflammation 3. Patients in poor general condition with unstable respiration or circulatory dynamics	

DBE double-balloon endoscopy, *NSAID* non-steroidal anti-inflammatory drug, *GIST* gastrointestinal stromal tumor, *ERCP* endoscopic retrograde cholangiopancreatography

For bile duct and pancreatic diseases, DBE is indicated for biliary tree treatment such as Roux-en-Y anastomosis after total gastrectomy and Billroth II surgery following partial gastrectomy. In such cases, other procedures such as ERCP, endoscopic drainage, stent placement, and lithotomy can also be performed. DBE is also indicated for removing foreign bodies such as dentures, needles, fish bones, and parasites from the small intestine.

Contraindications are the same as those for upper and lower gastrointestinal endoscopy, including patients with suspected perforation or severe inflammation, and those judged to be in poor general condition with unstable respiration or circulatory dynamics.

4.3.3 Pretreatment

4.3.3.1 Antegrade Insertion

When using the antegrade approach, insertion is usually possible as far as the middle small intestine or upper jejunum. Even without pretreatment, if the patient fasts from the previous evening, large amounts of food residue will not be present in the small intestine. Only a small amount of intestinal fluid is present in the ileum, posing no hindrance to observation. As for gastric fluoroscopy and per-oral contrast radiography of the small intestine, however, presence of a large amount of residual stool in the large intestine may cause pain or nausea during the examination. For this reason, although pretreatment is not required to the same extent as for lower gastrointestinal endoscopy, a small dose of laxative should be used to reduce the amount of residual stool.

Examples of pretreatment

Patients with normal defecatory habits: alosenn (Pursennid®) 2 T before sleep on the previous night. Patients with tendency toward constipation: Sodium picosulfate monohydrate (Laxoberon®) 1 unit dose before sleep on the previous night.

4.3.3.2 Retrograde Insertion

Pretreatment for retrograde insertion is basically the same as pretreatment for lower gastrointestinal endoscopy. A large amount of residue in the large intestine reduces the field of view for the endoscope and renders insertion difficult, preventing insertion as far as the ileum. Pretreatment with enteric lavage is therefore performed.

Examples of pretreatment

Sodium picosulfate monohydrate (Laxoberon®) 1 unit dose before sleep on the previous night.

PEG solution (Niflec®) 2 L on the morning of the examination

4.3.3.3 Patients with Stenosis

Pretreatment is omitted for patients with stenotic lesions in the jejunum for whom antegrade insertion is used.

Little residue remains after fasting alone. If the stenotic lesion is in the ileum, however, and retrograde insertion is used, stool is frequently retained in the large intestine if pretreatment has not been administered. In patients with mild stenosis and no symptoms of obstruction who are able to defecate, the same pretreatment as for normal retrograde insertion is frequently used. For patients with moderate to severe stenosis, pretreatment is adapted individually by means such as reducing the volume of PEG solution (Niflec®) or administering oral magnesium citrate (Magcorol®) on the previous day. Naturally, patients with severe stenosis carry a risk of perforation due to rapid increases in internal intestinal pressure, and provision of a full explanation to the patient and careful monitoring of their condition are vital. As such, hospitalization of patients is recommended for the purpose of examination.

4.3.3.4 Patients with Overt Bleeding

If obvious current bleeding continues from the small intestine, a balloon endoscope may be inserted via the antegrade approach without pretreatment. This is because there is a higher possibility of discovering the source of bleeding close to where blood is initially observed.

4.3.4 Premedication

Balloon endoscopy requires 1–3 h, longer than the time required for regular upper and lower gastrointestinal endoscopy, and causes correspondingly greater distress to the patient. The presence of continued symptoms, including abdominal pain or discomfort as well as pharyngeal discomfort, difficulty breathing, and nausea when applying an antegrade approach mean that we use premedication in almost all cases in our hospital. The level of consciousness used is typically conscious sedation, in which patients are able to communicate verbally when spoken to and are capable of indicating any distress during endoscopic treatment or OVT insertion. Premedication not only alleviates pain by decreasing the level of consciousness, but also eliminates anxiety and stabilizes respiratory and heart rates, creating an environment in which patients can undergo the procedure with great reliability.

Premedication frequently comprises the combined use of sedatives and analgesics. Sedatives include diazepam and midazolam, and pain relievers include buprenorphine hydrochloride, pentazocine, and pethidine hydrochloride. As an overdose of sedative may cause respiratory depression, respiration and circulatory dynamics must be monitored.

In our hospital, the method used is to administer midazolam 2–3 mg and buprenorphine hydrochloride 0.1 mg intravenously, increasing the dose little by little as required while observing the level of sedation. Even in long-drawn-out examinations, it is rare for the total doses to exceed midazolam 10 mg and buprenorphine hydrochloride 0.3 mg. Scopolamine butylbromide (Buscopan®) and glucagon are used as intestinal antispasmodics. During antegrade insertion, these agents are not normally used until the endoscope is inserted into the deepest region, since peristalsis assists with deeper insertion of the endoscope. These agents are used only if insertion is severely hampered by peristalsis of the large intestine.

4.4 Insertion Techniques

4.4.1 Antegrade and Retrograde Insertion Techniques

4.4.1.1 Antegrade Insertion (Fig. 4.6)

1. First insert the tip of the endoscope as far as the stomach, in the same way as a normal upper endoscopy. Immediately after entry to the stomach, suction out the gastric contents and air as much as possible to prevent aspiration and deflection of the stomach. The endoscopist holds the endoscope in this position while the assistant advances the OVT into the stomach.

   After this, the assistant holds the OVT as straight as possible to keep it from bending, while the endoscopist advances the endoscope toward the posterior end of the OVT.
2. If balloons are dilated in the stomach, because the lumen is large, the balloons will continue to dilate. For this reason, do not inflate the OVT balloon while inside the stomach. The posterior tip of the OVT can be inserted up to the 1,550 mm mark on the endoscope, so insert the endoscope as far as the horizontal limb of the duodenum before inflating the balloon at the tip of the endoscope.

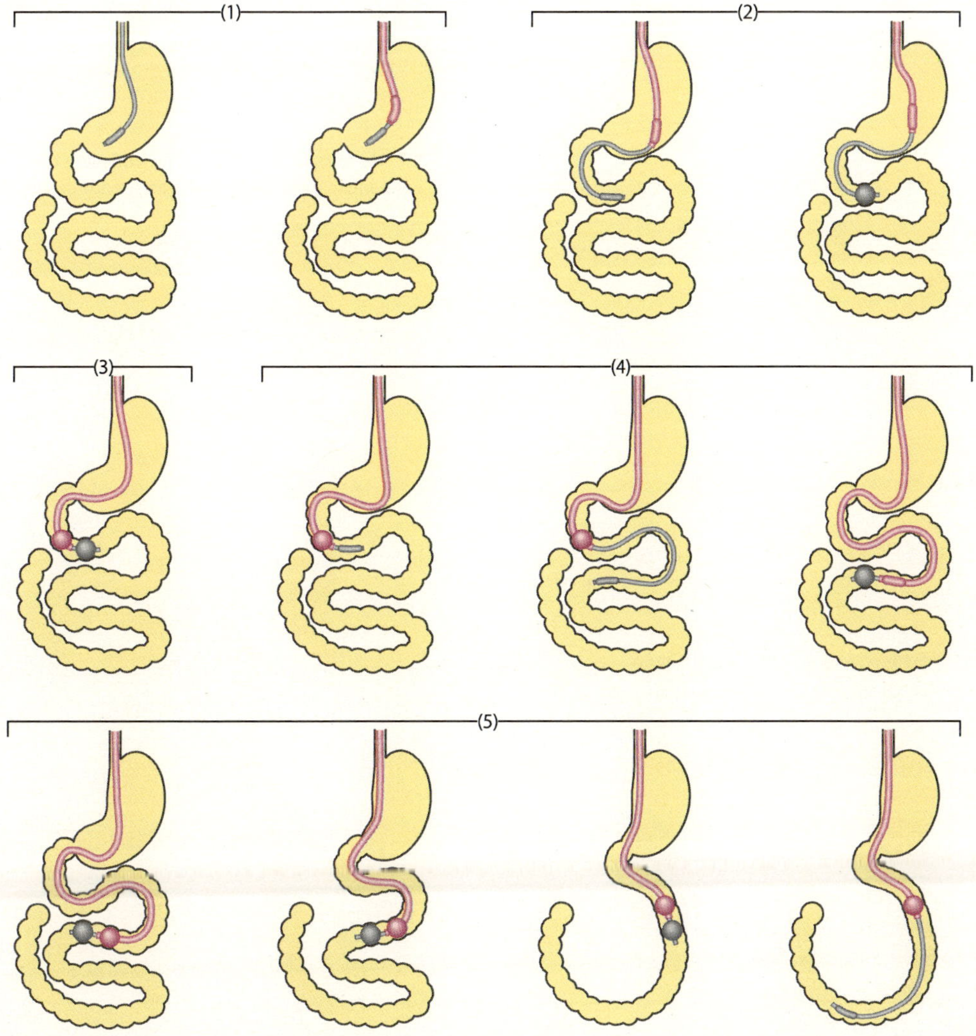

Fig. 4.6 Antegrade insertion

3. Insert the OVT along the endoscope, dilate the OVT balloon when the posterior end of the OVT has reached the 1,550 mm mark on the endoscope, and anchor the tip of the OVT in the duodenum. At this stage, with both balloons still dilated, pull back the entire system until stomach deflection is corrected.
4. Deflate the balloon at the tip of the endoscope, and insert the endoscope past the ligament of Treitz into the jejunum. Once the endoscope has been advanced as far as possible, dilate the endoscope balloon and advance the OVT after deflating the OVT balloon.
5. Dilate both balloons and grasp the intestine, withdrawing the entire system to completely correct the flexion of the stomach and shorten the jejunum. Next, deflate the balloon at the tip of the endoscope and insert it more deeply into the small intestine. From here on, basically repeat the same procedure, inserting the endoscope in concentric rings (Fig. 4.7).

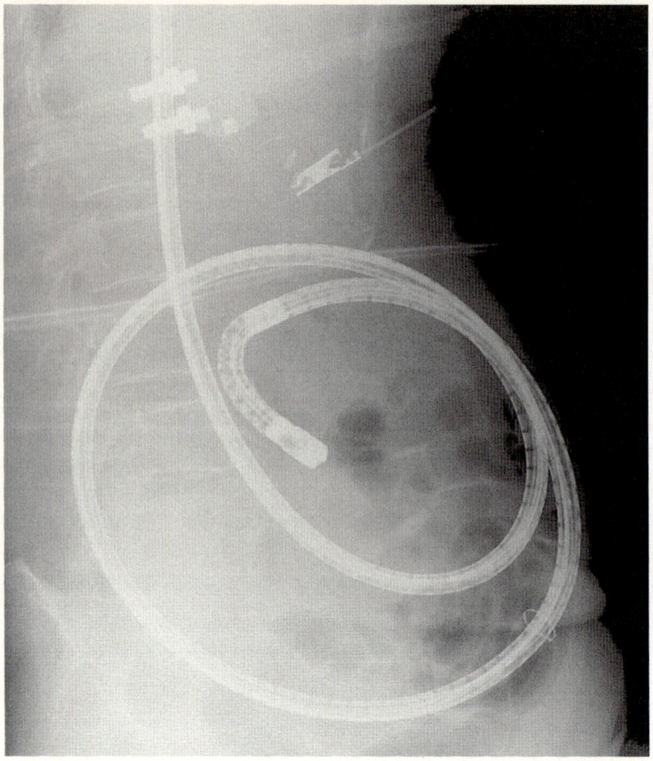

Fig. 4.7 Antegrade insertion. The endoscope is inserted in anticlockwise concentric circles using the antegrade insertion technique

4.4.1.2 Retrograde Insertion (Fig. 4.8)

1. As for regular lower gastrointestinal endoscopy, hold the tip of the endoscope and insert it into the anus, dilate the balloon at the tip of the endoscope in the sigmoid colon, and advance the OVT.
2. Dilate the OVT balloon, grasp the intestine with both balloons and withdraw the entire system for easy simplifica-

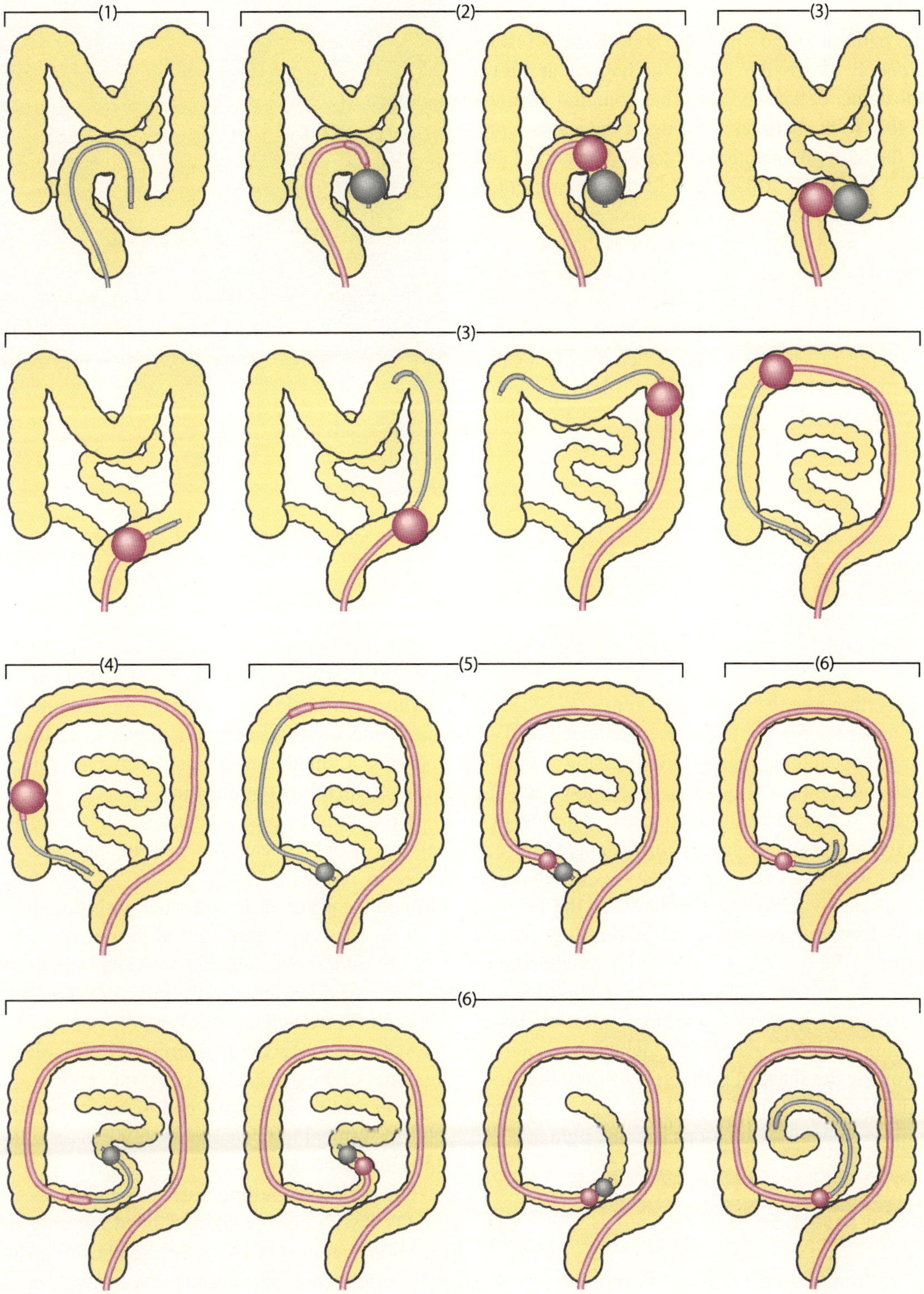

Fig. 4.8 Retrograde insertion

tion of the sigmoid colon loop. If straightening is difficult due to adhesion of the sigmoid colon, deflate the balloon at the tip of the endoscope and perform the next insertion even if the sigmoid colon is not completely straight. After this, the endoscopist advances the endoscope toward the posterior end of the OVT while the assistant holds the OVT.

3. Deflate the balloon at the tip of the endoscope, advance the tip as deeply as possible, dilate the balloon at the tip of the endoscope, deflate the OVT balloon, and advance the OVT close to the balloon at the tip of the endoscope.

   Repeat the balloon operations described in steps 2 and 3, anchoring the OVT at the sigmoid-descending colon junction, the splenic flexure, the transverse colon, and the hepatic flexure until the endoscope reaches the cecum.
4. After passing Bauhin's valve and reaching the terminus of the ileum, twist the endoscope to the left and move it at a slightly upward angle while watching Bauhin's valve at the 9 o'clock position on the screen. When Bauhin's valve appears at the 10–11 o'clock position, draw back the endoscope and insert it into the terminus of the ileum. After insertion, correct the left twist and upward angle, to facilitate insertion into the lower ileum.
5. Once the endoscope has been inserted into the ileum, advance it as far inside as possible, dilate the balloon at the tip of the endoscope, deflate the OVT balloon, and advance the OVT to close to the balloon at the tip of the endoscope. At this point, draw back the entire system slightly with both balloons dilated to straighten the intestine.

   When insertion into the terminal terminus of the ileum is difficult using the regular technique, advance the OVT balloon to the ascending colon before passing Bauhin's valve, dilate and anchor the colon, and draw back the entire system with both balloons to make insertion into the terminal ileum easier by decreasing the angle between this and the ascending colon. Other devices for enabling insertion include switching posture between the left and right lateral decubitus positions and performing manual compression on the right lower or right lateral abdomen.
6. Next, deflate the balloon at the tip of the endoscope and insert the endoscope deeper into the small intestine. Insert the endoscope so that it traces anticlockwise concentric circles following the shape of the large intestine (Fig. 4.9). If the endoscope is inserted clockwise, insertion often becomes more difficult as the loops become tighter.

4.4.2 Tips for Insertion

As for lower gastrointestinal endoscope insertion, it is also important when using DBE to keep insufflation as low as possible. Reducing insufflation prevents excessive extension or flexion of the intestine. According to Hirai et al., using carbon dioxide for insufflation is useful for assisting insertion and alleviating distress on the part of the patient [3].

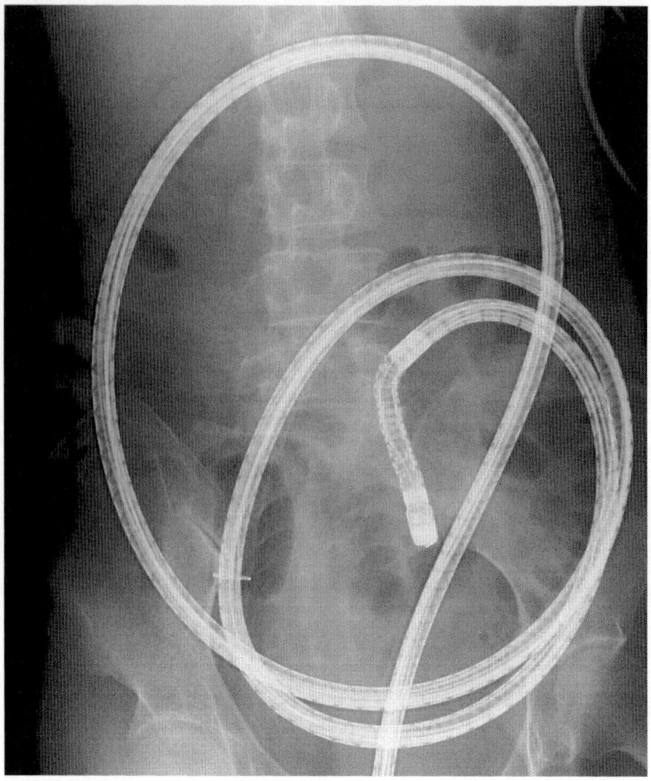

Fig. 4.9 Retrograde insertion. The endoscope is inserted in anticlockwise concentric circles using the retrograde insertion technique

During insertion, moving the endoscope slightly backwards and forwards and twisting it to right and left while applying a small upward angle enables efficient insertion without extending the intestine.

Attempting to pass through a point of flexion at the full angle will only stretch the loop of intestine; it is therefore better to return the angle as far as possible after passing through the point of flexion when inserting the endoscope.

A decrease in the amount of the water between the OVT and the endoscope will dramatically worsen how well the endoscope slides, and careful injection of additional water is important for efficient insertion.

At times when OVT insertion is difficult due to a tight flexion, slightly advance both the endoscope and OVT together and pull back the endoscope by a few centimeters. This movement may enable the OVT to pass slowly through the point of flexion.

The action of pulling back the endoscope together with the OVT with both balloons dilated not only folds back the intestine over the OVT in accordion fashion, but also enables the simplification of the next piece of intestine into which the endoscope will be inserted (Figs. 4.6(5) and 4.8(6)). The entire system should be pulled back to the point at which the endoscope disappears from the endoscope screen, and an endoscopist familiar with the procedure will come to recognize this point by looking at the endoscope screen even without the use of radiography. As the resistance felt while pulling back disappears once the loop is released, the point at which resistance disappears is also a sign to stop pulling back. Releasing the upward angle of the endoscope and freeing it also removes the flexion from the intestine during this simplification process, and prevents the next piece of intestine from forming a sharp curve at the end, like a walking stick.

If subsequent insertion is difficult even after the system has been pulled back some distance, in some cases inserting the endoscope after the OVT has been advanced without pulling back the entire system may enable passage through the difficult region, and attempting this maneuver is worthwhile.

4.5 Endoscopic Therapy Using DBE (Hemostasis, Polypectomy, Balloon Dilation Therapy)

4.5.1 Hemostasis [4]

Crohn's disease and other types of IBD that form ulcers, as well as angioectasia, hemangioma, arteriovenous malformation, and other vascular lesions may result in small intestinal bleeding leading to progressive anemia and shock. If elective DBE can be performed while carefully monitoring the general condition of the patient, hemostasis can be carried out using the EN-450T5 for treatment use (Fig. 4.10a, b). For lesions that are difficult to treat with endoscopic hemostasis, such as large hemangiomas and arteriovenous malformations, either a tattoo should be placed and preparations made for surgical treatment, or another non-endoscopic treatment such as vascular embolization should be chosen.

4.5.2 Polypectomy

Peutz-Jeghers syndrome (PJS) and inflammatory fibroid polyps (IFPs) frequently cause chronic intussusception or repeated intestinal obstruction. In cases of protrusive lesions and familial adenomatous polyposis (FAP), such small intestinal lesions may be removable by endoscopic polypectomy or endoscopic mucosal resection (Fig. 4.11a, b). In cases of PJS, the procedure may be performed several times to remove numerous polyps [5]. For polyps with a thick peduncle or wide base, the risk of hemorrhage during resection is high, and full-scale preparations for hemostasis are vital to ensure that bleeding can be stopped immediately. Rapid treatment is also required if bleeding occurs. This is because the fresh blood and blood clots from even a small-to-moderate hemorrhage in the narrow lumen of the small intestine render visibility extremely poor, making the point of bleeding difficult to identify.

4.5.3 Endoscopic Balloon Dilation (EBD)

EBD can be performed in many patients to treat benign stenosis of the small intestine in conditions such as Crohn's disease, intestinal tuberculosis, and chronic non-specific multiple ulcer of the small intestine (CNSU) (Fig. 4.12a–c). Intestinal stenosis due to Crohn's disease is the most frequent reason for surgery in Crohn's disease patients, and in our hospital around 80 % of patients who undergo surgery do so either because of stenosis or to treat fistula or ulceration associated with stenosis [6]. Flare-ups at lesion sites or recurrence at the site of anastomosis mean that recurrent intestinal stenosis is unavoidable in Crohn's disease. Relieving intestinal stenosis by EBD, which preserves the intestine and can be performed repeatedly, increases the possibility that quality of life and prognosis can be improved.

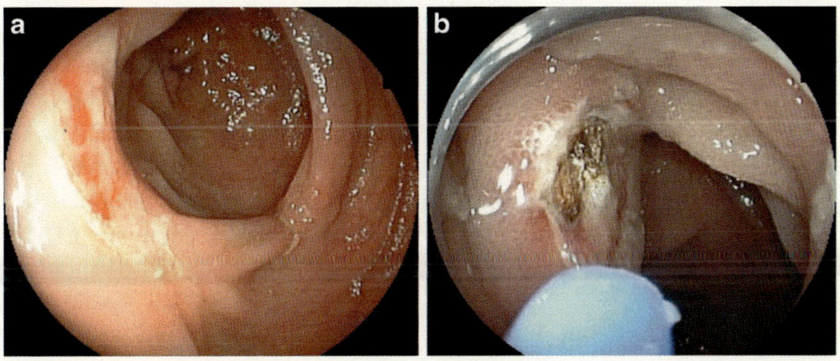

Fig. 4.10 Endoscopic hemostasis. (**a**) A man in his 1930s, who developed Crohn's disease (small intestinal) at 18 years old. He had been receiving maintenance administration of infliximab since 2007. Black stool appeared and progressive anemia (hemoglobin (Hb) 8.4 g/dL) was evident. Retrograde double-balloon endoscopy showed an open ulcer with appendant fresh blood and planar blood vessels on the ulcer floor, regarded as the source of bleeding, in the ileum on the proximal side of the iliocolic anastomosis. (**b**) As oozing bleeding from the vessels on the ulcer floor was evident during insufflation, ablation was performed by APC, and no further bleeding was observed

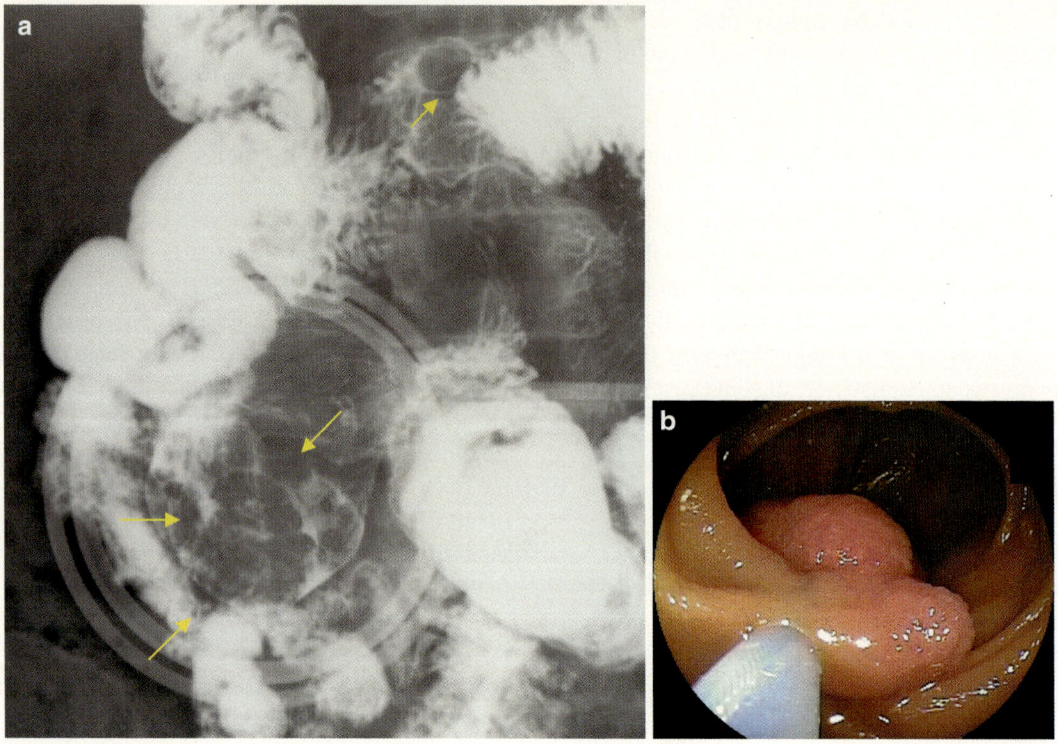

Fig. 4.11 Endoscopic polypectomy. (**a**) A woman in her 1930s, diagnosed with PJS at 2 years old. She was examined in our hospital for intermittent abdominal pain. Per-oral contrast radiography of the small intestine showed numerous polyps massed within the middle jejunum in the upper left of the abdomen, and the cause of pain was diagnosed as intussusception due to polyps. (**b**) The massed polyps within the jejunum were removed

Currently, lesions for which EBD is indicated to treat small intestinal stenosis in Crohn's disease at our hospital must meet the following conditions: (1) intestinal stenosis with symptoms of obstruction; (2) stenosis less than 3 cm long; (3) no tumor or fistula at the site of stenosis; (4) no deep ulceration at the site of stenosis; and (5) no sharp flexion due to the lesion. An analysis of 25 patients who were monitored for more than 6 months after initial EBD found a short-term success rate of 72 % and a cumulative surgery-free rate after 12 months of 72 %, both representing high figures. The only complications were acute pancreatitis alleviated by medical treatment in one patient and bleeding in one patient, with no occurrence of perforation [8].

The procedure for EBD comprises: (1) observation of the stenotic region; (2) diatrizoate meglumine (Gastrografin®) contrast enhancement; (3) guidewire placement; (4) insertion of a TTS balloon into the stenotic region; and (5) dilation of the balloon. The criterion for dilation pressure is that it should not exceed the specified pressure for each type of balloon, and dilation is performed under fluoroscopy while paying attention to how far the balloon is dilated and the speed at which the notch on top of the balloon disappears. The important point for ensuring that dilation is safe and does not cause perforation is to increase the pressure in the balloon very gradually during the initial stages of dilation. During dilation, the most important point to note is whether the patient complains of distress or pain, and if pain is felt then unnecessary inflation should be avoided. The time required for a single dilation is around 1–3 min, and the advantages and disadvantages of a second dilation should be considered after checking the condition of the lumen after dilation. At this point, a check must be made not only of how far the lumen has been extended, but also to see whether any complications such as bleeding or rupture are present.

The same indications for EBD as those for Crohn's disease also apply in cases of annular stenosis due to intestinal tuberculosis or CNSU. Surgical treatment must be considered in cases that do not meet these indication criteria.

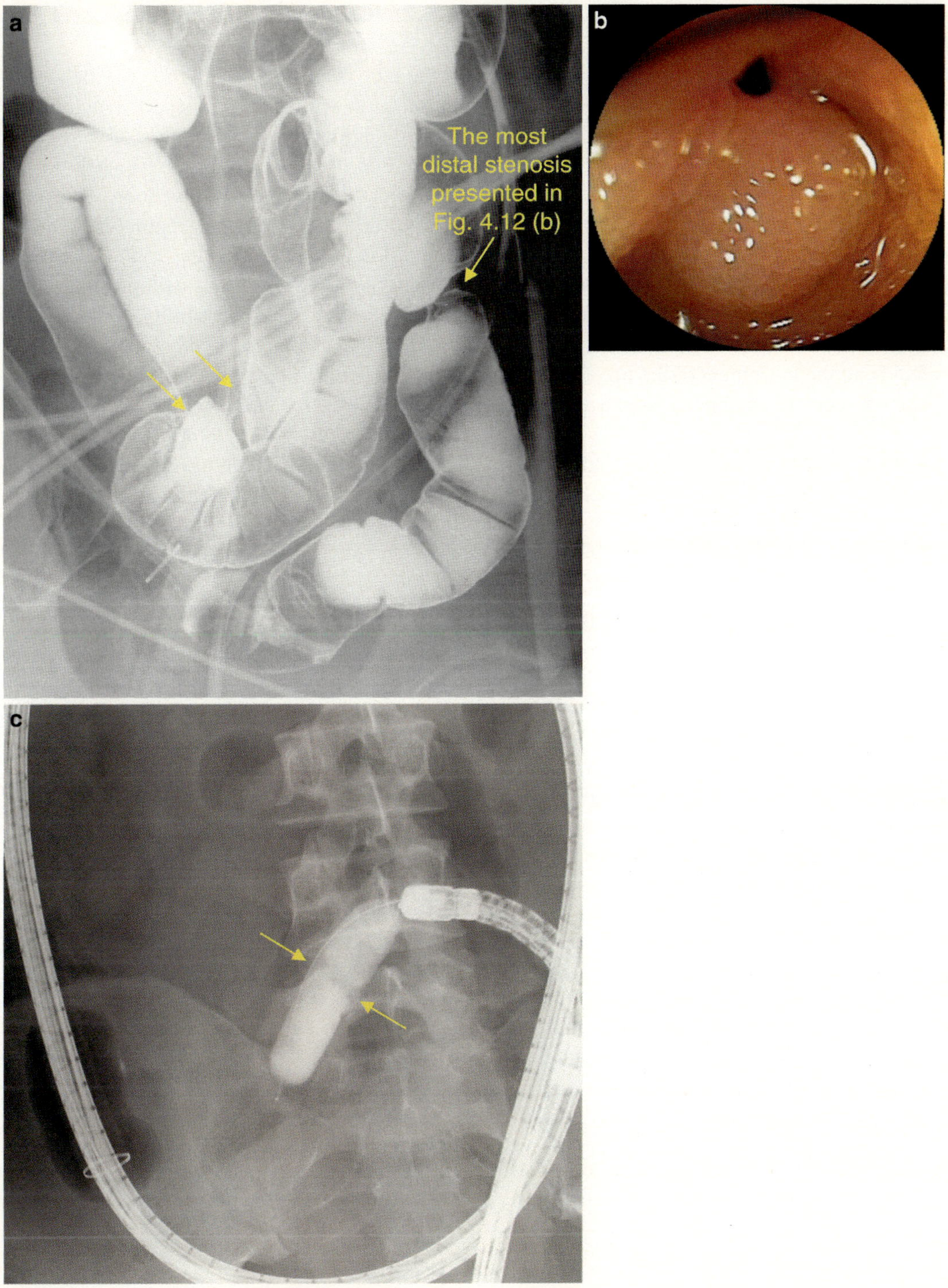

Fig. 4.12 Endoscopic balloon dilation. (**a**) A man in his 1920s, with small intestinal Crohn's disease, was referred with a diagnosis of ileus. Retrograde ileography of the ileum revealed ileal stenoses at three locations. The most distal stenosis was the most severe, with a further two sites of stenosis on the proximal side. All stenoses were less than 1 cm in length, and endoscopic dilation was regarded as indicated. (**b**) The most distal stenosis viewed by retrograde double-balloon endoscopy. Severe pinhole stenosis meant that the endoscope could not pass through. No ulceration was evident at the stenotic site. (**c**) A through the scope (TTS) balloon was dilated to 15–18 mm at 4.5 Atm for 1 min at the most distal stenosis observed by double-balloon endoscopy. The notch on the balloon was visible during the dilation process, but disappeared when dilation was complete, and the endoscope passed through the site of stenosis after dilation. Explanation in picture: site of stenosis in the most distal area observed by DBE

4.6 Complications

4.6.1 Complications Associated with Endoscope Insertion

One complication associated with insertion of the endoscope itself may occur in patients with severe adhesions, as application of excessive force to a severe adhesion may result in tissue damage, and possibly perforation. Care must be taken not to push too hard if the tip of the endoscope stops moving as if anchored at an adhesion site, or if the movement of the endoscopist's hand and the movement of the tip of the endoscope on the screen seem to become disconnected during insertion.

In Crohn's disease, longitudinal ulcers surround the edges of the endoscope from the 10 o'clock to the 12 o'clock direction, and reports have described the edge of the endoscope tip coming into contact with the bottom of a longitudinal ulcer and causing perforation as a result of insertion alone [8]. As identification of longitudinal ulcers may not be possible until the endoscope is being withdrawn, great care is required to try and insert the endoscope with great delicacy while remaining constantly focused on the lesion.

During antegrade insertion, long examination time or excessive simplification or straightening of the esophagus, stomach, or jejunum may cause acute pancreatitis by a mechanism such as imposition of abnormal force on the pancreas from the outside, compression of the papilla, or flexion of the pancreatic duct. We are therefore currently shortening examination times and administering pancreatic enzyme inhibitors to all patients undergoing antegrade insertion on the morning of the examination to prevent the onset of pancreatitis.

Aspiration pneumonia may also easily occur when antegrade insertion is used, particularly in elderly patients, although the use of sedatives is also a factor, and care must be taken with both examination time and frequent suction of sputum.

4.6.2 Ovt-Induced Complications

If the tube is advanced with the OVT balloon widely dilated in a region with plenty of space (such as the stomach or dilated angioectasia), perforation of the small intestine may result, and if resistance is sensed when the tube is inserted then deflation of the OVT balloon must be confirmed by X-ray fluoroscopy. Various reports have described perforation of longitudinal ulcers in Crohn's disease, particularly as a result of dilating the OVT balloon [9].

As there is also the possibility of mucosal damage should the mucosa become trapped between the tube and the endoscope, as well as of perforation due to tearing of adhesions by OVT insertion, careful operation is required. Because emergency surgical laparotomy may become necessary should perforation occur, informed consent must be obtained from patients and their families on the basis of sufficient information.

References

1. Yamamoto H et al. Total enteroscopy with a nonsurgical steerable double-balloon method. Gastrointest Endosc. 2011;53:216–20.
2. Pennazio M et al. Outcome of patients with obscure gastrointestinal bleeding after capsule endoscopy: report of 100 consecutive cases. Gastroenterology. 2004;126:643–53.
3. Hirai F et al. Efficacy of carbon dioxide insufflation inendoscopic balloon dilatation therapy using double balloon endoscopy. Gastrointest Endosc. 2007;66(Suppl):S26–9.
4. Ohmiya N et al. Diagnosis and treatment of obscure GI bleeding at double balloon endoscopy. Gastrointest Endosc. 2007;66:S72–7.
5. Sakamoto H et al. Nonsurgical management of small-bowel polyps in Peutz-Jeghers syndrome with extensive polypectomy by using double-balloon endoscopy. Gastrointest Endosc. 2011;74:328–33.
6. Arima S et al. The history of surgery for Crohn's disease at Chikushi Hospital. Med Bull Fukuoka Univ. 2002;29:113–9.
7. Hirai F et al. Endoscopic balloon dilatation using double-balloon endoscopy is a useful and safe treatment for small intestinal strictures of Crohn's disease. Dig Endosc. 2010;22:200–4.
8. Ohmiya N et al. Small-bowel obstruction: diagnostic comparison between double-balloon endoscopy and fluoroscopic enteroclysis, and the outcome of enteroscopic treatment. Gastrointest Endosc. 2009;69:84–93.
9. Oshitani N et al. Evaluation of deep small bowel involvement by double-balloon enteroscopy in Crohn's disease. Am J Gastroenterol. 2006;101:1484–9.

Part II

Specific Findings of Small Intestinal Lesions

Protruded Lesions

5

Naoki Ohmiya

5.1 Findings-Based Diagnostic Approach

If protruded lesions are observed, the first step is to distinguish between epithelial and non-epithelial lesions. The marginal rising appearance of epithelial lesions is comparatively steep, and the surface of the protrusion exhibits an abnormal structure. The marginal rising appearance of non-epithelial lesions is comparatively smooth, sometimes with a bridging fold. The surface of the protrusion is either covered in normal mucosa, or mucosal lesions such as villus swelling due to the expression effect, engorgement, or ulceration may be present.

The next step is to investigate whether protruded lesions are localized or diffuse. For localized lesions, it must be determined whether they are single or multiple (Table 5.1).

5.2 Procedure for Differential Diagnosis of Epithelial Tumors and Polyps

5.2.1 Small Intestinal Carcinoma

The morphology of most early-stage carcinomas comprises protrusions, flat elevations, or what in the large intestine are described as laterally spreading tumors (LSTs). As they progress, these lesions are categorized as protruded or ulcerated [1], with ulcerated carcinomas further classified into non-stenotic, extraintestinal, or annular stenotic types.

Protruded carcinomas comprise clearly demarcated elevations with a papillary or regular pattern, and erosion or ulceration may form on the surface due to peristaltic stimulation or ischemic changes during intestinal intussusception.

N. Ohmiya (✉)
Department of Gastroenterology, Nagoya University Graduate School of Medicine, 65 Tsurumai-cho, Showa-ku, Nagoya 466-8550, Japan
e-mail: nohmiya@med.nagoya-u.ac.jp

Ulcerated carcinomas are characterized by irregular borders with a dentate appearance, but may sometimes be difficult to differentiate from malignant lymphoma if the irregularity is slight.

Annular stenotic carcinomas often produce a short annular stenosis called a "napkin-ring sign," and the intestinal tract is frequently dilated on the proximal side of the tumor [2].

At the border between the tumor and non-tumorous tissue, the tumor compresses the mucosa downward as if spilling onto the mucosal surface, with an overhanging edge and an irregular boundary surface.

5.2.2 Carcinoid

The frequency of small intestinal carcinoid is extremely low in Japan compared with that in Europe and the United States. Although it is an epithelial tumor, carcinoid originates in the deep mucosal layer and expands into the submucosa, meaning that it appears as a somewhat yellowish submucosal tumor covered in normal to smooth mucosa. The surface frequently shows depression, and may have a tongue-like external appearance. Erosion and ulceration may be present. Vascular proliferation may be evident on the surface [3].

Carcinoid is frequently found in the ileum, particularly closer to the terminus of the ileum, and multiple occurrences are common.

5.2.3 Adenoma

Protruded and flat elevated lesions are common. The surface is nodular-granular, sometimes with a depression in the center [4]. Adenomas are classified histologically as tubular, tubular-villous, or villous. Lesion size ranges from 0.5 to 5.0 cm, with more villous structures tending to be larger.

In familial colorectal adenoma, multiple adenomas occur in the jejunum within 100 cm of the duodenum and the

T. Matsui et al. (eds.), *Endoscopy in the Diagnosis of Small Intestine Diseases*, DOI 10.1007/978-4-431-54352-7_5, © Springer Japan 2014

Table 5.1 Small intestinal diseases causing protruded lesions

Localized		
Single	Malignant	Malignant lymphoma, small intestinal carcinoma, metastatic small intestinal tumor, gastrointestinal stromal tumor (GIST), carcinoid
	Benign	Hamartoma, adenoma, aberrant pancreas, hemangioma, lipoma, lymphangioma, inflammatory fibroid polyp (IFP), leiomyoma
Multiple	Malignant	Malignant lymphoma,[a] small intestinal carcinoma,[b] metastatic small intestinal tumor, GIST,[c] carcinoid
	Benign	Hamartoma,[d] adenoma,[e] aberrant pancreas, hemangioma,[f] lipoma, lymphangioma
Diffuse	Malignant	Malignant lymphoma,[a] metastatic small intestinal tumor

[a]Immunoproliferative small intestinal disease (IPSID) (including MALT lymphoma), follicular lymphoma, T-cell lymphoma
[b]May be associated with disorders such as familial adenomatous polyposis (FAP), hereditary non-polyposis colorectal carcinoma, Peutz-Jeghers syndrome, and Crohn's disease
[c]May be present with von Recklinghausen's disease (*VRD*)
[d]Peutz-Jeghers syndrome, juvenile polyposis, Cowden's disease
[e]Familial adenomatous polyposis (FAP)
[f]Blue rubber bleb nevus syndrome
GIST gastrointestinal stromal tumor, *IFP* inflammatory fibroid polyp

ligament of Treitz and in the ileum within 60 cm of the ileocecal valve [5, 6]. Multiple adenomas are also seen in the distal ileum, including the ileal pouch, following total colectomy for familial colorectal adenoma, showing a higher frequency of occurrence with longer time since surgery [7].

5.2.4 Hamartoma

Hamartoma occurs when a tumor-like hyperplasia arises in the characteristic component tissue of an organ. Small intestinal hamartomas can be broadly divided into systemic hamartomatous polyposis and solitary hamartoma. The former includes Peutz-Jeghers syndrome, juvenile polyposis, Cowden's disease [8], and neurofibromatosis (von Recklinghausen's disease, VRD) [9], while the latter includes conditions such as solitary Peutz-Jeghers-type polyp, myoepithelial hamartoma (aberrant pancreas), Brunner's gland hamartoma, and juvenile polyp.

Peutz-Jeghers-type polyp is a lobulated or nodular semipedunculated or pedunculated protrusion, with twisting of the peduncle or intussusception occurring in large lesions, and an *erosion* or ulceration may form on the surface due to ischemic changes [10]. Myoepithelial hamartoma (aberrant pancreas) takes on the morphology of a sessile, smooth-surfaced submucosal tumor. Brunner's gland hamartoma usually occurs as a semi-pedunculated or pedunculated polyp covered in normal mucosa. Primary occurrence of a juvenile polyp in the small intestine is extremely rare, and is seen as a reddish semi-pedunculated or pedunculated polyp exhibiting gland duct dilatation on its surface.

5.2.5 Treatment

Adenoma, mucosal carcinoma, Peutz-Jeghers-type polyp, and juvenile polyp are indications for endoscopic treatment [10]. They may, however, cause severe chronic intussusception, and large Peutz-Jeghers-type polyps with broad peduncles may envelop the serosa, posing a high risk of producing a fistula when they are removed. In such cases they can be more safely resected by laparoscopic surgery.

Small intestinal carcinomas and carcinoids that have infiltrated below the submucosa are resected surgically.

In cases of multiple carcinoid, detailed observation is carried out preoperatively by BE and the lesion boundaries on the proximal and distal sides are marked. If this is not possible, intraoperative endoscopy is performed, as it is important that no small lesions be overlooked for resection.

Chemotherapy for small intestinal carcinoma usually follows one of the regimens used for colorectal carcinoma, such as FOLFOX or FOLFIRI. If complications occur such as hemorrhage in myoepithelial hamartoma (aberrant pancreas), a main location in the submucosa should be considered.

References

1. Honda W et al. Enteroscopic and radiologic diagnoses, treatment, and prognoses of small-bowel tumors. Gastrointest Endosc. 2012;76:344–54.
2. Partridge BJ et al. Small bowel cancers diagnosed device-assisted enteroscopy at a U.S. referral center: a five-year experience. Dig Dis Sci. 2011;56:2701–5.

3. Scherübl H et al. Neuroendocrine tumors of the small bowels are on the rise: early aspects and management. World J Gstrointest Endosc. 2010;2:325–34.
4. Matsumoto T et al. Small-intestinal involvement in familial adenomatous polyposis: evaluation by double-balloon endoscopy and intraoperative enteroscopy. Gastrointest Endosc. 2008;68:911–9.
5. Ohsato K et al. Small-intestinal involvement in familial polypopsis diagnosed by operative intestinal fiberscopy: report of four cases. Dis Colon Rectum. 1977;20:414–20.
6. Iida M et al. Diagnostic value of intraoperative fiberscopy for small intestinal polyps in familial adenomatous coli. Endoscopy. 1980;12: 161–5.
7. Iida M et al. Ileal adenomas in postcolectomy patients with familial adenomatous coli/Gardner's syndrome:incidence and endoscopic appearance. Dis Colon Rectum. 1989;32:1034–8.
8. Thomson M et al. Double balloon enteroscopy in children: diagnosis, treatment, and safety. World J Gastroenterol. 2010;16:56–62.
9. Hirashima K et al. Multiple gastrointestinal stromal tumors in neurofibromatosis type 1: report of a case. Surg Today. 2009; 39:979–83.
10. Ohmiya N et al. Management of small-bowel polyps in Peutz-Jeghers syndrome by using enteroclysis, double-balloon enteroscopy, and videocapsule endoscopy. Gastrointest Endosc. 2010;72: 1209–16.

Submucosal Elevations

6

Shotaro Nakamura

6.1 Findings-Based Diagnostic Approach

Submucosal elevation is a general term for lesions in which the main lesion is covered in the same mucosa as the surrounding mucosa and protrudes into the intestinal lumen as a hemisphere or sphere. These lesions themselves are located below the submucosa, with the majority comprising non-epithelial tumors or tumorous lesions, but carcinoids, which are derived from the deep mucosal layer and inflammatory fibroid polyps (IFPs) must also be considered during differentiation (Fig. 6.1) (Table 6.1).

Radiography and endoscopy reveal protruded lesions covered with normal mucosa with a smooth surface. Factors such as the number, size, color, surface properties, and hardness of lesions are important for qualitative diagnosis.

If there are multiple lesions with the same properties, malignant lymphoma, pneumatosis cystoides intestinalis, and systemic disorders such as neurofibromatosis must be considered during differentiation.

For solitary submucosal elevations, differentiation proceeds by estimating the main location of the lesion from its size and morphology. Soft tumors can be differentiated by color into lipomas, lymphangiomas, and hemangiomas.

Among hard lesions, IFPs and carcinoids arise in the deep mucosal layer, whereas erosion or irregular ulceration is frequently present at the apex. These two lesions are difficult to distinguish on the basis of images, but the former is pedunculate or semi-pedunculate, while the latter often forms a yellowish hemispherical protrusion. GIST is a hard tumor arising from a deeper layer, and is frequently multinodular with extraintestinal growth. This kind of lesion has a smooth surface, and ulceration tends to be comparatively smaller in diameter and deeper.

Malignant lymphoma exhibits a wide range of morphologies, and is not as hard as carcinoma or GIST. As it is derived from the deep mucosal layer to the shallow submucosal layer, granular changes on the surface, reddening, and small vessel proliferation are observed, and erosion or ulceration is frequently present.

S. Nakamura (✉)
Department of Medicine and Clinical Science, Graduate School of Medical Sciences, Kyushu University, 3-1-1, Maidashi, Higashi-ku, Fukuoka City 812-8582, Japan
e-mail: shonaka@intmed2.med.kyushu-u.ac.jp

T. Matsui et al. (eds.), *Endoscopy in the Diagnosis of Small Intestine Diseases*,
DOI 10.1007/978-4-431-54352-7_6, © Springer Japan 2014

Fig. 6.1 Radiological/endoscopic differential diagnostic procedure for small intestinal submucosal elevations

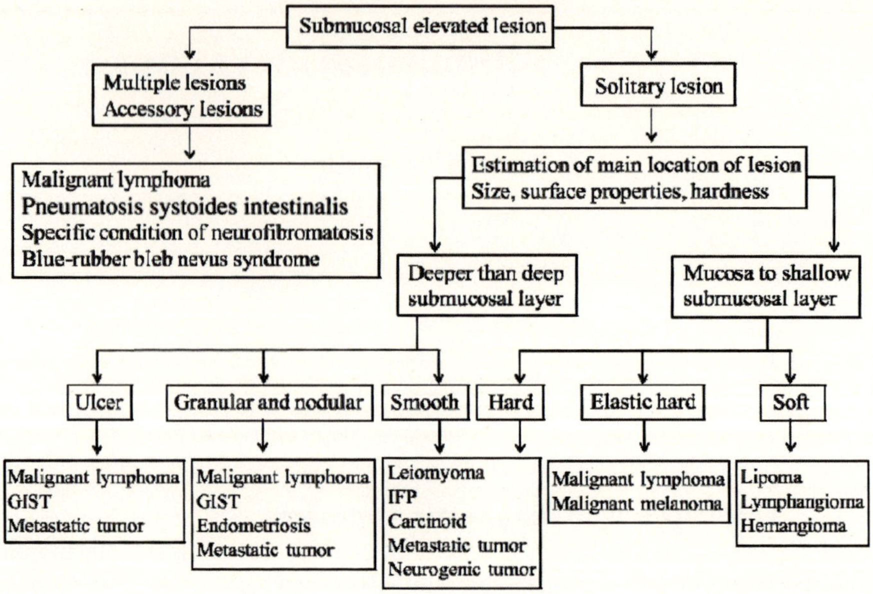

Table 6.1 Small intestinal diseases causing submucosal elevations

Comparatively common conditions	Uncommon conditions
Malignant	
Malignant lymphoma	Malignant lymphoma
Diffuse large B-cell lymphoma	Mantle cell lymphoma
Mucosa-associated lymphoid tissue (MALT) lymphoma	Burkitt lymphoma
Follicular lymphoma	T-cell lymphoma
GIST	Leiomyosarcoma
Carcinoid	Kaposi sarcoma/angiosarcoma
Metastatic small intestinal tumor	Malignant melanoma
Benign	
Lipoma	Schwannoma/neurofibroma
Lymphangioma	Intestinal endometriosis
Hemangioma	Pneumatosis cystoides intestinalis
Inflammatory fibroid polyp (IFP)	
Leiomyoma	

References

1. Shephard NA et al. Tumours of the small intestine. In: Bosman FT, et al, editors. WHO classification of tumours of the digestive system. 4th ed. Lyon: IARC; 2010. p. 95–118.
2. Nakamura S et al. A clinicopathologic study of primary small intestine lymphoma: prognostic significance of mucosa-associated lymphoid tissue-derived lymphoma. Cancer. 2000;88:286–94.
3. Rondonotti E et al. Small-bowel neoplasms in patients undergoing video capsule endoscopy: a multicenter European study. Endoscopy. 2008;40:488–95.
4. Mitsui K et al. Role of double-balloon endoscopy in the diagnosis of small-bowel tumors: the first Japanese multicenter study. Gastrointest Endosc. 2009;70:498–504.
5. Hirano A et al. Comparison of capsule endoscopy and double balloon endoscopy for the diagnosis of submucosal tumor of the small bowel. Dig Endosc. 2012;24:287.

Ulcerative Lesions

7

Kunihiko Aoyagi

7.1 Findings-Based Diagnostic Approach

Ulcerative lesions can be broadly divided into tumorous and non-tumorous ulceration.

When ulceration occurs due to an ulcerative disorder, this is frequently noticed as ulcerated protrusions, including primary carcinoma, metastatic intestinal carcinoma, malignant lymphoma, and GIST.

The most common form of metastatic carcinoma is lung cancer metastasis.

Causes of non-tumorous ulceration include inflammatory bowel disease, vasculitis/allergy, infection, ischemia, medication, and amyloidosis.

Morphology, size, distribution, depth, and multiplicity are taken into consideration when differentiating ulcerative lesions. In terms of morphology, lesions are determined to be circular, long, or irregular. For long ulcers, whether they are longitudinal or annular with respect to the long axis of the intestine is important, as is the relationship with the mesenterium.

Care is required when differentiating between ulcerated protruded lesions and ulcerative lesions with localized edema. Marginal rising appearance, surface properties, morphology and hardness of the protrusion, and irregularity or otherwise of the ulcer margin contribute to the diagnosis.

If differentiation by endoscopy alone is problematic, radiography, biopsy, CT, MRI, and serology tests are performed.

In Churg-Strauss syndrome and polyarteritis nodosa, symptoms of systemic vasculitis contribute to the diagnosis, while specific skin lesions are taken into account in Schönlein-Henoch purpura and Behçet's disease.

7.2 Diagnostic Procedure for Differential Diagnosis of Basic Lesions

For large or long lesions, other modalities such as radiography also contribute to the diagnosis. (Tables 7.1, 7.2, 7.3 and 7.4)

K. Aoyagi (✉)
Department of Gastroenterology and Medicine, Fukuoka University Faculty of Medicine, 7-45-1 Nanakuma, Jonan-ku, Fukuoka 814-0180, Japan
e-mail: kaoyagi@fukuoka-u.ac.jp

T. Matsui et al. (eds.), *Endoscopy in the Diagnosis of Small Intestine Diseases*,
DOI 10.1007/978-4-431-54352-7_7, © Springer Japan 2014

Table 7.1 Ulcerative lesions and frequency

Comparatively common conditions	Uncommon conditions
Malignant	
Malignant lymphoma	Small intestinal carcinoma
GIST	
Carcinoid	
Benign	
Crohn's disease	Behçet's disease
Drug-induced enteropathy	Simple ulcer
Intestinal tuberculosis	Cytomegalovirus (CMV) infection
Schönlein-Henoch purpura	Strongyloidiasis
	Churg-Strauss syndrome
	Polyarteritis nodosa
	Systemic lupus erythematosus
	Chronic non-specific multiple ulcers of the small intestine (CNSU)
	Intestinal amyloidosis
	Graft-versus-host disease
	Ischemic enteritis
	Radiation enteritis
	Inflammatory fibroid polyp (IFP)

Table 7.2 Differentiation of comparatively common types of ulceration

	Crohn's disease	Intestinal tuberculosis	Drug-induced enteropathy
Ulcer morphology	Longitudinal[a]	Annular/girdle-like	Irregular
Ulcer distribution	Cobblestone appearance	Irregular	Annular
Intervening mucosal findings	Irregular ulceration Aphtha-like ulceration	Stepping stone-like appearance	Erosion Scattered
Affected site	Stepping stone-like appearance	Areas of atrophic scarring Ileum>jejunum	Ileum>jejunum
Cause			
	Inflammatory polyps Ileum>jejunum Unknown	*Mycobacterium tuberculosis*	NSAIDs, oral aspirin

[a]Mainly located on the mesenteric side. Meets main diagnostic criteria if ≥4–5 cm along the long axis of the intestine.

Table 7.3 Differentiation of punched-out ulceration

	Behçet's disease/simple ulcer	CMV enteritis	Polyarteritis nodosa/Churg-Strauss syndrome
Intervening mucosal findings	Reddening	Reddening, edema	Reddening, edema
Affected site	Mainly in the ileocecal region	Jejunum/ileum	Jejunum/ileum
Lesion distribution	Single, scattered	Scattered (immune deficiency)	Scattered
Extraintestinal findings	Signs of Behçet's disease		Vasculitis syndrome

Table 7.4 Differentiation of annular ulceration

	Intestinal tuberculosis	Chronic non-specific multiple ulcers of the small intestine (CNSU)	Drug-induced enteropathy	Ischemic enteritis
Ulcer morphology	Annular	Annular/oblique	Circular, annular, membranous	Girdle-like/regional
Ulcer depth	Shallow	Shallow	Shallow	Deep
Affected site	Ileum>jejunum	Ileum>jejunum	Ileum>jejunum	Ileum>jejunum
Lesion distribution	Scattered	Scattered	Scattered	Single, scattered

References

1. Esaki M et al. Intraoperative enteroscopy detects more lesions but is not predictive of postoperative recurrence in Crohn's disease. Surg Endosc. 2001;15:455–9.
2. Matsumoto T et al. Endoscopic features of chronic nonspecific multiple ulcers of the small intestine: comparison with nonsteroidal anti-inflammatory drug-induced enteropathy. Dig Dis Sci. 2006;51: 1357–63.
3. Sato S et al. Colonoscopy in the diagnosis of intestinal tuberculosis in asymptomatic patients. Gastrointest Endosc. 2004;59:362–8.
4. Iida M et al. Postoperative recurrence in patients with intestinal Behçet's disease. Dis Colon Rectum. 1994;37:16–21.

8 Aphthous Lesions

Fumihito Hirai

8.1 Findings-Based Diagnostic Approach

Aphthae are normally understood as the smallest type of lesion to possess mucosal defects.

When carrying out differential diagnosis, matters such as the morphology, distribution, density, uneven distribution, and arrangement of aphthae must be taken into account.

Aphthae commonly occur in inflammatory disorders, frequently in conjunction with major lesions, but may also occur on their own.

Aphthae resemble lymph follicles, and may take on a wide range of morphologies, ranging from lesions with a small central depression to those close to small ulcers. In Crohn's disease, somewhat coarse aphthae with obvious white coating are frequently evident.

Aphthae are known to display characteristic distributions in a number of disorders, in terms of arrangement (longitudinal, transverse, etc.) and unevenness of distribution (presence or absence on the side of mesenteric adhesions). For example, longitudinal aphthae are frequently present on the side of mesenteric adhesions in Crohn's disease, but in intestinal tuberculosis they occur from the distal ileum to the ileocecal region, as areas rich in lymphatic tissue, and tend to be aligned with the flow of lymph along the transverse axis of the intestinal tract.

Biopsy of aphthae is frequently useful in the differentiation of inflammatory disorders, such as the detection of non-caseating epithelioid cell granuloma in Crohn's disease.

Characteristic lesions may develop from aphthae, and endoscopic observations should be performed over time as required.

If aphthae are present together with tumorous lesions, this may either be due to tumor infiltration or secondary due to mechanical stimulation or other cause.

Aphthae caused by vasculitis or allergy frequently occur as a result of vascular collapse or mucosal weakening.

Aphthae due to systemic disorders are frequently accessory lesions, with the characteristics of various different disorders commonly appearing as the main lesions, such as the severe edema evident in systemic lupus erythematosus.

Aphthae are non-specific lesions, and as such are frequently of little significance. They may, however, be extremely important as early lesions in the early-stage morphology of a disease. Other findings must also be taken into account for differentiation to be carried out efficiently. (Table 8.1)

F. Hirai (✉)
Department of Gastroenterology, Fukuoka University Chikushi Hospital, 1-1-1 Zokumyoin, Chikushino, Fukuoka 818-8502, Japan
e-mail: fuhirai@cis.fukuoka-u.ac.jp

T. Matsui et al. (eds.), *Endoscopy in the Diagnosis of Small Intestine Diseases*,
DOI 10.1007/978-4-431-54352-7_8, © Springer Japan 2014

Table 8.1 Aphthous lesions

Inflammatory disorders	Vasculitis: allergic disorder
Crohn's disease[a]	Systemic lupus erythematosus
Behçet's disease/simple ulcer[a]	Periarteritis nodosa
Intestinal tuberculosis[a]	Churg-Strauss syndrome
NSAID-induced enteropathy[a]	Schönlein-Henoch purpura
Drug-induced enteropathy (non-NSAID)	Eosinophilic enteritis
Infectious enteritis[a]	
Chronic non-specific multiple ulcers of the small intestine (CNSU)	
Ulcerative colitis (pouchitis)	
Tumorous disorders	**Others**
Malignant lymphoma	Intestinal amyloidosis[a]
Benign lymphoproliferative disease	Parasitic disorders
	Radiation enteritis
Metastatic tumor	Ischemic enteritis[a]
	Graft versus host disease
	Anastomotic ulcer

[a]Disorders in which aphthae are frequently associated.

References

1. Laufer I et al. Early lesions of Crohn's disease. Am J Roentgenol. 1978;130:307–11.
2. Simpkins KC. Aphthoid ulcers in Crohn's colitis. Clin Radiol. 1977;28:601–8.
3. Yao T. Double contrast enterolysis with air. In: Freeny PC, Stevenson GW, editors. Malgulis and Burhenne's alimentaly tract radiology. St Louis: Mosby; 1994. p. 548–51.
4. Matsumoto T et al. Crohn's disease of aphthous type: serial changes in intestinal lesions. Br J Radiol. 2000;73:1046–51.

Stenotic Lesions

9

Takahiro Beppu

9.1 Findings-Based Diagnostic Approach

Stenotic lesions can be broadly divided into those caused by inflammatory disorders and those due to tumors.

Among inflammatory disorders, fibrosis due to chronic inflammation and stenosis due to edema in ulcers occur in diseases such as Crohn's disease, small intestinal tuberculosis, chronic non-specific multiple ulcers of the small intestine, NSAID-induced enteropathy, Behçet's disease/simple ulcer, ischemic enteritis, and radiation enteritis.

Crohn's disease is characterized by longitudinal and annular ulceration, small intestinal tuberculosis by annular ulceration, chronic non-specific multiple ulcers of the small intestine by oblique ulceration, and NSAID-induced enteropathy by annular ulceration and membranous stenosis. Longitudinal stenosis also appears in tuberculosis and ischemic enteritis.

Stenosis due to edema of the small intestine may also occur. This finding may be evident in the acute phase of infectious enteritis, anisakiasis, eosinophilic enteritis, T-cell lymphoma, and other disorders.

T. Beppu (✉)
Department of Gastroenterology, Fukuoka University Chikushi Hospital, 1-1-1 Zokumyoin, Chikushino, Fukuoka 818-8502, Japan
e-mail: bouzutb@yahoo.co.jp

In tumorous disorders, stenosis frequently occurs when tumor growth into the lumen is severe, and the probability of malignancy also rises. Large tumors may also be partly ulcerated. Stenosis occurs with primary small intestinal carcinoma among epithelial tumors, and with malignant lymphoma, GIST, metastatic small intestinal carcinoma, lipoma, inflammatory fibroid polyp (IFP), Peutz-Jeghers syndrome, and other non-epithelial tumors. In circumferential malignant tumorous stenosis, although lesions tend to be larger in malignant lymphoma than in adenoma, extension of the intestinal tract is usually better.

When IFP and Peutz-Jeghers syndrome tumors become advanced, they may cause intussusception due to introversion of Meckel's diverticulum, producing secondary stenosis (Table 9.1).

9.2 Stenosis Score (Fukuoka Index)

The Fukuoka Index was developed to quantify radiographic findings in Crohn's disease. In this index, stenosis score is: (1) if there is no dilatation on the proximal side of the stenosis and the width of the intestinal tract lumen is at least half that of the neighboring healthy intestinal tract lumen; (2) if there is no dilatation on the proximal side and the width of the narrow part of the intestinal lumen is less than half that of the neighboring healthy intestinal tract lumen; and (3) if there is pronounced narrowing of the intestinal lumen with dilatation of the intestinal tract on the proximal side (Fig.9.1).

T. Matsui et al. (eds.), *Endoscopy in the Diagnosis of Small Intestine Diseases*,
DOI 10.1007/978-4-431-54352-7_9, © Springer Japan 2014

Table 9.1 Stenotic lesions

Inflammatory disorders	Tumorous disorders
Crohn's disease, small intestinal tuberculosis, chronic non-specific multiple ulcers of the small intestine (CNSU), NSAID-induced enteropathy, Behçet's disease/simple ulcer, ischemic enteritis, acute phase of infectious enteritis, anisakiasis, eosinophilic enteritis, Satoyoshi syndrome, radiation enteritis, etc.	Primary small intestinal carcinoma, malignant lymphoma, GIST, metastatic small intestinal carcinoma, lipoma, inflammatory fibroid polyp (IFP), Peutz-Jeghers syndrome, etc.
	Others
	Postoperative adhesion, postoperative anastomosis, introversion of Meckel's diverticulum, chronic pseudo-obstruction, etc.

Fig. 9.1

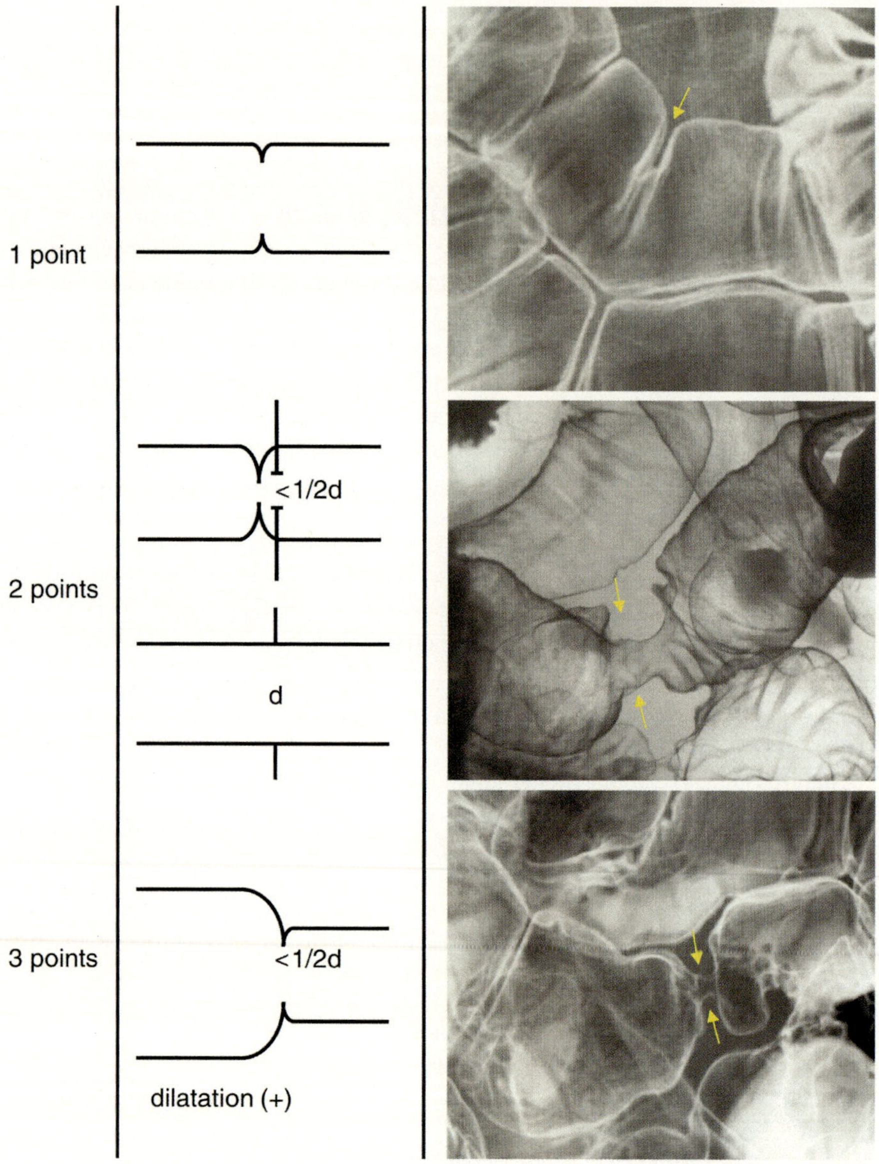

*Yellow arrows indicate sites of stenosis.

References

1. Sou S et al. Clinical and endoscopic healing after infliximab treatment in patients with Crohn's disease. Digest Endosc. 2006;18:29–33.
2. Fukumoto A et al. Diagnosis and treatment of small-bowel stricture by double balloon endoscopy. Gastrointest Endosc. 2007;66:S108–12.
3. Naganuma M et al. Safety and usefulness of balloon endoscopy in Crohn's disease patients with postoperative ileal lesions. J Crohns Colitis. 2011;5:73–4.
4. Sunada K et al. Advances in the diagnosis and treatment of small bowel lesions with Crohn's disease using double-balloon endoscopy. Therap Adv Gastroenterol. 2009;2:357–66.
5. Matsumoto T et al. Endoscopic features of chronic nonspecific multiple ulcers of the small intestine: comparison with nonsteroidal anti-inflammatory drug-induced enteropathy. Dig Dis Sci. 2006;51:1357–63.
6. Matsumoto T et al. Double-contrast barium enteroclysis as a patency tool for nonsteroidal anti-inflammatory drug-induced enteropathy. Dig Dis Sci. 2011;56:3247–53.
7. Ohmiya N et al. Small-bowel obstruction: diagnostic comparison between double-balloon endoscopy and fluoroscopic enteroclysis and the outcome of enteroscopic treatment. Gastrointest Endosc. 2009;69:84–93.
8. Yamagami H et al. Usefulness of double-balloon endoscopy in the diagnosis of malignant small-bowel tumors. Clin Gastroenterol Hepatol. 2008;6:1202–5.
9. Ohmiya N et al. Management of small-bowel polyps in Peutz-Jeghers syndrome by using enteroclysis, double-balloon enteroscopy, and videocapsule endoscopy. Gastrointest Endosc. 2010;72:1209–16.

10 Hemorrhagic Lesions

Tomonori Yano

10.1 Findings-Based Diagnostic Approach

1. If the source of bleeding cannot be identified by upper and lower gastrointestinal endoscopy, a lesion may have been overlooked, and repeat examination should therefore be considered if there may have been problems with timing or accuracy.
2. As a basic rule, stool color is blacker the closer the source of bleeding is to the *proximal side of GI tract* and redder the closer it is to the distal side. As red stool may pass from lesions in the duodenum and beyond, however, depending on the amount of bleeding and the amount of time that has elapsed, patients must always be asked about frequency of evacuation as well as stool color.
3. Sources of bleeding may be vascular, neoplastic, or ulcerative lesions or diverticula of the small intestine.
4. Vascular lesions account for a large proportion of bleeding sources among elderly patients and those with underlying heart, liver, or kidney disease.
5. If dynamic contrast-enhanced CT reveals findings of lesions such as small intestinal tumor, thickened bowel wall, or stenosis, balloon-assisted endoscopy (BAE) should be considered in light of the possibility of tumor or IBD.
6. If leakage of contrast agent into the intestine is evident in contrast-enhanced CT or symptoms indicate the possibility of continuous bleeding, emergency BAE should be performed, as this enables hemostasis to be performed simultaneously with diagnosis. As the location of bloody intestinal fluid offers a clue as to which insertion route to use, in principle the antegrade route is used without pretreatment. However, if the source of bleeding can be identified as located near the terminus of the ileum, then the retrograde route with pretreatment should be considered.
7. If there are no findings on CT and bleeding has already stopped spontaneously, or in the case of chronic iron-deficiency anemia with no overt bleeding, CE should be performed first, and BAE considered once the location and type of lesion have been identified.
8. As the rate of positive findings decreases the longer the time between final hemorrhage and examination, endoscopy should be performed quickly.
9. The most important task is to identify lesion location, but this is also the most difficult, and a long transparent hood should be fitted to the tip of the BAE when searching for lesions, to minimize blind spots behind folds or on the inside of flexions.
10. As the small intestine lacks landmarks, it is easy to lose sight of bloody intestinal fluid and lesions. Marking clips should be utilized as landmarks.
11. If flowing blood is an obstacle preventing lesion observation, underwater endoscopy should be used.
12. Lesions should be observed while noting whether bleeding is pulsatile, recording findings on the basis of the endoscopic classification of vascular lesions of the small intestine, and selecting a method of treatment.
13. In the event that no lesions are evident from examination of the entire small intestine despite obvious heavy small intestinal bleeding, or if only Type 1a angiodysplasia can be found, the possibility of spontaneous hemostasis of Type 2a lesions should be kept in mind, and emergency BAE should be considered in the event of recurrent hemorrhage (Table 10.1).

T. Yano (✉)
Division of Gastroenterology, Department of Internal Medicine, Jichi Medical University, 3311-1 Yakushiji, Shimotsuke 329-0498, Japan
e-mail: tomonori@jichi.ac.jp

T. Matsui et al. (eds.), *Endoscopy in the Diagnosis of Small Intestine Diseases*,
DOI 10.1007/978-4-431-54352-7_10, © Springer Japan 2014

Table 10.1 Small intestinal diseases causing hemorrhagic lesions

Type of lesion	Frequent	Infrequent
Vascular lesions	Type 1a	Type 2b
	Type 1b	Type 3
	Type 2a	Type 4 (unclassified)
		Varices
Neoplastic lesions	GIST	Lymphoma
	Cancer	Hemangioma
		Lymphangioma (hemorrhagic lesions are rare)
		Hamartoma
Ulcerative lesions	Crohn's disease	Behçet disease
	NSAID-induced enteropathy	Simple ulcer
		Chronic non-specific multiple ulcers of the small intestine
		Cytomegalovirus enteritis
		Blind loop syndrome
		Anastomotic ulcer
Diverticulum	Meckel's diverticulum	Jejunal diverticulum
	Duodenal diverticulum	Ileal diverticulum

Table 10.2 Endoscopic classification of vascular lesions of the small intestine

Type 1a	Punctate (<1 mm), reddish, either not bleeding or only oozing
Type 1b	Macular (several millimeters), reddish, either not bleeding or only oozing
Type 2a	Punctate (<1 mm), with pulsatile hemorrhage
Type 2b	Pulsating red protrusions without surrounding venous dilation
Type 3	Pulsating red protrusions with surrounding venous dilation
Type 4	Not classified as any of the above

10.2 Points for Differential Diagnosis

Vascular lesions should be diagnosed according to the endoscopic classification of vascular lesions of the small intestine, noting whether lesions are pulsatile (Table 10.2).

Type 1 lesions have venous or capillary characteristics, and can be regarded as corresponding to angiectasia. Such lesions are appropriately treated with APC or other electroablation therapy.

Type 2 lesions have arterial characteristics, and can be regarded as corresponding to Dieulafoy's lesion. Such lesions are appropriately treated with hemostatic clipping.

Type 3 lesions have both venous and arterial characteristics, and can be regarded as corresponding to arteriovenous malformation (AVM). If the lesions are small, appropriate treatment is with hemostatic clipping of the feeding artery. If lesions are large, appropriate treatment is with abdominal transcatheter arterial embolization or surgical resection.

With respect to diverticula, problems may be caused by Meckel's diverticulum and duodenal diverticulum. Meckel's diverticulum occurs in 2–4 % of the population, and in adults this lesion is found on the mesenteric side of the cecum ileum approximately 60–100 cm proximal to the ileocecal valve. As false-negative results may occur, this pathology cannot be ruled out even if results from scintigraphy for Meckel's diverticulum are negative. Likewise, even if Meckel's diverticulum or duodenal diverticulum is evident on balloon endoscopy, the diverticulum cannot be confirmed as the source of bleeding in the absence of ulceration, erosive lesions, or exposed blood vessels, and a proactive search for other sources of bleeding should be undertaken.

References

1. Yano T et al. Endoscopic classification of vascular lesions of the small intestine (with videos). Gastrointest Endosc. 2008;67:169–72.
2. Iwamoto M et al. Double-balloon endoscopy for jejunal hemangioma (with video). Gastrointest Endosc. 2007;66:184–5.
3. Shinozaki S et al. Long-term outcome of patients with obscure gastrointestinal bleeding investigated by double-balloon endoscopy. Clin Gastroenterol Hepatol. 2010;8:151–8.

Diffuse Lesions

11

Takayuki Matsumoto

11.1 Findings-Based Diagnostic Approach

1. Non-neoplastic diseases of the small intestine frequently cause diffuse lesions (Table 11.1). Among neoplastic diseases, lymphoproliferative diseases causing diffuse lesions should always be kept in mind during differential diagnosis.
2. Findings of diffuse lesions comprise swelling of folds, loss of folds, multiple nodules, granular mucosa, or a combination thereof (Fig. 11.1).
3. Swelling of the folds is evident in acute diseases, intestinal amyloidosis, and intestinal lymphoangiectasia. Neoplastic diseases rarely cause swelling of the folds alone, although the finding may be prominent in adult T-cell lymphoma. Edematous changes to the full thickness of the intestine are pronounced in the far-advanced stages of acute disorders, causing severe swelling of the folds. Distensibility is not poor in intestinal amyloidosis or lymphangiectasia, but multiple nodules and granular mucosa are frequently present in addition to swelling of the folds, although distensibility is not poor in intestinal amyloidosis or lymphangiectasia.
4. Multinodular changes constitute histological changes to the submucosa that are visualized as nodular shadows, whereas granular mucosa reflects the enlargement or atrophy of small intestinal villi. Multiple nodules are evident in AL-type intestinal amyloidosis, intestinal lymphangiectasia, and pneumatosis cystoides intestinalis. Neoplastic diseases that should be distinguished are gastrointestinal polyposis and mantle-cell lymphoma, with swelling of the folds apparent in intestinal amyloidosis and intestinal lymphangiectasia.
5. Granular mucosa is evident in cases of protozoal or parasitic infections and type AA intestinal amyloidosis, frequently in association with loss of folds. Immunoproliferative small intestinal disease (IPSID) and enteropathy-associated T-cell lymphoma are types of malignant lymphoma that must be differentiated.
6. The fine granular mucosa evident in chronic-phase strongyloidiasis and isosporiosis is caused by villous atrophy, and the granules are heterogeneous in size. In contrast, granular mucosa is minor in giardiasis, and the folds are preserved. In type AA intestinal amyloidosis, the deposition of amyloid fibrous proteins in the lamina propria alters the villous structure. This disturbance of the villous structure results in granular mucosa. In severe cases, the shape of folds may be blunted or lost.

T. Matsumoto (✉)
Department of Medicine and Clinical Science, Graduate School of Medicine, Kyushu University, 3-1-1 Maidashi, Higashi-ku, Fukuoka 812-8582, Japan
e-mail: matane@intmed2.med.kyushu-u.ac.jp

T. Matsui et al. (eds.), *Endoscopy in the Diagnosis of Small Intestine Diseases*,
DOI 10.1007/978-4-431-54352-7_11, © Springer Japan 2014

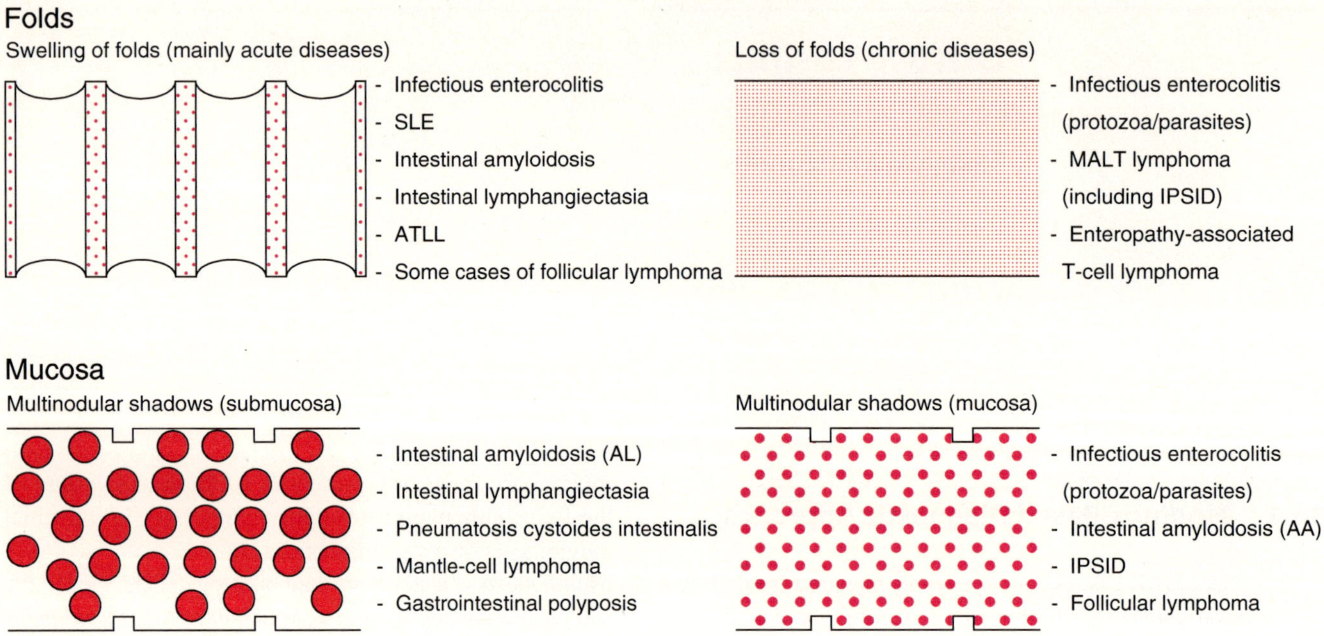

Fig. 11.1 (**a–d**) Differential diagnosis of diffuse lesions (p53)

Table 11.1 Small intestinal diseases causing diffuse lesions

Acute inflammatory diseases
(1) Infections
Parasitic infections
Nematode infection (anisakiasis)
Strongyloidiasis
Giardiasis
Bacterial infection
(2) Other inflammatory diseases
Systemic lupus erythematosus (SLE)
Eosinophilic gastroenteritis
Chronic non-neoplastic diseases
(1) Infections
Strongyloidiasis
Giardiasis
Isosporiosis
Mycobacterium avium complex infection
(2) Other diseases
Intestinal amyloidosis
Intestinal lymphangiectasia
Scleroderma
Portal hypertensive enteropathy
Intestinal lesions of Satoyoshi disease
Neoplastic diseases
(1) Lymphoproliferative disease
Adult T-cell lymphoma
Enteropathy-associated T-cell lymphoma
IPSID (including MALT lymphoma)
Follicular lymphoma
(2) Metastatic small intestinal cancer

References

1. Tada S et al. Endoscopic features in amyloidosis of the small intestine: clinical and morphologic differences between chemical types of amyloid protein. Gastrointest Endosc. 1994;40:45–50.
2. Aoyagi K et al. Characteristic endoscopic features of intestinal lymphangiectasia: correlation with histological findings. Hepatogastroenterology. 1997;44:133–8.
3. Endo H et al. Capsule endoscopic evaluation of eosinophilic enteritis before and after treatment. Digestion. 2011;83:134–5.
4. Nakamura S et al. A clinicopathologic study of primary small intestine lymphoma: prognostic significance of mucosa-associated lymphoid tissue-derived lymphoma. Cancer. 2000;88:286–94.
5. Matsumoto T et al. Performance of antegrade double-balloon enteroscopy. Comparison with push enteroscopy. Gastrointest Endosc. 2005;62:392–8.

12 Reddish Lesions

Kunihiko Aoyagi

12.1 Findings-Based Diagnostic Approach

1. Diseases causing reddish lesions can be broadly divided into neoplastic and non-neoplastic ulceration.

K. Aoyagi (✉)
Department of Gastroenterology and Medicine, Fukuoka University Faculty of Medicine, 7-45-1 Nanakuma, Jonan-ku, Fukuoka 814-0180, Japan
e-mail: kaoyagi@fukuoka-u.ac.jp

2. When neoplastic diseases cause redness, this is due to erosion by tumor infiltration or mechanical irritation at the borders of the tumor.
3. Possible non-neoplastic causes of redness comprise vasculitis/allergy, infection, ischemia, drugs, and others.
4. Granular and nodular mucosa is frequently associated with chronic infection and intestinal amyloidosis.
5. Small areas of redness that are recognizable as angiectasia must not be biopsied for diagnostic purposes (Tables 12.1, 12.2 and 12.3).

T. Matsui et al. (eds.), *Endoscopy in the Diagnosis of Small Intestine Diseases*,
DOI 10.1007/978-4-431-54352-7_12, © Springer Japan 2014

Table 12.1 Diseases causing reddish lesions

Comparatively frequent disease	Infrequent disease
Benign	Vasculitis/allergy
Eosinophilic enteritis	Systemic lupus erythematosus
Drug-induced enteritis	Churg-Strauss syndrome
Schönlein-Henoch purpura	Polyarteritis nodosa
Angiectasia	Infection
Bacterial infection (*Salmonella*, *Yersinia*, *Vibrio parahaemolyticus*)	Cytomegalovirus infection
	Intestinal anisakiasis
	Giardiasis
	Strongyloidiasis
	Bacterial infection (typhoid fever, Whipple's disease)
	Tumor
	Small intestinal cancer
	Malignant lymphoma (particularly T-cell lymphoma)
	Pyogenic granuloma
	Others
	Behçet disease
	Simple ulcer
	Portal hypertensive enteropathy
	Ischemic enteritis
	Chronic non-specific multiple ulcers of the small intestine
	Graft-versus-host disease

Table 12.2 Points for differential diagnosis of basic lesions

	Schönlein-Henoch purpura	Eosinophilic gastroenteritis	Systemic lupus erythematosus	Drug-induced enteritis	Angiectasia
Affected area	Jejunum/ileum	Jejunum/ileum	Jejunum/ileum	Ileum > jejunum	Jejunum/ileum
Mucosal findings	Redness, *erosion*, submucosal hemorrhage	Redness	Redness	Redness, *erosion*	Angiectasia
Edema	+	+	+	+ to –	–
Ulceration	+ to –	– to +	– to +	+ to –	–
Morphology	Irregular	Irregular	Irregular	Irregular/annular	
Cause	Vasculitis	Allergy	Vasculitis	NSAID, aspirin	Acquired degenerative lesions

Table 12.3 Chronic infectious diseases causing reddish lesions

	Intestinal tuberculosis	Strongyloidiasis	Giardiasis	Isosporiosis
Affected area	Ileum > jejunum	Jejunum > ileum	Jejunum > ileum	Jejunum > ileum
Mucosal findings	Atrophic scarring area	Granular mucosa, *erosion*	Normal to Fine granular mucosa	Granular mucosa
Edema	– to +	+ to –	+ to –	+ to –
Ulceration	+ to –	– to +	–	–
Morphology	Irregular, annular or girdle-like	Irregular		
Cause	*Mycobacterium tuberculosis*	*Strongyloides*	*Giardia lamblia*	*Isospora*

References

1. Esaki M et al. GI involvement in Henoch-Schönlein purpura. Gastrointest Endosc. 2002;56:920–3.
2. Sato S et al. Colonoscopy in the diagnosis of intestinal tuberculosis in asymptomatic patients. Gastrointest Endosc. 2004;59:362–8.
3. Kinoshita Y et al. Clinical characteristics of Japanese patients with eosinophilic esophagitis and eosinophilic gastroenteritis. J Gastroenterol. 2013;48(3):333–9.
4. Yanai S et al. Endoscopic findings of enteropathy-type T-cell lymphoma. Endoscopy. 2007;39 Suppl 1:E339–40.

13 Edematous Lesions

Kunihiko Aoyagi

13.1 Findings-Based Diagnostic Approach

1. Edematous changes are recognizable as swelling of the folds. Diseases causing swelling of the folds can be broadly divided into neoplastic and non-neoplastic diseases.
2. Possible non-neoplastic causes of edema include vasculitis/allergy, infection, ischemia, and drugs.
3. In neoplastic diseases such as cancer infiltration/metastasis and malignant lymphoma, the folds are thickened by tumor cell infiltration, and frequently appear hard because they are poorly distensible by air.
4. The distribution of edema may be localized/segmental or diffuse.
5. The intestinal margins exhibit an irregular dentate shape under radiography known as a dentate appearance, reflecting acute-phase submucosal edema and intestinal spasm.
6. Diseases that exhibit peripheral eosinophilia in addition to swelling of the folds are eosinophilic enteritis, Churg-Strauss syndrome, polyarteritis nodosa, and parasitosis (Tables 13.1, 13.2, and 13.3).

K. Aoyagi (✉)
Department of Gastroenterology and Medicine, Fukuoka University Faculty of Medicine, 7-45-1 Nanakuma, Jonan-ku, Fukuoka 814-0180, Japan
e-mail: kaoyagi@fukuoka-u.ac.jp

T. Matsui et al. (eds.), *Endoscopy in the Diagnosis of Small Intestine Diseases*,
DOI 10.1007/978-4-431-54352-7_13, © Springer Japan 2014

Table 13.1 Edematous lesions and frequency

Comparatively frequent	Infrequent
Malignant	Vasculitis / allergy
Cancer infiltration/metastasis	Systemic erythematosus
Malignant lymphoma	Churg-Strauss syndrome
	Polyarteritis nodosa
Benign	Infection
Eosinophilic enteritis	Cytomegalovirus infection
Schönlein-Henoch purpura	Intestinal anisakiasis
Crohn's disease	Giardiasis
Drug-induced enteritis	Strongyloidiasis
Intestinal tuberculosis	*Bacterial infection* (*Salmonella*, *Yersinia*, typhoid fever, *Vibrio parahaemolyticus*, Whipple's disease)
	Ischemia
	Ischemic enteritis
	Radiation enteritis
	Others
	Behçet disease
	Simple ulcer
	Ischemic enteritis
	Chronic non-specific multiple ulcers of the small intestine
	Graft-versus-host disease
	Intestinal amyloidosis
	Intestinal lymphangiectasia
	Celiac disease
	Hypoganglionosis

Table 13.2 Points for differential diagnosis of basic lesions

	Schönlein-Henoch purpura	Eosinophilic enteritis	Systemic lupus erythematosus	Intestinal anisakiasis	Ischemic enteritis
Affected area	Jejunum/ileum	Jejunum/ileum	Jejunum/ileum	Jejunum/ileum	Jejunum/ileum
Mural localization	Mucosa or submucosa	Mucosa to serosa	Submucosa to serosa	Submucosa	Mucosa, submucosa
Folds findings	Swelling	Swelling	Swelling	Swelling, thumbprinting sign	Thumbprinting sign
Regularity	Comparatively irregular	Comparatively irregular	Comparatively irregular	Irregular	Irregular
Mucosal findings	Redness, erosion, ulceration, submucosal hemorrhage	Redness, ulceration	Almost normal to redness	Almost normal to redness	Redness, segmental ulceration, granular mucosa
Cause	Vasculitis	Allergy	Vasculitis	Infection	Ischemia

Table 13.3 Diseases causing diffuse edema

	Giardiasis	Strongyloidiasis	AA-type intestinal amyloidosis	AL-type intestinal amyloidosis
Affected area	Jejunum > ileum	Jejunum > ileum	Jejunum	Jejunum
Mural localization	Mainly mucosa	Mainly mucosa	Mainly mucosa	Submucosa
Folds findings	Swelling, loss	Swelling, loss	Granular swelling, loss	Multitumor-like thickening
Regularity	Regular	Comparatively regular	Comparatively regular	Irregular
Mucosal findings	Normal to fine granular	Granular mucosa, *erosion*	Granular mucosa, *erosion*	Submucosal tumor-like protrusion
Cause	Infection	Infection	AA-type amyloid deposition	AL-type amyloid deposition

References

1. Esaki M et al. GI involvement in Schönlein-Henoch purpura. Gastrointest Endosc. 2002;56:920–3.
2. Kinoshita Y et al. Clinical characteristics of Japanese patients with eosinophilic esophagitis and eosinophilic gastroenteritis. J Gastroenterol. 2013;48(3):333–9.
3. Hizawa K et al. Double-contrast radiographic assessment of lupus-associated enteropathy. Clin Radiol. 1998;53:825–9.
4. Matsui T et al. Intestinal anisakiasis: clinical and radiologic features. Radiology. 1985;157:299–302.
5. Tada S et al. Endoscopic features in amyloidosis of the small intestine: clinical and morphologic differences between chemical types of amyloid protein. Gastrointest Endosc. 1994;40:45–50.

14 Case Presentations: Flat/Small Protrusions

Yuji Maehata, Atsushi Hirano, Shunichi Yanai, and Hiroshi Kawano

14.1 Case 1, 2 [1]

14.1.1 Female, 20s (Fig. 14.1a, b)

Principle complaint: Anemia

- Father suffered from adenomatous polyposis.
- Per-oral DBE showed a semi-pedunculated protrusion in the jejunum. The surface was nodular and whitish.
- Tiny non-pedunculated protrusions were also scattered in the jejunum.

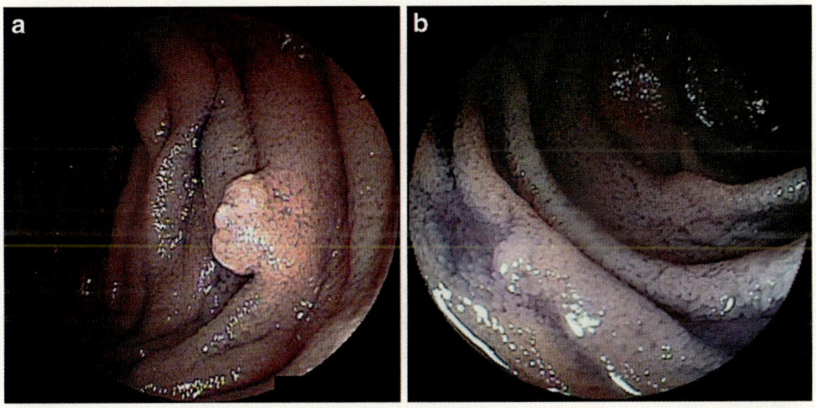

Fig. 14.1

14.1.2 Male, 20s (Fig. 14.2a, b)

Principle complaints: Anemia, fecal occult bleeding

- Multiple adenomatous polyps were evident at the terminus of the ileum. Positive results were obtained for the APC genetic mutation.
- CE showed whitish flat elevations scattered in the jejunum.
- Tiny whitish protrusions were evident in the central jejunum.

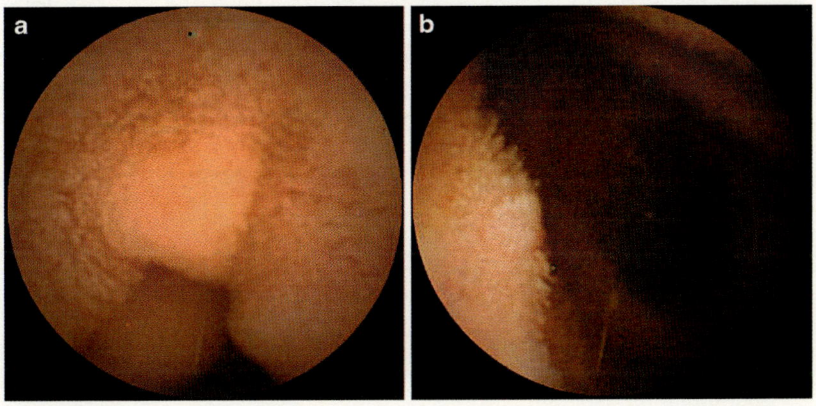

Fig. 14.2

Y. Maehata (✉) • A. Hirano
Department of Medicine and Clinical Science, Graduate School of Medical Sciences, Kyushu University, 3-1-1 Maidashi, Higashi-ku, Fukuoka 812-8582, Japan
e-mail: ymaehata@intmed2.med.kyushu-u.ac.jp

S. Yanai
Japan Seamen's Relief Association Moji Hospital, 1-3-1 Kiyotaki, Moji-ku, Kitakyushu 801-8550, Japan

H. Kawano
Dicision of Gastroenterology, Department of Medicine, Kurume University School of Medicine, 67 Asahi-machi, Kurume 830-0011, Japan

T. Matsui et al. (eds.), *Endoscopy in the Diagnosis of Small Intestine Diseases*,
DOI 10.1007/978-4-431-54352-7_14, © Springer Japan 2014

14.1.3 Small Intestinal Adenoma (Figs. 14.3 and 14.4)

- Small intestinal adenomas are present in around 60 % of patients with familial adenomatous polyposis (FAP). In disorders other than this, however, the prevalence of adenoma is low. The majority of cases are asymptomatic, but large tumors may cause intestinal hemorrhage, obstruction, or intussusception. The rate at which they become cancerous is unknown.
- Most small intestinal adenomas are discovered as protruded lesions. On radiography, they are visualized as small, translucent structures, but visualization of tiny lesions is no easy task.
- On small intestinal endoscopy, they are observed as non-pedunculate or pedunculated protrusions. The surface is granular or nodular, and the lesions are frequently whitish in color. They may only be noticed after dye spraying.

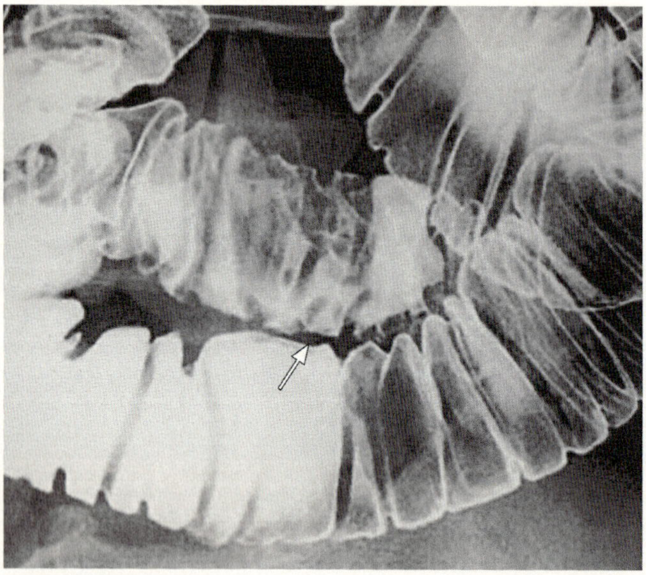

Fig. 14.3 On radiography, a small translucent structure (*arrow*) was evident in the jejunum

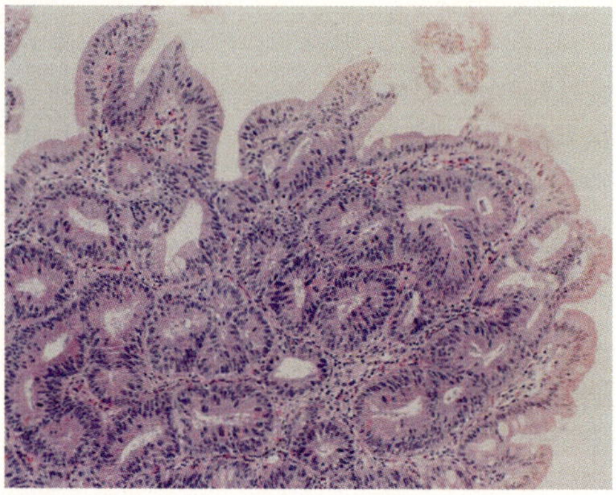

Fig. 14.4 Histopathological image of a biopsy specimen. This shows findings of tubular adenoma with moderate dysplasia

14.2 Case 3 [2]

14.2.1 Female, 80s (Fig. 14.5a–d)

Principle complaint: Upper abdominal pain

- A small intestinal tumor was identified on abdominal ultrasonography.
- Per-oral DBE showed a brownish, low, circumferential flat elevation in the jejunum with coarse nodules in the center of the lesion.
- There was no clear ulcer formation, but pronounced narrowing of the jejunum tract was present in the central area and the scope was unable to pass through.
- Intra- and postoperative endoscopic observation of the area of the lesion from the distal side revealed a circumferential, coarse nodular protrusion continuous with a flat elevation.

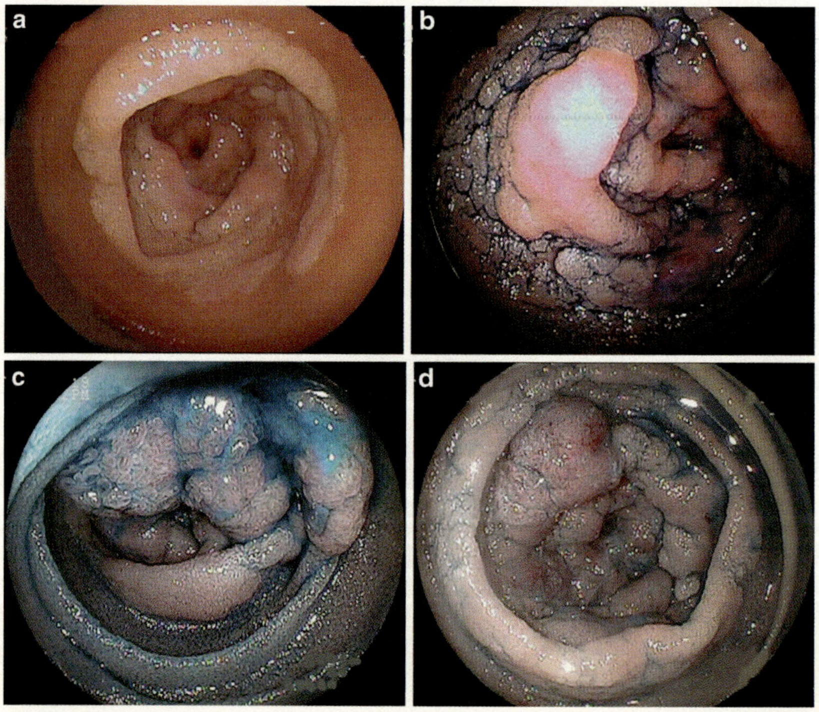

Fig. 14.5

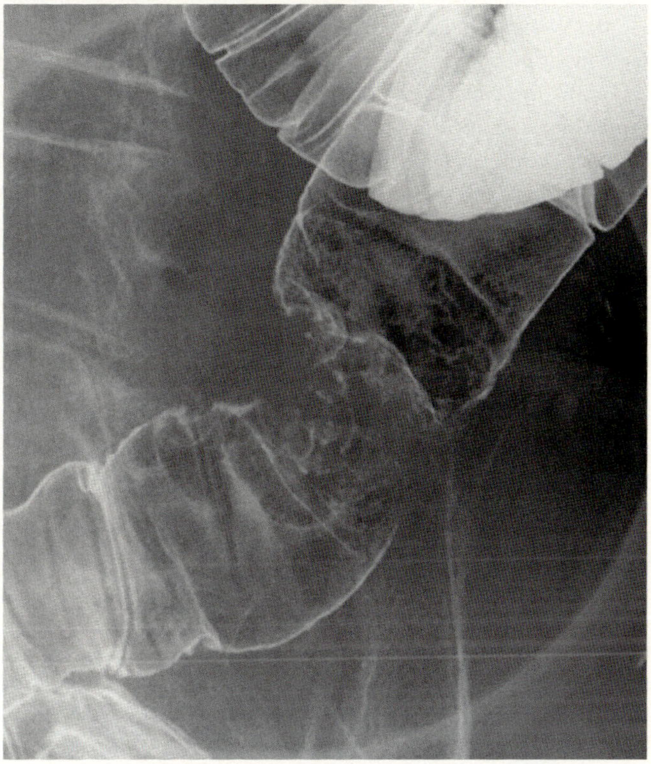

Fig. 14.6 Radiography showed narrowing of the tract lumen in the jejunum, with a fine granular filling defect on the proximal side, and a coarse nodular filling defect on the distal side

14.2.2 Small Intestinal Carcinoma (Figs. 14.6 and 14.7a, b)

- Many small intestinal carcinomas comprise ulcerated localized lesions, but some also take the same form as the laterally spreading tumors (LSTs) found in the large intestine.
- In this case, radiography revealed an obvious applecore-like finding. This was regarded as due to a fine small intestinal tract lumen and visualization of the coarse nodules in the center as a filling defect due to consolidation.
- Pathologically (Fig. 14.7b), mixed adenoma and well differentiated adenocarcinoma were present, and the lesion was conjectured to represent the process of cancerous transformation in the adenoma-carcinoma sequence. Infiltration was evident as far as the muscularis propria (arrow).

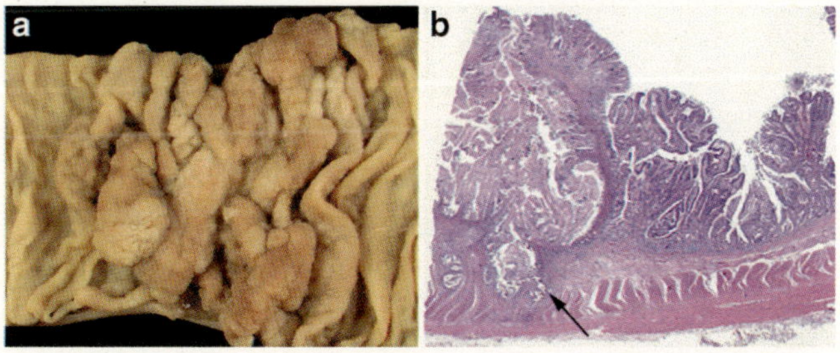

Fig. 14.7

14.3 Case 4 [3]

14.3.1 Male, 60s (Fig. 14.8a–d)

Principle complaint: Repeated abdominal pain, symptoms of ileus

- Per-anal DBE showed annular stenosis of the ileum. The scope was unable to pass through to the proximal side.
- A narrow annular ulcer was observed in a location consistent with the stenosis.
- Regional rough mucosa was present in the ileum on the distal side of the stenosis, and the villi in that area were enlarged and/or flattened.
- Very slight mucosal defects were also present in the same area.

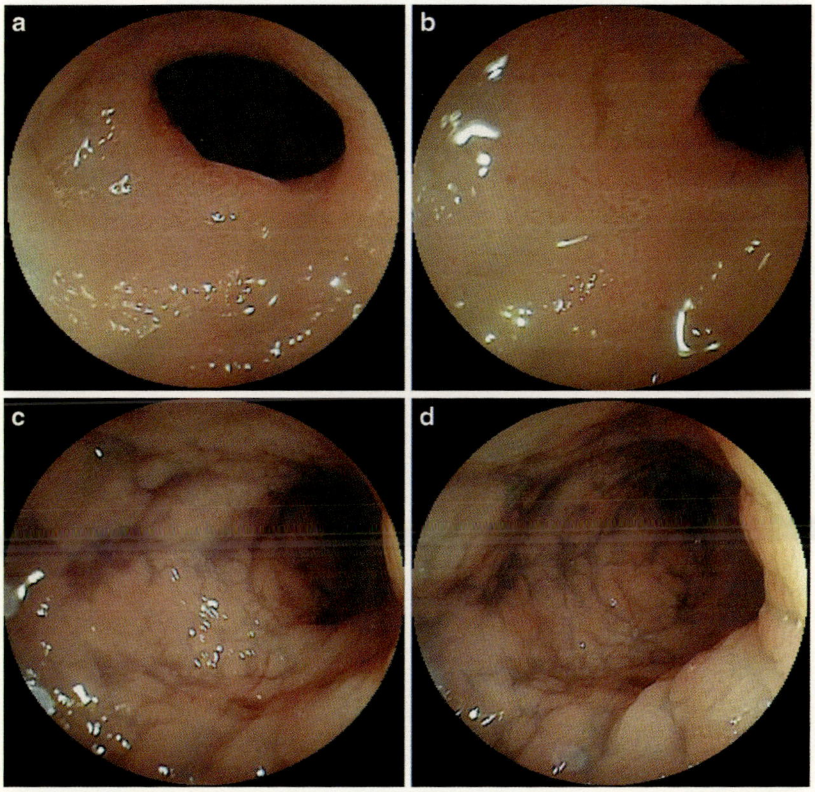

Fig. 14.8

14.3.2 MALT Lymphoma (Figs. 14.9 and 14.10)

- MALT lymphoma is a low-grade lymphoma derived from marginal-zone B cells in mucosa-associated lymphoid tissue (MALT), which forms in extranodal organs in the context of chronic inflammation.
- Reports of small intestinal MALT lymphoma are comparatively rare, but poorly demarcated rough mucosa is regarded as one of its features. Cases in which this entity has caused stenosis have also been reported.
- Small intestinal diseases that can cause rough mucosa with annular ulceration include intestinal tuberculosis, ischemic enteritis, and NSAID-induced enteropathy.
- In this case, as apoptotic bodies were observed on the epithelium of the stenosis when the patient discontinued oral NSAIDs, this may have been a case of combined NSAID-induced enteropathy and MALT lymphoma.

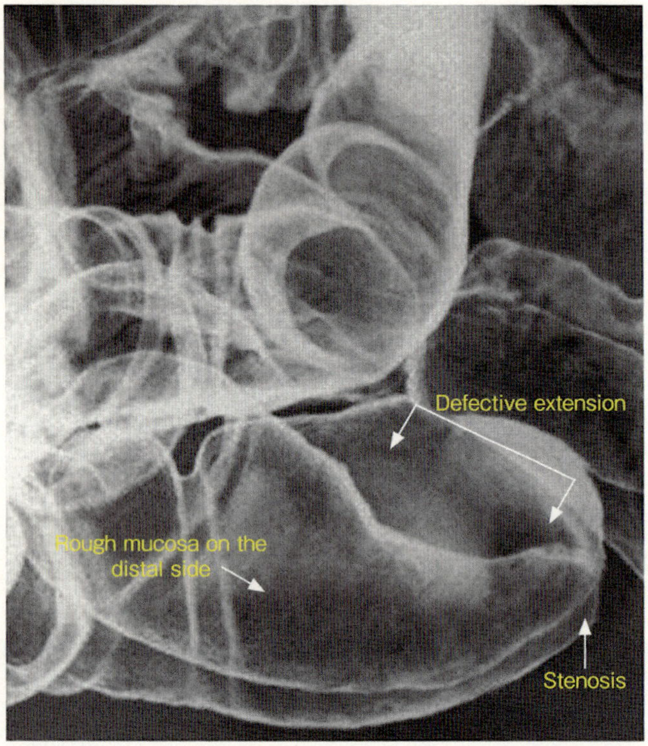

Fig. 14.9 The proximal side of the ileal stenosis is somewhat dilated, and rough mucosa and findings of defective extension are visible on the distal side of the stenosis

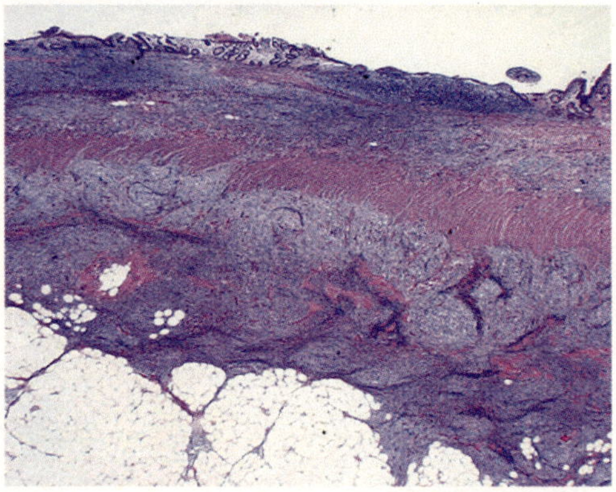

Fig. 14.10 Histopathological image of resected specimen: MALT lymphoma that has infiltrated beyond the serosa into the adipose tissue of the mesenterium

15 Case Presentations: Depression

Takayuki Matsumoto

15.1 Case 1, 2 [1]

15.1.1 Male, 20s (Fig. 15.1a, b)

Principle complaint: Bloody stools

- Observation of the small intestine by colonoscopy revealed over 1,000 adenomatous polyps.
- The resected large intestine contained around 2,500 polyps, and a diagnosis of adenomatous polyposis was made. Colorectal carcinoma was not present.
- Genetic analysis showed a nonsense mutation in exon 10 of the APC gene.
- DBE showed scattered whitish small protrusions in the jejunum.

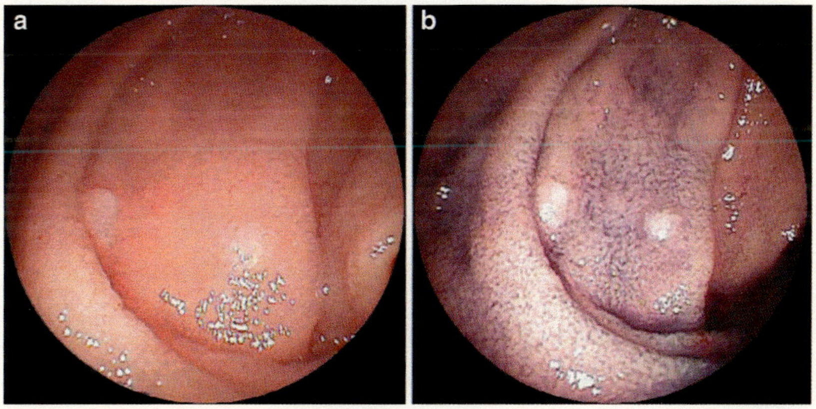

Fig. 15.1

15.1.2 Male, 30s (Fig. 15.2a, b)

Principle complaint: Fecal occult bleeding

- Observation of the small intestine by colonoscopy identified multiple adenomatous polyps.
- No mutation of the APC gene was identified, and no tumors were evident outside the colon.
- DBE showed tiny brownish flat elevations (a) and a small concave lesion that was made visible by dye spraying (b, arrow).

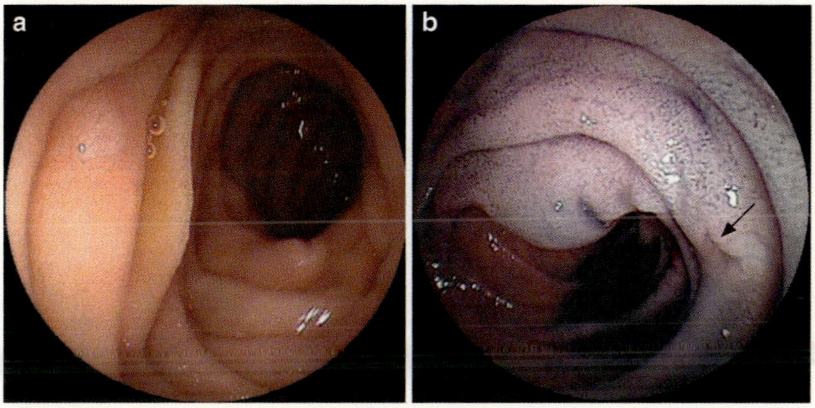

Fig. 15.2

T. Matsumoto (✉)
Department of Medicine and Clinical Science, Graduate School of Medicine, Kyushu University, 3-1-1 Maidashi, Higashi-ku, Fukuoka 812-8582, Japan
e-mail: matane@intmed2.med.kyushu-u.ac.jp

T. Matsui et al. (eds.), *Endoscopy in the Diagnosis of Small Intestine Diseases*, DOI 10.1007/978-4-431-54352-7_15, © Springer Japan 2014

15.1.3 Intestinal Adenoma (Associated with FAP) (Fig. 15.3)

- Familial adenomatous polyposis is a genetic disorder in which multiple adenomas occur in the large intestine, and colorectal cancer always develops if left untreated.

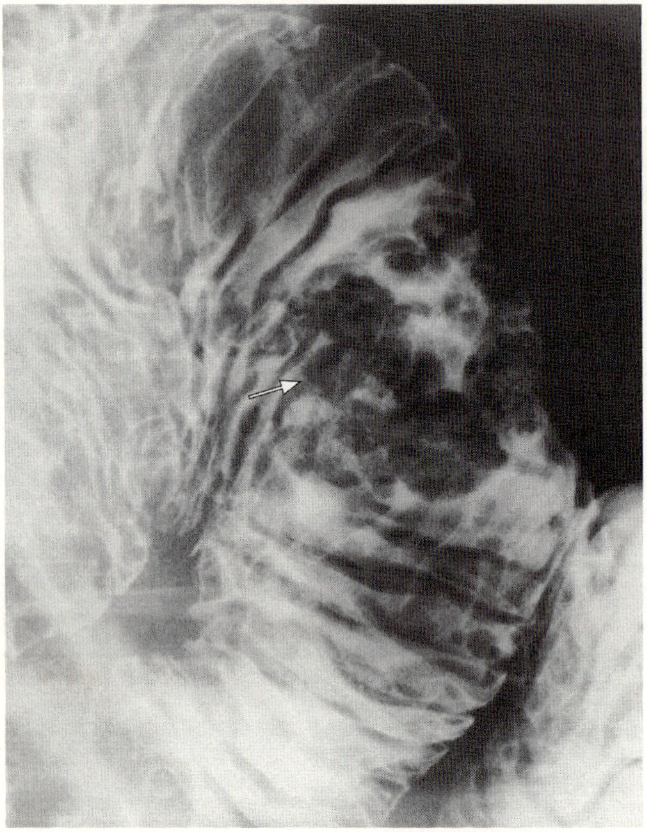

Fig. 15.3 Nodular-aggregating lesion in another case of FAP (*arrow*)

In most cases, the cause is a heterozygous mutation of the APC gene on the fifth chromosome, but FAP may also occur due to a homozygous mutation in the oxidative DNA repair gene MUTYH.
- The presence of duodenal adenomas in this condition has been known for some time. Recently, small intestinal adenomas have also been found to tend to occur, some of which turn cancerous.
- Small intestinal adenomas also occur with a frequency of around 60 %, commonly in the upper jejunum, and appear as small white protrusions or small depressions on endoscopy.
- Enlarged nodular-aggregating lesions of the small intestine can be visualized by radiography, but small intestinal endoscopy is far more useful for the diagnosis of tiny lesions.

Reference

1. Matsumoto T et al. Small intestinal involvement in familial adenomatous polyposis: evaluation by intraoperative enteroscopy and double-balloon endoscopy. Gastrointest Endosc. 2008;68:911–9.

Case Presentations: Protrusions of Submucosal Elevations

16

Yuho Sato, Yoshihiko Karashima, Sadahiro Funakoshi, Kazeo Ninomiya, Tomonori Yano, Hideki Ishibashi, and Issei Egashira

16.1 Case 1 [1]

16.1.1 Female, 50s (Fig. 16.1a–d)

Principle complaint: Nothing in particular

- Observation of the small intestine by colonoscopy showed a small protrusion, 4 mm in size, in the terminal ileum with a comparatively smooth marginal rising appearance. The lesion had a smooth surface that was somewhat more yellowish in color compared with the surrounding mucosa.
- Dye spraying showed clear demarcation of the margin with the surrounding mucosa, with no depression or surface erosion.
- The morphology of the protrusion did not vary when the volume of air was reduced.
- 20-MHz balloon ultrasonography (c): A comparatively internally homogenous hypoechoic tumor was present, mainly located in the third layer. There was no continuity with the fourth layer.
- Endoscopic mucosal resection: A transparent cap was fitted to the tip of the scope, and the endoscopic mucosal resection with cap method was used for total resection of the carcinoid (d).

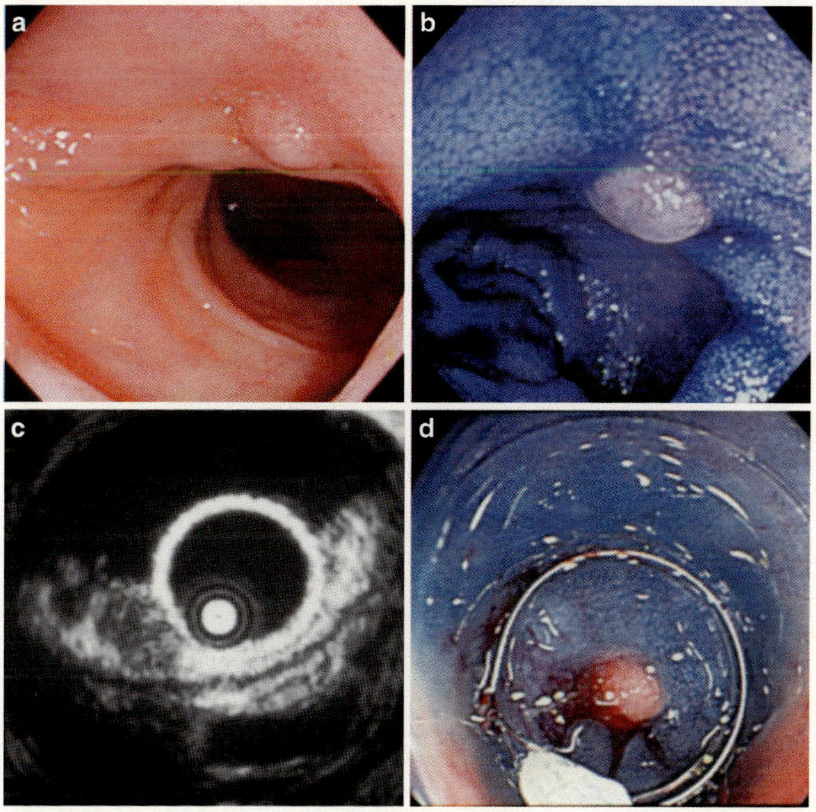

Fig. 16.1

Y. Sato (✉) • Y. Karashima • K. Ninomiya
Department of Gastroenterology, Fukuoka University Chikushi Hospital, 1-1-1 Zokumyoin, Chikushino 818-8502, Japan
e-mail: ufosato@hotmail.co.jp

S. Funakoshi • H. Ishibashi
Department of Gastroenterology and Medicine, Fukuoka University Faculty of Medicine, 7-45-1 Nanakuma, Jonan-ku, Fukuoka 814-0180, Japan

T. Yano
Department of Internal Medicine, Division of Gastroenterology, Jichi Medical University, 3311-1 Yakushiji, Shimotsuke 329-0498, Japan

I. Egashira
Department of Medicine and Clinical Science, Graduate School of Medical Sciences, Kyushu University, 3-1-1, Maidashi, Higashi-ku, Fukuoka 812-8582, Japan

T. Matsui et al. (eds.), *Endoscopy in the Diagnosis of Small Intestine Diseases*, DOI 10.1007/978-4-431-54352-7_16, © Springer Japan 2014

16.1.2 Carcinoid (Figs. 16.2 and 16.3)

- Carcinoid is more common in men, with the age of onset usually in the 50s. Principle complaints include abdominal pain, diarrhea, and melena. As such lesions are composed of endocrine cells, symptoms including rubeosis and asthmatic attacks may sometimes arise (carcinoid syndrome).
- Other than in the duodenum, small intestinal carcinoid is rare, but when it does occur this is commonly in the ileum, particularly the terminal ileum.
- Carcinoid is generally regarded as low grade, but tumors larger than 20 mm have an increased possibility of metastasis to the liver and lymph nodes.

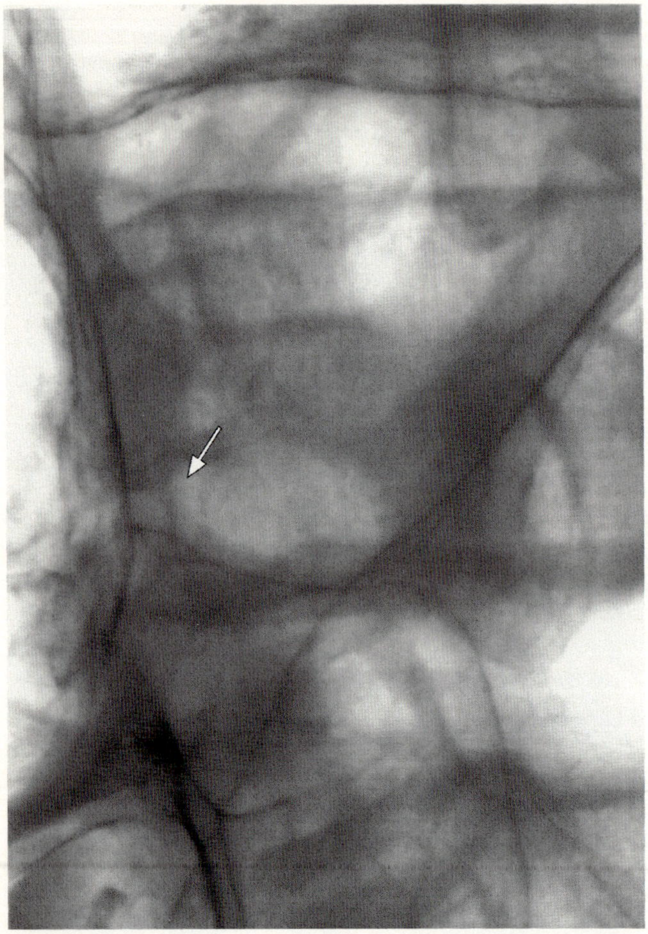

Fig. 16.2 A 4-mm-diameter protrusion with a smooth surface and a comparatively smooth marginal rising appearance of the tumor is present in the terminal ileum (*arrow*)

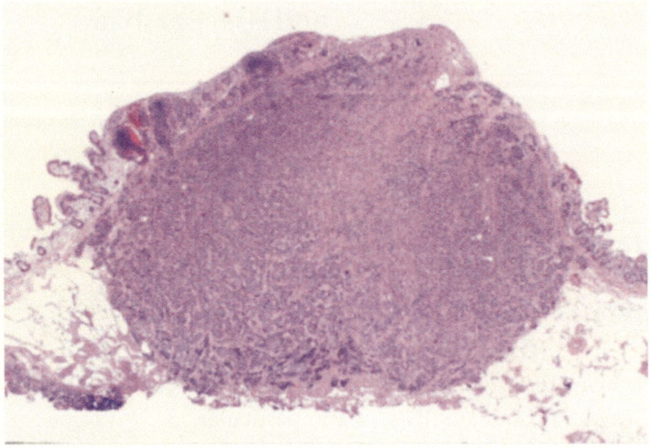

Fig. 16.3 Low-magnification image with hematoxylin and eosin staining. The tumor is limited to the submucosa, with a maximum diameter of 4 mm

16.2 Case 2 [2]

16.2.1 Male, 30s (Fig. 16.4a–d)

Principle complaint: Persistent fecal occult blood, iron deficiency anemia

- Per-oral DBE revealed a 10-mm long, narrow protruded lesion 20 cm on the distal side of the ligament of Treitz. Dye spraying showed that the surface was covered with normal small intestinal epithelium. The lesion was soft.
  Protrusions of submucosal tumor
- Per-anal DBE showed multiple long, narrow polyps with a maximum size of 5–6 mm in the terminus of the ileum. These were soft lesions, with the surface covered in normal small intestinal mucosa.

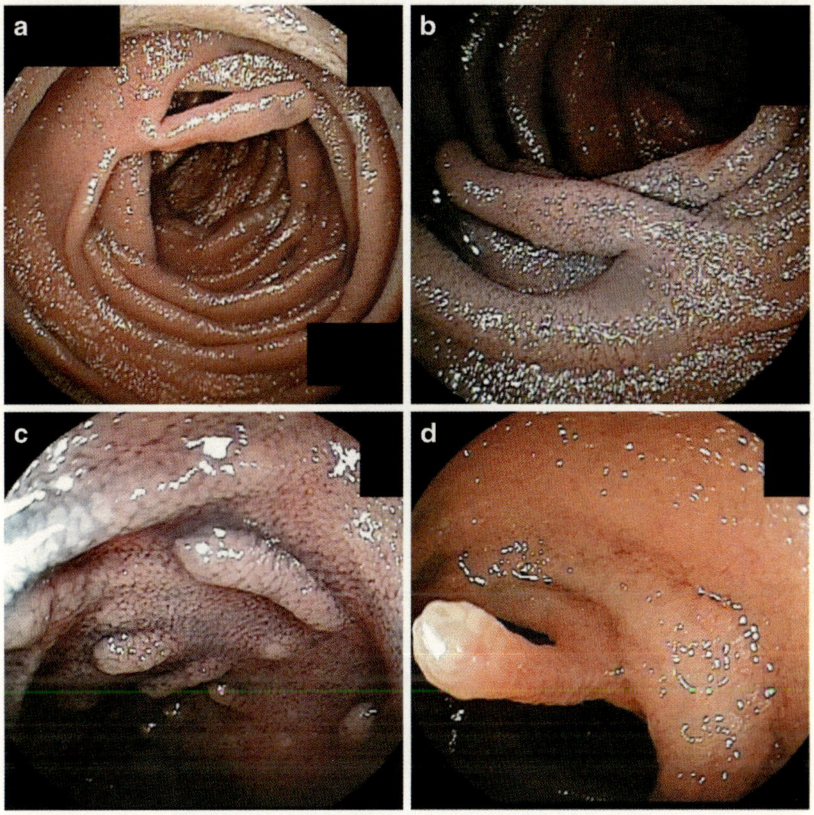

Fig. 16.4

16.2.2 Muco-Submucosal Elongated Polyp (MSEP) (Figs. 16.5 and 16.6)

- This is a protruded lesion with a morphology similar to that of the colonic MSEP (CMSEP) found in the colon, and is long and narrow, covered in normal small intestinal mucosa, and soft.
- In terms of histopathological findings, this lesion is characterized by submucosa containing edematous loose connective tissue under normal mucosa, with dilated lymph ducts and blood vessels.
- The etiology is unknown, but a mechanism is conjectured whereby a disconnection occurs in the mucosa and submucosa due to some sort of mechanical action, causing dilatation of the lymph ducts and veins into the lumen. Protrusions of submucosal tumor
- In this case, resection was performed as diagnostic treatment.
- Inflammatory polyp is one disorder for which differentiation is required.

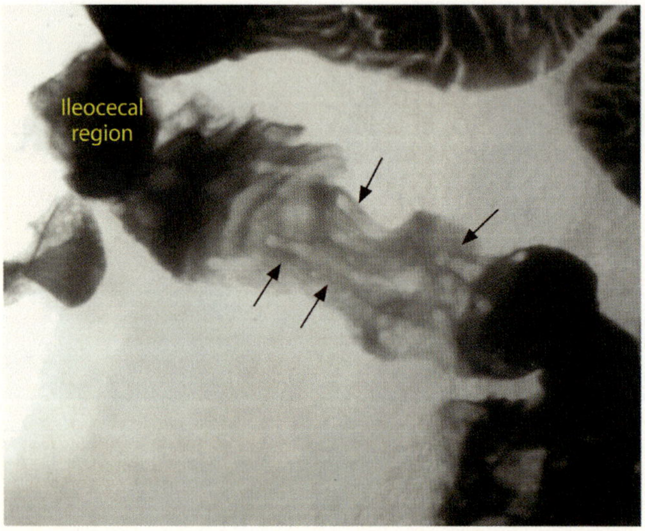

Fig. 16.5 Radiography. Long and narrow, translucent structures (*arrows*) are scattered around the terminus of the ileum (*arrows*)

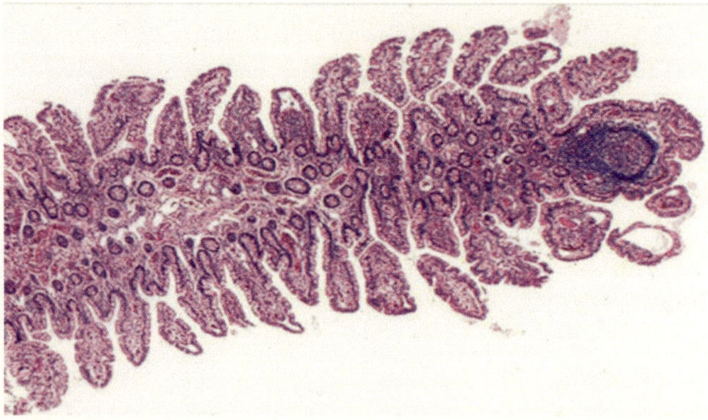

Fig. 16.6 In histopathological findings, the lesion comprised a normal mucosal layer with no atypical gland ducts or hyperplasia and mildly edematous submucosa. There was no infiltration of inflammatory cells into the mucosa or submucosa, and MSEP was diagnosed

16.3 Case 3 [3]

16.3.1 Female, 50s (Fig. 16.7a–d)

Principle complaint: Tarry stool, anemia

- A submucosal tumor with a somewhat steep marginal rising appearance of the tumor was present, occupying around half the circumference of the jejunal tract lumen.
- A bridging fold was evident, with ulceration at the apex.

CT revealed narrowing of the small intestinal lumen, thickened bowel wall, and a tumor with intraluminal enhancement.

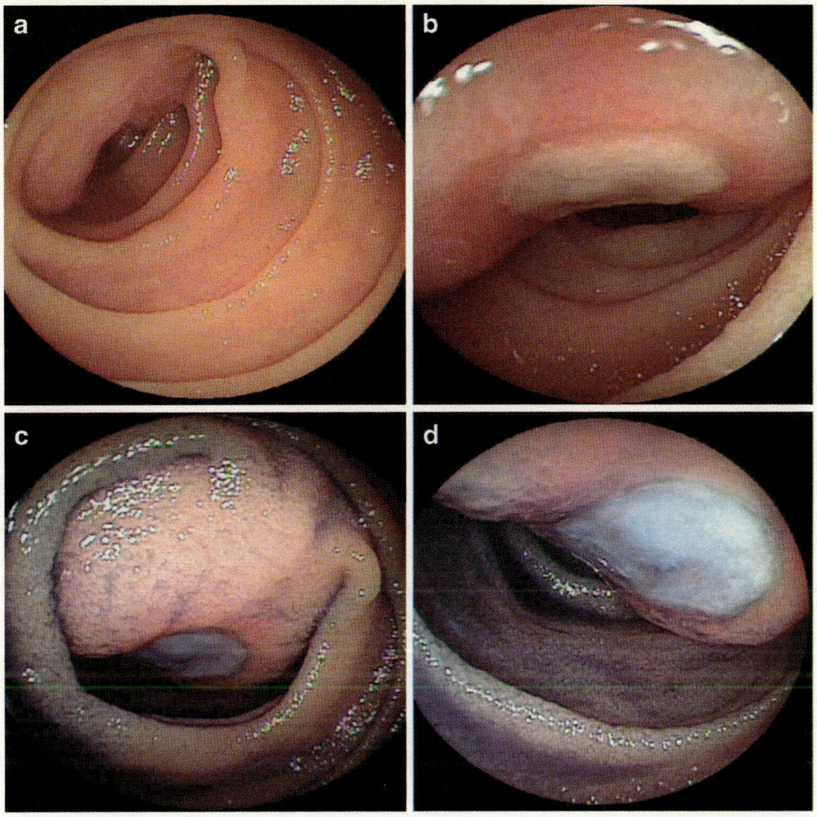

Fig. 16.7

16.3.2 GIST (Figs. 16.8 and 16.9a, b)

- GIST accounts for the majority of mesenchymal tumors of mesodermal origin among gastrointestinal mesenchymal tumors, and exhibits the morphology of a submucosal tumor.
- GIST may occur from the esophagus to the rectum, with a frequency of around 50–60 % in the stomach and 20–30 % in the small intestine.
- GIST is classified as intraluminal (occurring within the gastrointestinal lumen), extraluminal (growing outside the intestinal wall), or a combination.
- In patients with tumors around 2 cm in size, the morphology is often that of a protrusion with a smooth surface and smooth marginal rising.
- As the diameter of the tumor enlarges, a range of different morphologies may arise, such as delle or ulceration at the apex or multinodular tendencies.

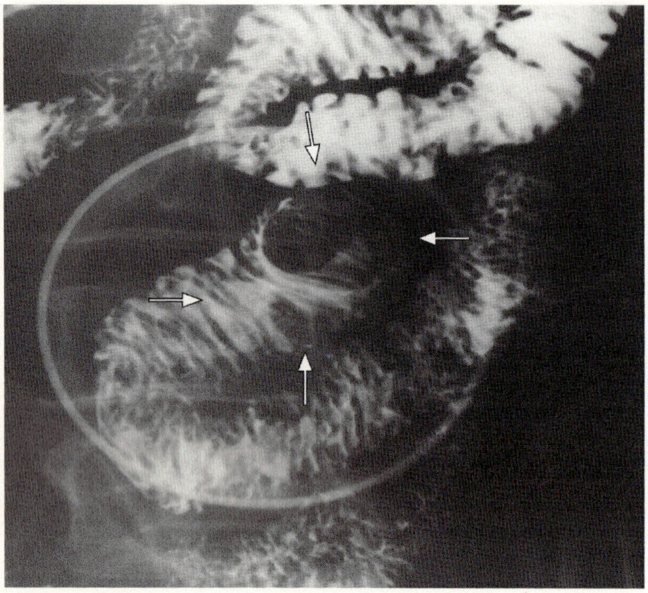

Fig. 16.8 A protruded lesion with a smooth surface is evident in the upper small intestine

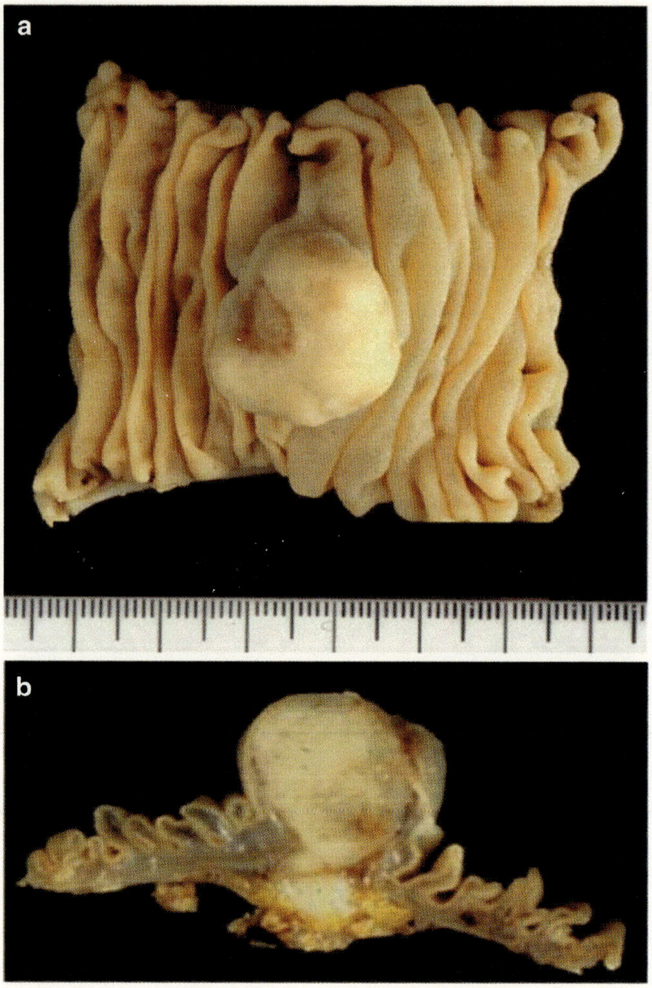

Fig. 16.9 (**a**, **b**) A 25×22×20 mm tumor, with pronounced growth into the intestinal lumen, was present 45 cm from the ligament of Treitz

16.4 Case 4 [4]

16.4.1 Male, 40s (Fig. 16.10a–d)

Principal complaint: Tarry stool

- Mother suffered from von Recklinghausen disease. Skin lesions were also identified on the patient since early childhood.
- Antegrade DBE revealed an elastic-hard twin-crested submucosal elevation in the upper jejunum.
- The protrusion showed a comparatively steep marginal rising appearance, and its surface was covered with normal small intestinal villi. Linear open ulcers and a stria-like depression were present at the peak.
- CE showed a smooth-surfaced lesion in the upper small intestine, similar to a submucosal tumor together with vascular ectasia (c).
- A slight indentation (d, arrow) was seen at the peak of the protrusion, suggesting the presence of an ulcer or depression.

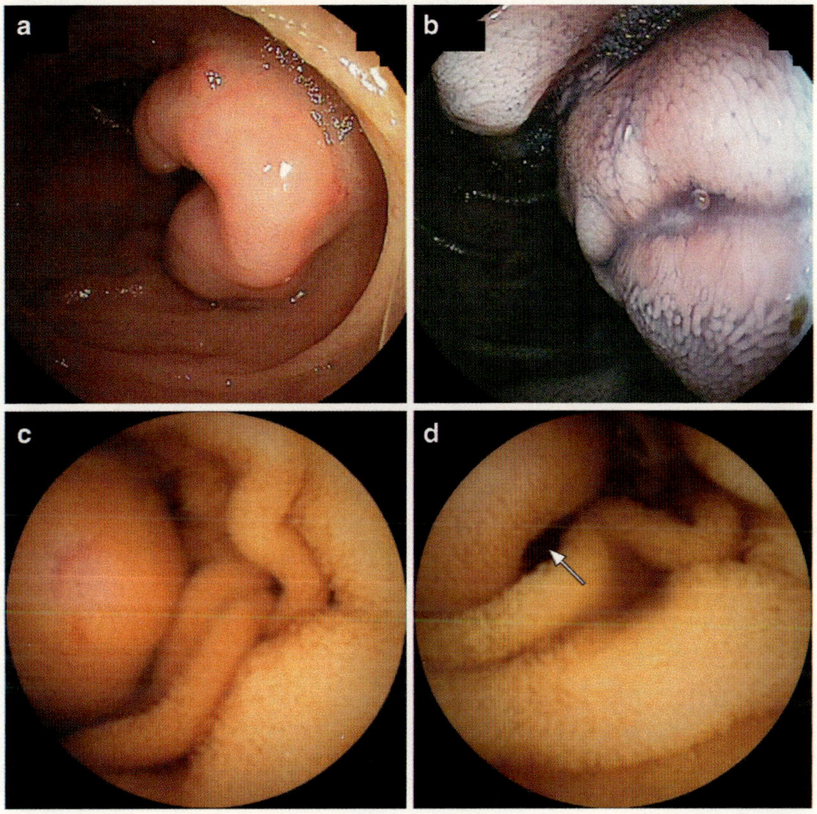

Fig. 16.10

16.4.2 GIST (Figs. 16.11, 16.12 and 16.13)

- GISTs are submucosal tumors composed of mesenchymal-cell-derived spindle-shaped cells that are positive for c-kit and CD34 expression. They often arise in the small intestine, and are generally categorized as intraluminal, dumbbell-shaped and extraluminal growths.
- GIST frequently occurs as multiple tumors in von Recklinghausen disease.
- Intraluminal growths are visualized on radiography as distinct, smooth filling defects. Ulceration or depression at the peak of the protrusion can be observed on compression or double-contrast images.
- GISTs are visible under endoscopy as elastic-hard submucosal elevation with associated ulceration or depression. Biopsy frequently does not lead to a confirmed diagnosis. These tumors frequently occur in the jejunum, and so are often overlooked during CE.

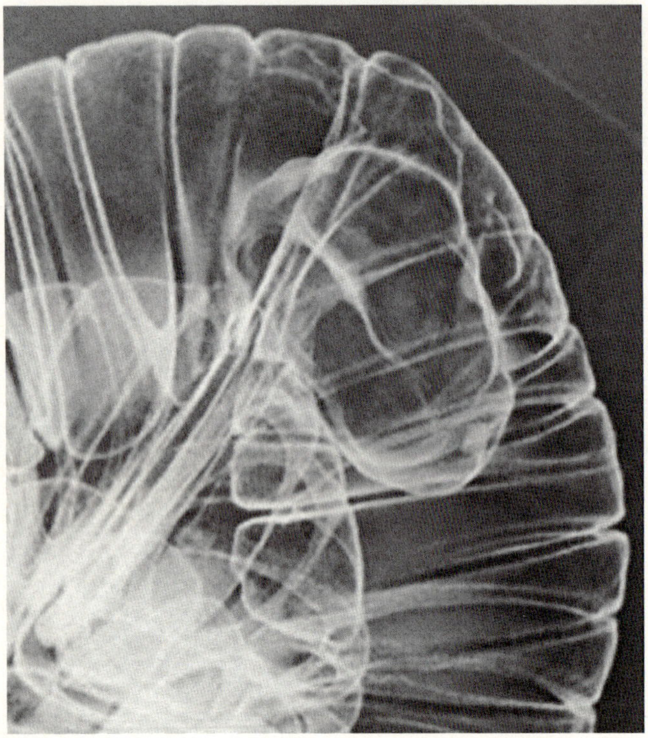

Fig. 16.11 Radiography revealed a smoothly demarcated elevated lesion in the upper jejunum, with a distinct linear barium patch

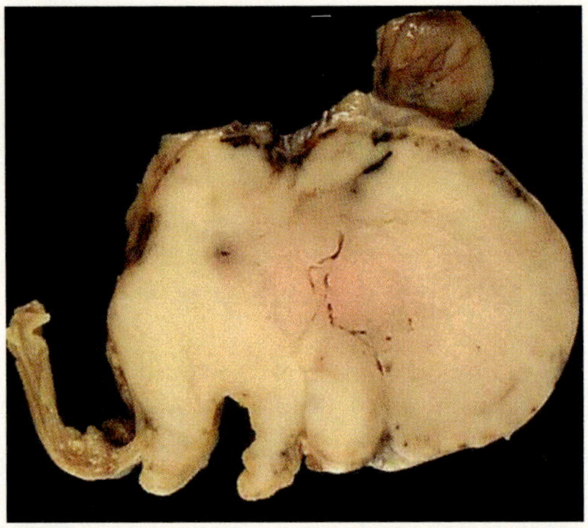

Fig. 16.12 Histopathology showed proliferation of c-kit-positive spindle-shaped tumor cells

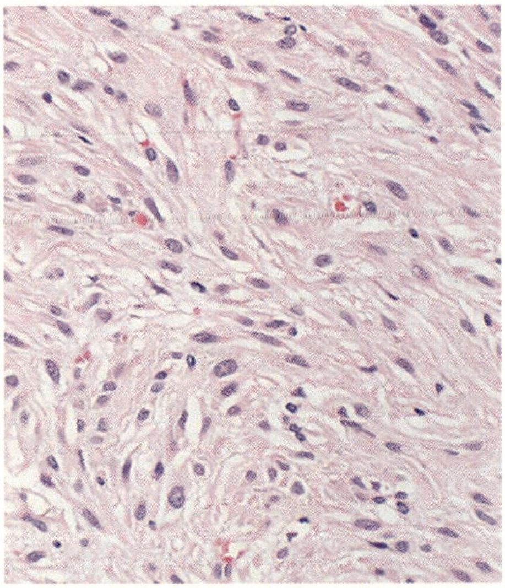

Fig. 16.13 Macroscopic examination of the resected specimen showed an ash-gray solid tumor arising from the intrinsic muscle layer, covered with non-atypical small intestinal mucosa

16.5 Case 5, 6 [5]

16.5.1 Male, 60s (Fig. 16.14a, b)

Principal complaint: Obscure gastrointestinal bleeding (OGIB)

- Two white submucosal tumors with smooth surfaces were evident in the jejunum.
- Left: Comparatively flat lesion.
- Right: Nodular lesion with bridging folds.

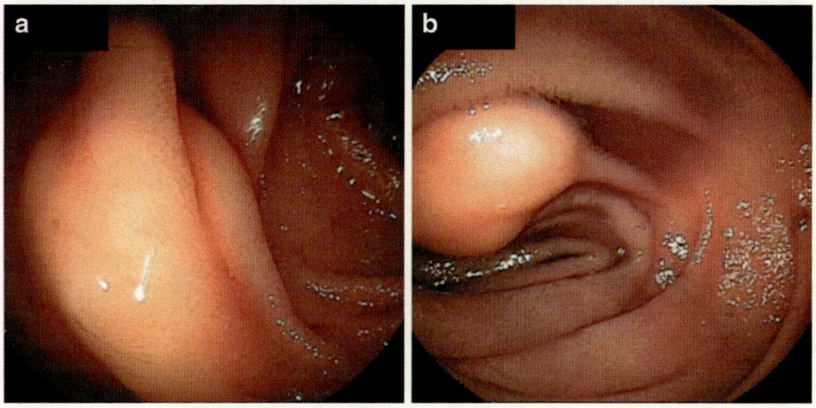

Fig. 16.14

16.5.2 Female, 80s (Fig. 16.15a, b)

Principal complaint: OGIB

- A translucent, white submucosal tumor was apparent.
- White fine granules were present on the surface.

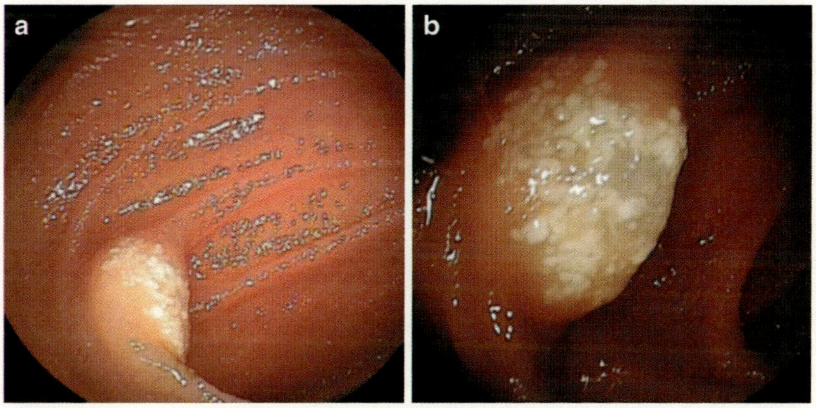

Fig. 16.15

16.5.3 Lymphangioma (Figs. 16.16 and 16.17)

- Lymphangiomas are visible under endoscopy as smooth-surfaced, translucent protrusions. These lesions are yellowish-white when the principal location is in the submucosal layer, and white and granular when in the lamina propria.
- They are visualized on radiography as comparatively distinct oval filling defects in filled images, and as smooth, sessile protrusions in double-contrast images.

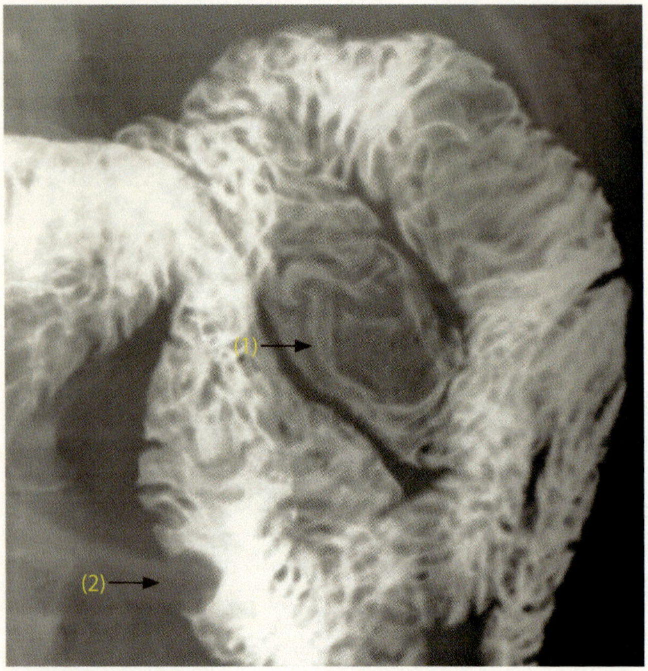

Fig. 16.16 Case 5: An elevated lesion with a distinct marginal rising appearance was evident in the jejunum. The lesion displayed a smooth surface, and easily changed shape under pressure (*arrow 1*). A soft, round filling defect was also apparent on the distal side (*arrow 2*)

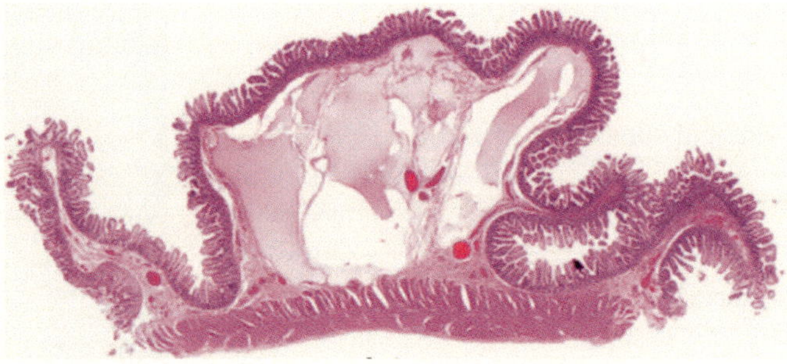

Fig. 16.17 Case 5: A dilated lymph duct containing an accumulation of lymph was visible in the submucosal layer, backed by a single layer of endothelial cells

16.6 Case 7

16.6.1 Male, 40s (Fig. 16.18a–d)

- Onset with symptoms of anemia with no bleeding, admitted to hospital with Hb 4.4 g/dl. No particular underlying condition.
- A 5-cm sessile protrusion was evident in the proximal jejunum, with a small amount of bleeding.
- Water-immersion endoscopy revealed a mixture of white-spotted/white villi and blood-filled villi.
- The center of the lesion was somewhat depressed, with a yellow ulcer mound, and the entire lesion was covered with countless white villi interspersed in places with blood-filled villi.

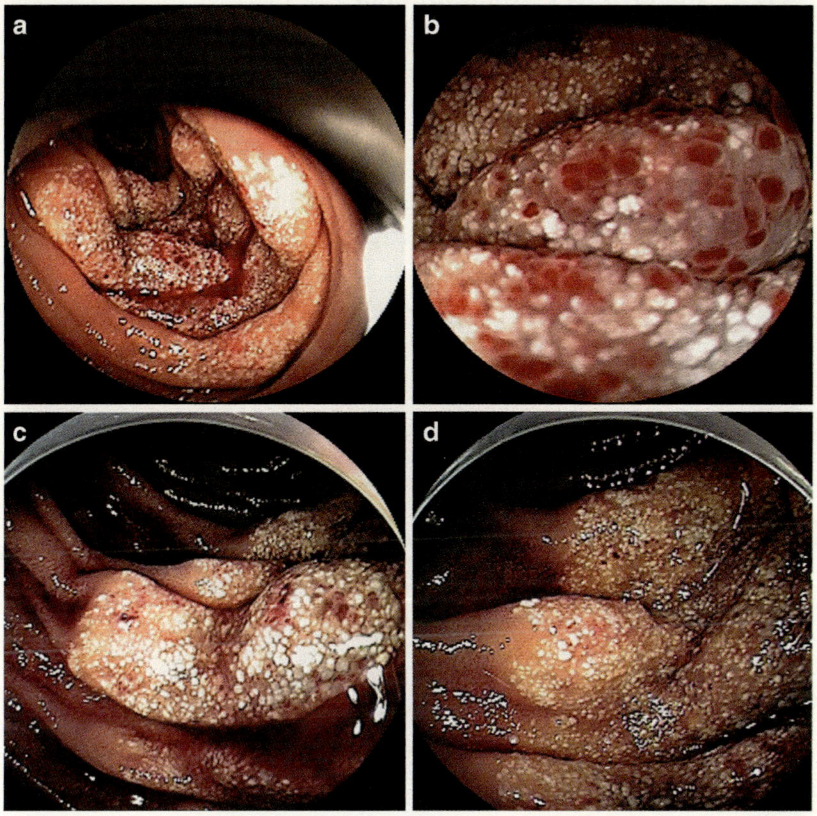

Fig. 16.18

16.6.2 Cavernous Lymphangioma (Figs. 16.19 and 16.20)

- Cavernous lymphangiomas are yellowish-white, translucent protrusions with a smooth surface characterized by surface white-spotted/white villi.
- They range from small lesions a few millimeters in diameter to massive ones up to 20 cm in size. Small lesions resemble gastric xanthoma at first glance and are asymptomatic, frequently being discovered incidentally during small intestinal endoscopy and posing few clinical problems. Large lesions, however, can cause intestinal intussusception, abdominal pain, or hemorrhage, and may require treatment.
- These lesions are visualized by contrast radiography as round to oval or semi-pedunculated submucosal tumors with a smooth surface. The lesions are soft, and easily change shape under pressure.

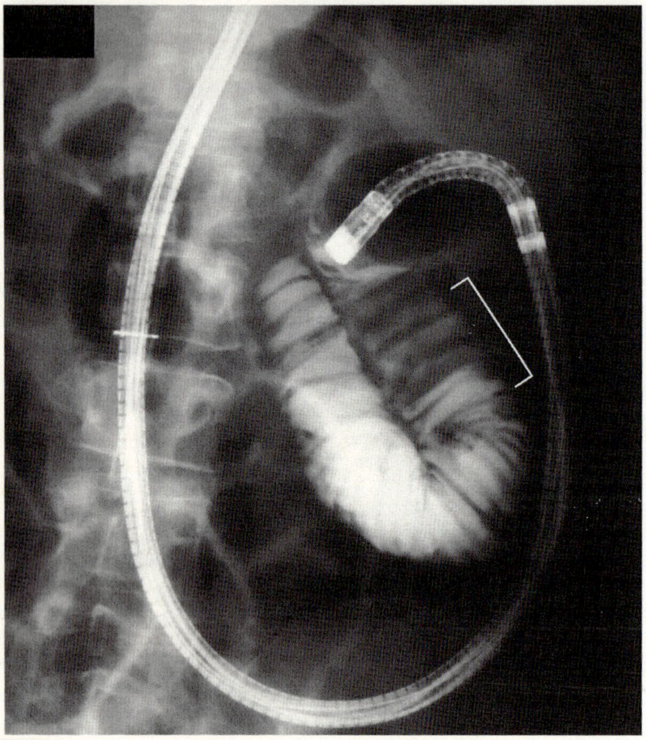

Fig. 16.19 Selective contrast enhancement with dilation of the balloon at the tip of the endoscope visualized a sessile protrusion extending 5 cm from the endoscope tip

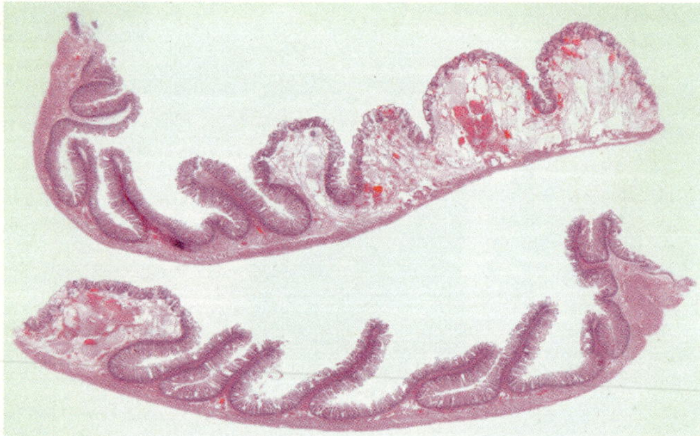

Fig. 16.20 Dilated lymph ducts are evident in the submucosal layer, with bleeding into some lymph ducts

16.7 Case 8

16.7.1 Male, 70s (Fig. 16.21a–d)

Principal complaint: Tarry stool

- Antegrade DBE showed a pedunculated submucosal tumor in the jejunum. The soft lesion had a smooth surface and was pale yellow in color.
- Small ulcers were evident at the base (left) and peak (right) of the submucosal tumor.

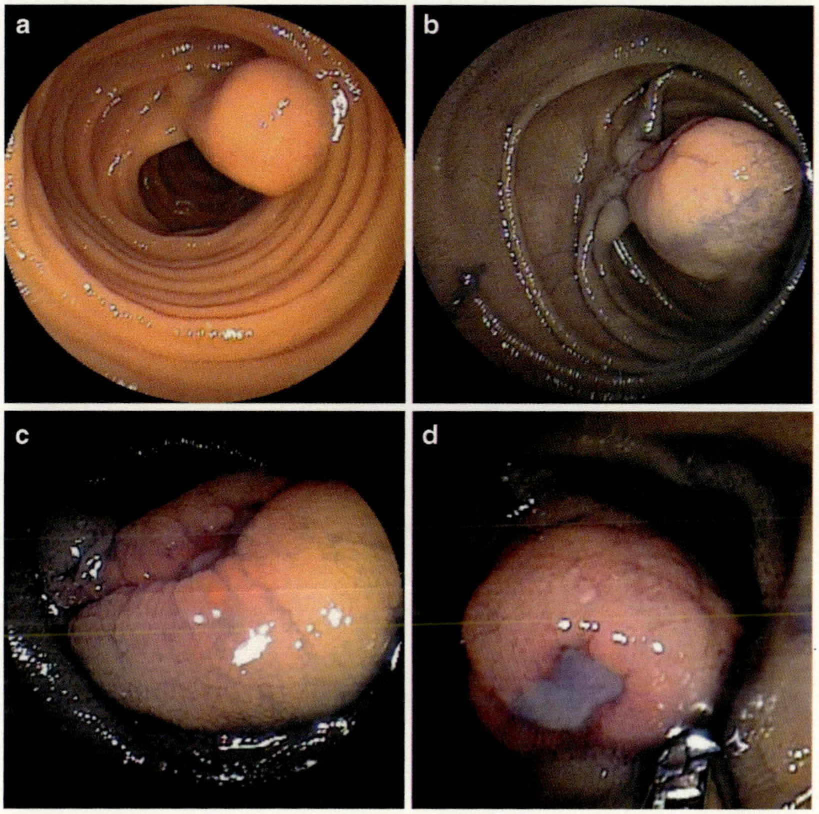

Fig. 16.21

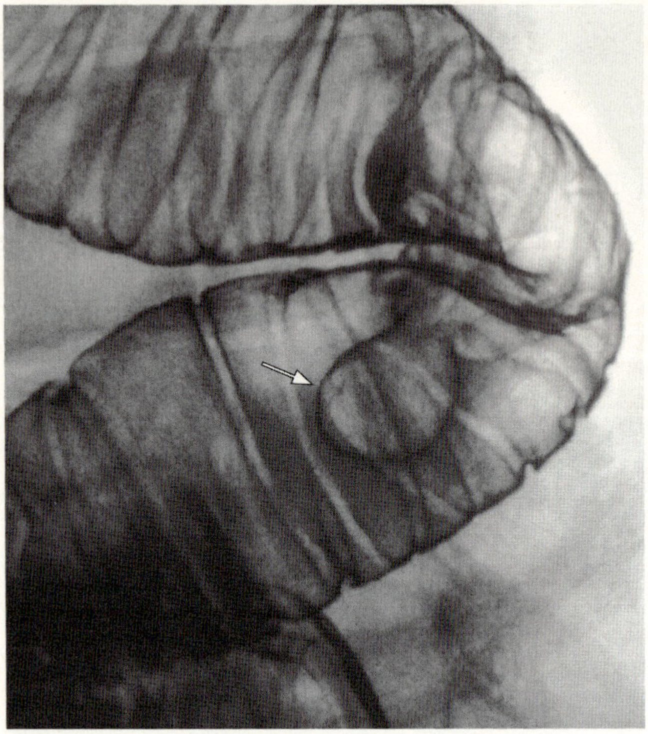

Fig. 16.22 Radiography revealed a pedunculated elevated lesion, showing the form of a submucosal tumor with a smooth surface, with a barium fleck at the peak due to a small ulcer (*arrow*)

16.7.2 Lipoma (Figs. 16.22 and 16.23a, b)

- Lipomas are a comparatively common type of benign small intestinal tumor, and are asymptomatic while they remain small, but can cause intestinal intussusception when they grow larger. Erosion or ulceration of the tumor surface may also occur, causing gastrointestinal bleeding.
- Endoscopically, these lesions characteristically take the form of sessile to pedunculated submucosal tumors, with a smooth, pale-yellow surface. They are soft when pushed with forceps.

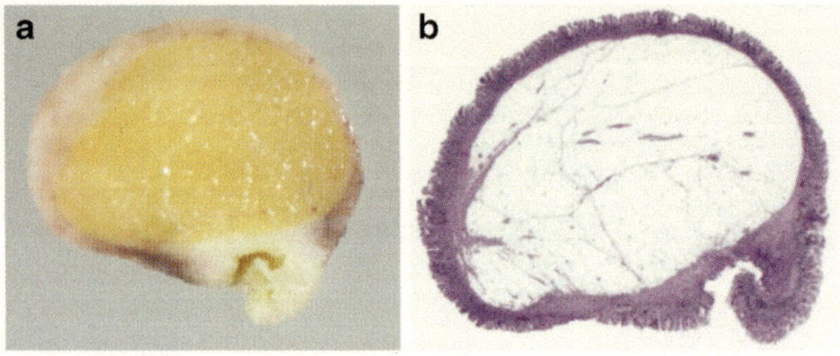

Fig. 16.23 (**a**, **b**) The majority of the tumor was covered with normal mucosa and it was composed of fully mature adipose tissue, leading to a diagnosis of lipoma

16.8 Case 9 [6]

16.8.1 Male, 70s (Fig. 16.24a–d)

Principal complaints: Bloody stool, anemia

- Underlying conditions: anti-coagulation therapy and pacemaker implantation for bradycardic atrial fibrillation, aortic valve insufficiency, and mitral valve insufficiency.
- A 5-mm semi-pedunculated polyp-shaped lesion was evident in the distal ileum.
- No villous structures were evident on the surface, and the lesion was somewhat irregular and oozing bleeding.
- Local injection of physiological saline with added epinephrine into the base produced good swelling, and endoscopic mucosal resection (EMR) was performed.

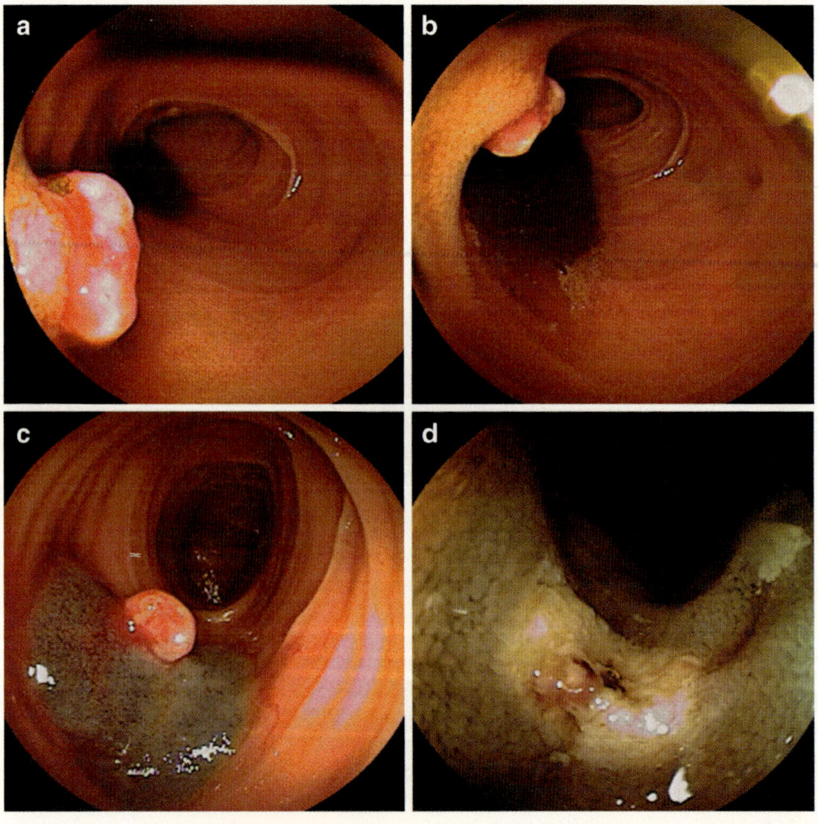

Fig. 16.24

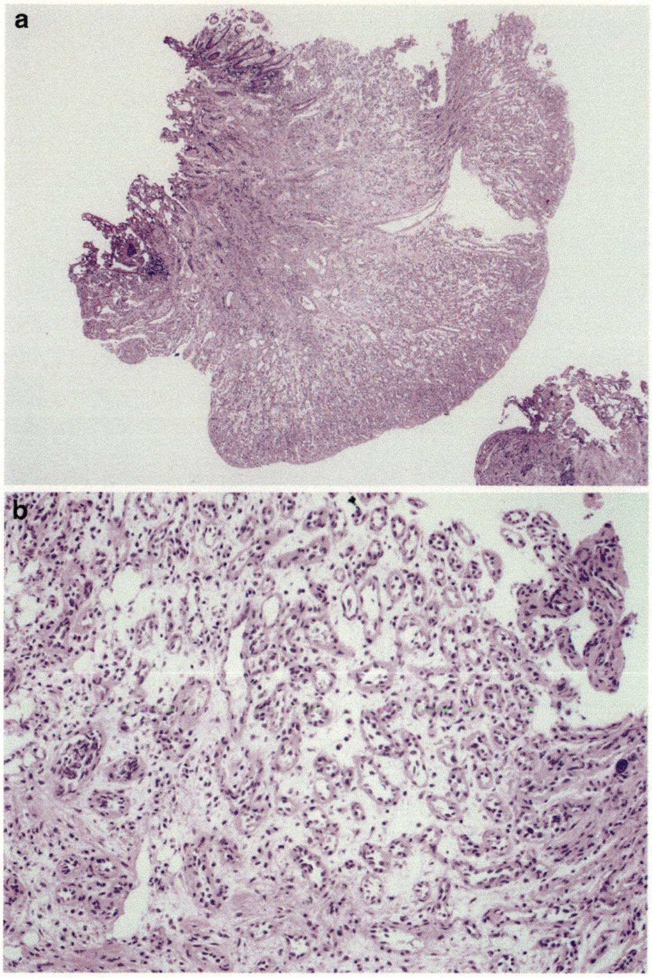

Fig. 16.25 (**a**, **b**) The inside of the lesion was densely packed with capillary vessels

16.8.2 Hemangioma (Fig. 16.25a, b)

- Hemangiomas are benign lesions that stem from the proliferation of blood vessels, with the majority occurring in the skin, although they may arise anywhere in the body. They are broadly categorized on the basis of proliferated blood vessel morphology and type into capillary hemangioma, cavernous hemangioma, and mixed type, in addition to pyogenic granuloma. Cavernous hemangioma is the most common type in the digestive tract, followed by capillary hemangioma (approximately 5–10 %). The most common symptom of small intestinal hemangioma is gastrointestinal bleeding, which occurs in 66 % of cases, followed by abdominal pain in 19 %, as well as intestinal obstruction and intestinal intussusception.
- Capillary hemangioma can be recognized endoscopically as a bright scarlet lesion, and mostly occurs as a single lesion. This lesion ranges in size from several millimeters to several centimeters. Histopathologically, dense proliferation of capillary vessels is evident in the submucosa. Individual vessels are formed from the small vascular lumen with a single layer of flat endothelium, and are filled with red blood cells.

16.9 Case 10 [7]

16.9.1 Male, 60s (Fig. 16.26a–d)

Principal complaint: OGIB

- A submucosal tumor with a comparatively steep marginal rising appearance and bridging folds was evident in the upper jejunum (a).
- The tumor was dark blue in color and white at the peak, with central redness (b).
- Normal villous structures were evident, even at the tumor peak. No formation of erosive lesions or ulcers was seen (c, d).

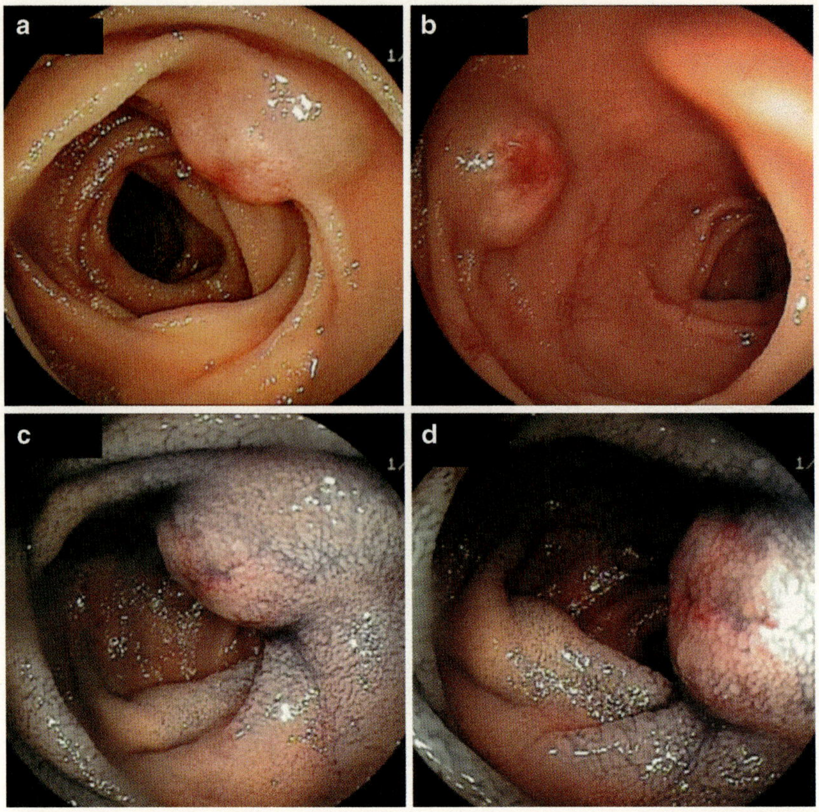

Fig. 16.26

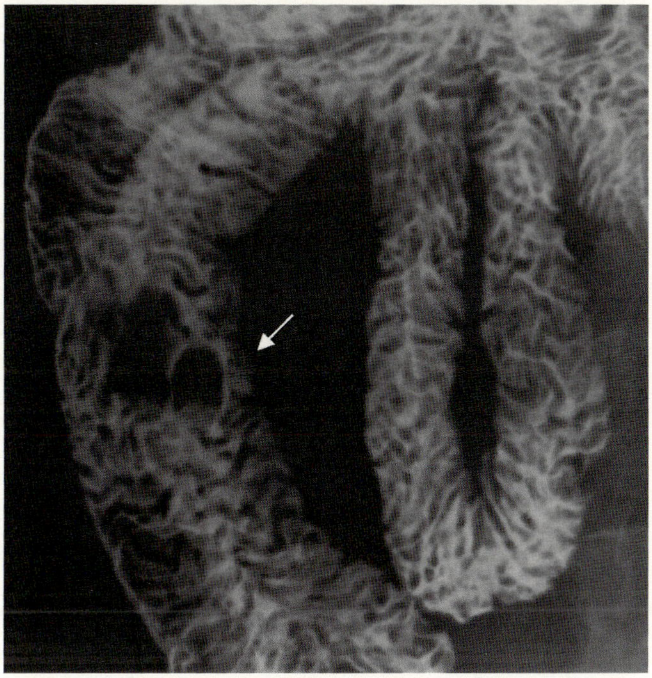

Fig. 16.27 An elevated lesion with a distinct marginal rising appearance was evident in the upper jejunum (*arrow*). The protrusion on the left was an adjacent lymphangioma

16.9.2 Cavernous Hemangioma (Figs. 16.27 and 16.28)

- In Japan, cavernous hemangioma is somewhat more common in men, and is frequently discovered from symptoms of gastrointestinal bleeding.
- Various shapes are seen on radiography, including oval and nodular.
- On endoscopy, the lesion appears bluish-white or dark red.

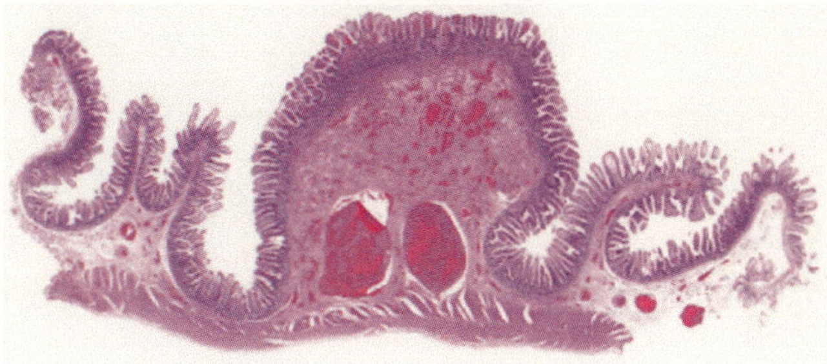

Fig. 16.28 A markedly dilated blood vessel containing an accumulation of red blood cells was visible within the submucosal layer. Large organized blood clots were apparent

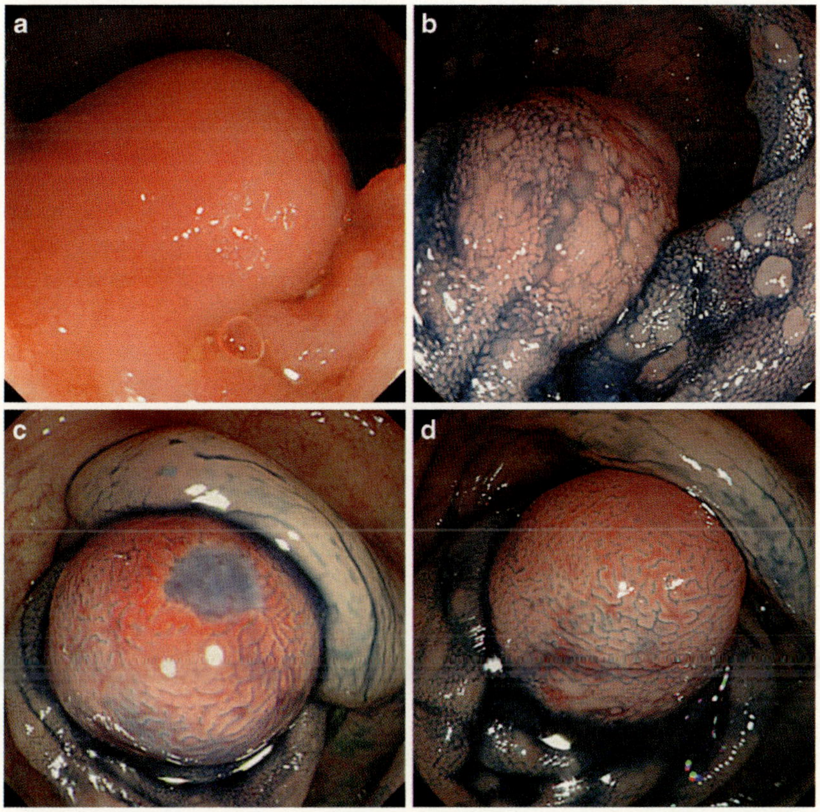

Fig. 16.29

16.10 Case 11 [8]

16.10.1 Male, 60s (Fig. 16.29a–d)

Principal complaint: Symptom free

- A comparatively hard, semi-pedunculated submucosal tumor with a smooth surface 20 mm in size was evident in the terminal ileum.
- The lesion was a tumor with sufficient mobility to shift from the small intestine to the cecum and back.
- Observation within the cecum showed a reddish surface of the protrusion, with shallow ulceration.

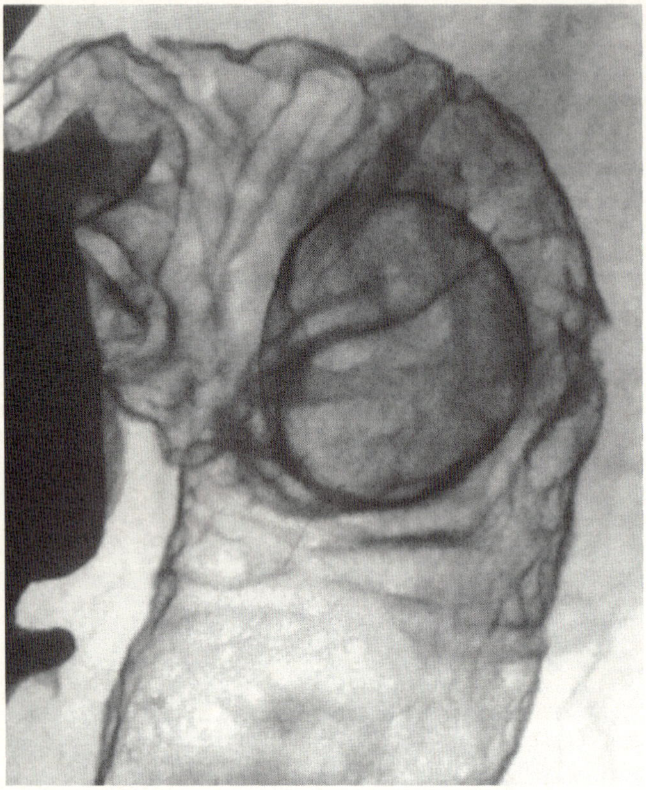

Fig. 16.30 Radiography showed a semi-penduncuIated, elevated lesion with a smooth surface in the terminal ileum

16.10.2 Inflammatory Fibroid Polyp (IFP) (Figs. 16.30 and 16.31)

- Around 70 % of IFPs in the small intestine occur within 150 cm on the proximal side of the ileocecal valve.
- Endoscopically, they are characteristically semi-pedunculated or pedunculated submucosal tumors with a smooth surface, and are comparatively hard when pushed with forceps. Gastrointestinal bleeding may result if mechanical irritation at the peak causes loss of surface mucosa, resulting in erosion and ulcer formation.

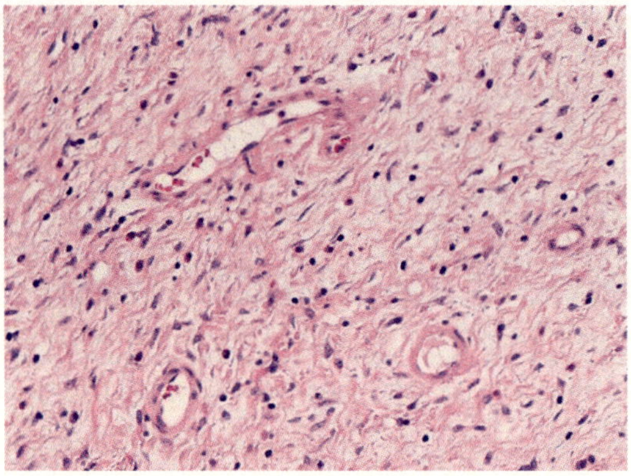

Fig. 16.31 Histopathology (hematoxylin and eosin (HE) staining) revealed small blood vessel growth, interspersed with spindle-shaped cell proliferation and collagen fiber growth. Inflammatory cells (mature lymphocytes, plasmacytes, eosinophils) were also present in the same area. Immunostaining showed positive results for CD34 and vimentin, and IFP was diagnosed

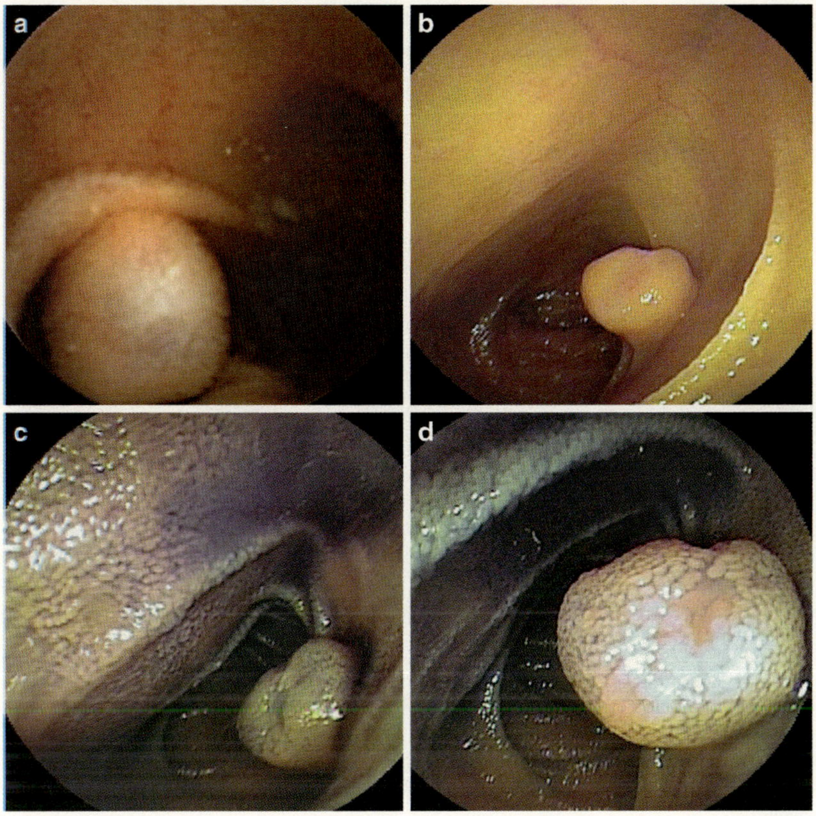

Fig. 16.32

16.11 Case 12 [9]

16.11.1 Female, 40s (Fig. 16.32a–d)

Principal complaint: Abdominal pain

- CE (a) showed a semi-pedunculated submucosal tumor in the middle small intestine.
- The surface of the protrusion was covered in normal mucosa, with no ulcer formation or erosion.
- Retrograde DBE (b, c, d) showed an elevated lesion in the middle small intestine, approximately 10 mm in diameter.
- The lesion was covered with normal mucosa, with a shallow depression at the peak.
- The lesion was elastic-hard when pushed with forceps.

16.11.2 Heterotopic Pancreas (Figs. 16.33 and 16.34)

- Heterotopic pancreas is defined as the presence of pancreatic tissue that lacks anatomic or vascular continuity with the tissue of the main pancreas.
- In most cases, this condition is asymptomatic, and is frequently discovered incidentally during testing or other abdominal surgery or at autopsy.
- If symptoms are present, this is frequently due to ileal heterotopic pancreas, where intestinal intussusception or bleeding may result.
- Radiography typically shows a smooth, non-pedunculated protrusion.
- Endoscopically, heterotopic pancreas appears as a clearly demarcated, elastic-hard semihemispherical submucosal tumor. Surface depressions may be present.

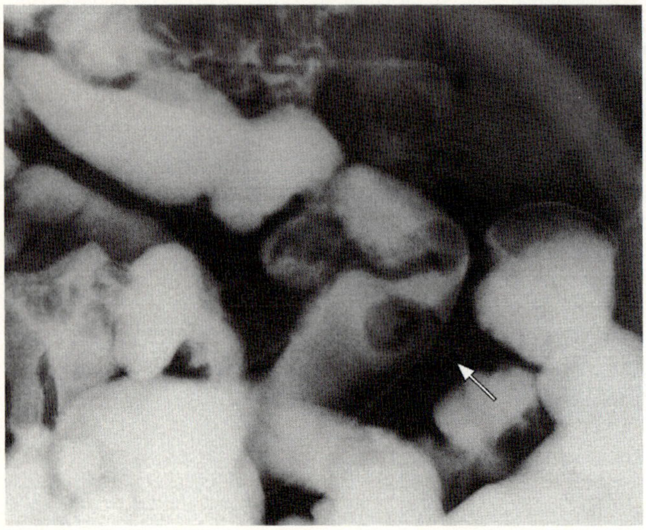

Fig. 16.33 A filling defect around 1 cm in diameter was evident in the middle pelvic small intestine (*arrow*)

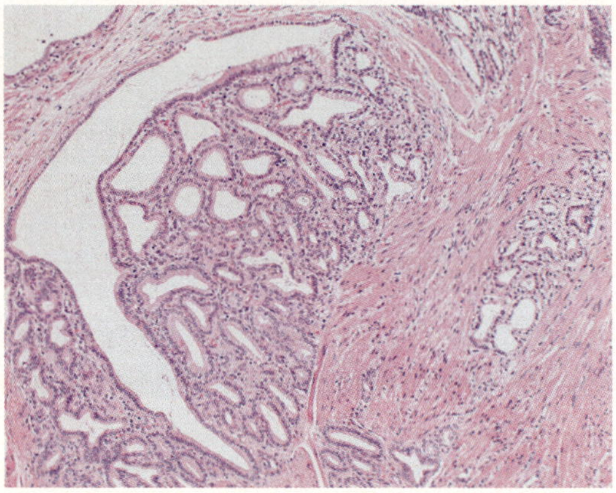

Fig. 16.34 Glandular ducts resembling pancreatic ducts were evident within increased growth of smooth muscle fibers immediately under non-atypical small intestinal mucosa

References

1. Scherübl H et al. Neuroendocrine tumors of the small bowels are on the rise: early aspects and management. World J Gstrointest Endosc. 2010;2:325–34.
2. Matake H et al. Long pedunculated colonic polyp composed of mucosa and submucosa: proposal of a new entity, colonic muco-submucosal elongated polyp. Dis Colon Rectum. 1998;41:1557–61.
3. Matsui N et al. Endosonographic detection of dumbbell-shaped jejunal GIST using double balloon enteroscopy. Endoscopy. 2008;40 Suppl 2:E38–9.
4. Spada C et al. Video capsule endoscopy in small-bowel tumours: a single centre experience. Scand J Gastroenterol. 2008;43:497–505.
5. Shigematsu A et al. Endoscopic diagnosis of lymphangioma of the small intestine. Am J Gastroenterol. 1988;83:1289–93.
6. Iwamoto M et al. Double-balloon endoscopy for jejunal hemangioma (with video). Gastrointest Endosc. 2007;66:184–5.
7. Chen CH et al. Profound iron deficiency anemia caused by a small-intestinal cavernous hemangioma. Gastrointest Endosc. 2009;69: 1392–3.
8. Miyata T et al. A case of inflammatory fibroid polyp causing small-bowel intussusception in which retrograde double-balloon enteroscopy was useful for the preoperative diagnosis. Endoscopy. 2004; 36:344–7.
9. Pang LC et al. Pancreatic heterotopia: a reappraisal and clinicopathologic analysis of 32 cases. South Med J. 1988;81:1264–75.

17 Case Presentations: Protrusion with Ulcer

Sadahiro Funakoshi, Takao Kanemitsu, Noritaka Takatsu, Masashi Yamaguchi, Shotaro Nakamura, Takayuki Matsumoto, Haruhiko Takahashi, and Kohei Fujita

17.1 Case 1 [1]

17.1.1 Female, 20s (Fig. 17.1a–d)

Principal complaint: Abdominal tumor, black stool

- An elevated lesion with a coarse nodular surface occupying around half the circumference of the lumen was present 120 cm distal to the ligament of Treitz.
- An ulcer with a thick white coat was present on the surface.
- CT and MRI showed a metastatic tumor with contrast-enhanced margins in the liver, as well as an irregularly shaped, heterogeneously densely stained tumor adjacent to the uterus. Internal necrotic changes were also evident.

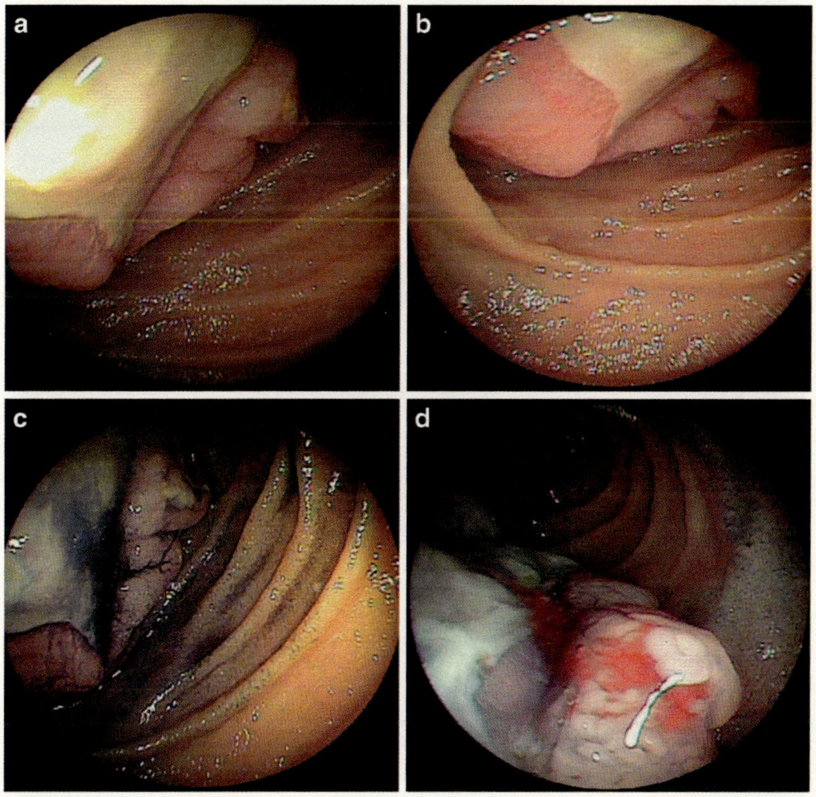

Fig. 17.1

S. Funakoshi (✉) • M. Yamaguchi
Department of Gastroenterology and Medicine, Fukuoka University Faculty of Medicine, 7-45-1 Nanakuma, Jonan-ku, Fukuoka 814-0180, Japan
e-mail: smctw605@ybb.ne.jp

T. Kanemitsu • N. Takatsu • H. Takahashi
Department of Gastroenterology, Fukuoka University Chikushi Hospital, 1-1-1 Zokumyoin, Chikushino 818-8502, Japan

S. Nakamura • T. Matsumoto
Department of Medicine and Clinical Science, Graduate School of Medicine, Kyushu University, 3-1-1, Maidashi, Higashi-ku, Fukuoka 812-8582, Japan

K. Fujita
Department of Gastroenterology, Fukuoka Red Cross Hospital, 3-1-1 Ookusu, Minami-ku, Fukuoka 815-8555, Japan

T. Matsui et al. (eds.), *Endoscopy in the Diagnosis of Small Intestine Diseases*,
DOI 10.1007/978-4-431-54352-7_17, © Springer Japan 2014

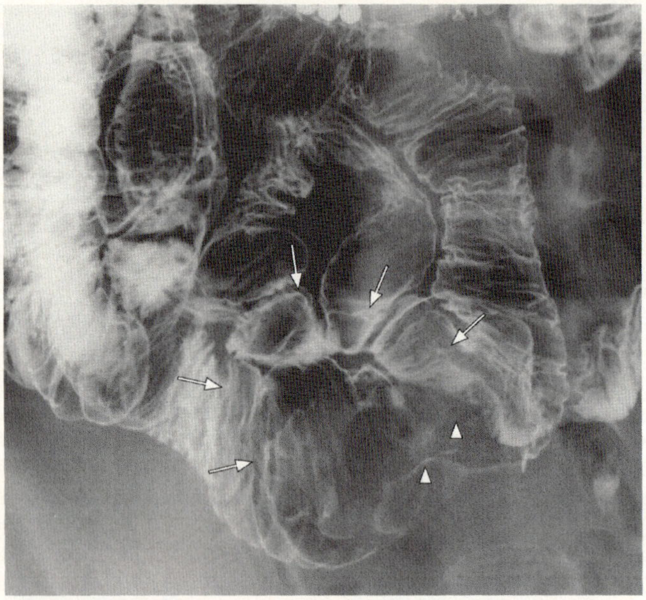

Fig. 17.2

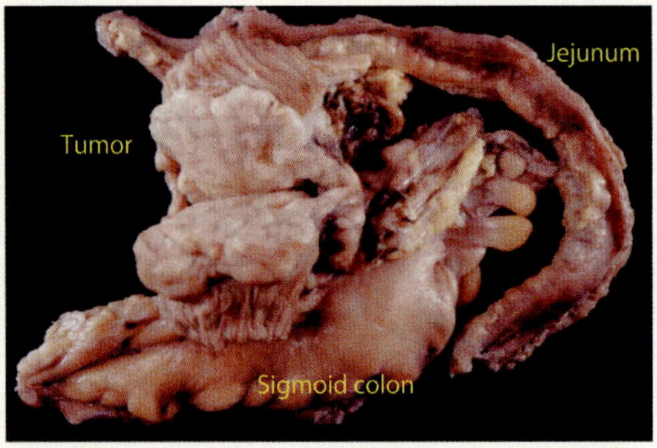

Fig. 17.3 A tumor 65×60×50 mm in size was evident 100 cm from the ligament of Treitz, with strong adhesion to and infiltration of the sigmoid colon. As the lesion was ≥5 cm and <10 cm in size with signs of necrosis, the patient was regarded as showing high risk, with an MIB-1 index of around 15 %

17.1.2 GIST (Figs. 17.2 and 17.3)

- In general, GIST in the duodenum or small intestine shows greater malignant potential than gastric GIST, and the prognosis is frequently poor.
- Lesions with a tumor diameter ≥5 cm are expected to have high malignant potential.
- Other findings suggesting malignancy include ulcer formation, rapid growth, and multiple nodules.
- Lesions showing inhomogenous internal echogenicity on EUS and irregular margins can be expected to show high malignant potential.
- In addition to tumor diameter, the presence of tumor necrosis and an MIB-1 index ≥10 % are regarded as indicative of higher risk.
- Imatinib is the established standard pharmacotherapy (as postoperative adjuvant chemotherapy).

Elevated lesions with coarse surface nodules (arrows) were evident in the jejunum, with barium flecks on the peaks (arrowheads). The tumor was anchored within the pelvis.

17.2 Case 2 [2]

17.2.1 Female, 40s (Fig. 17.4a–d)

Principal complaints: Stomach pain, black stool, anemia

- A submucosal elevation covered in normal mucosa with a steep marginal rising appearance was evident in the jejunum. Ulcer formation was present at the peak.
- The ulcer was covered in a thick white coat, with no irregular invasion evident at the margins.
- Palpation with forceps showed that the lesion was mobile, but the cushion sign was negative.

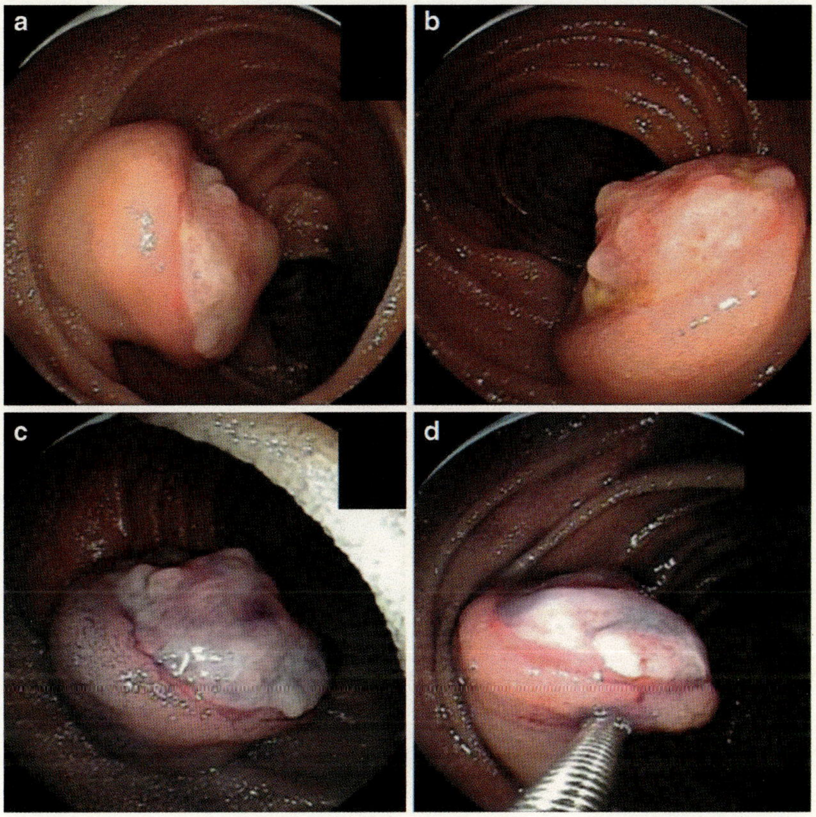

Fig. 17.4

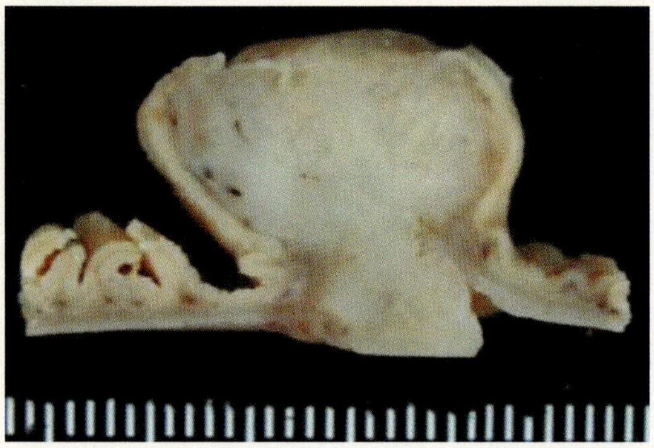

Fig. 17.5 Tumor section. Intra- and extraluminal proliferation of a white solid tumor (mixed type) were evident

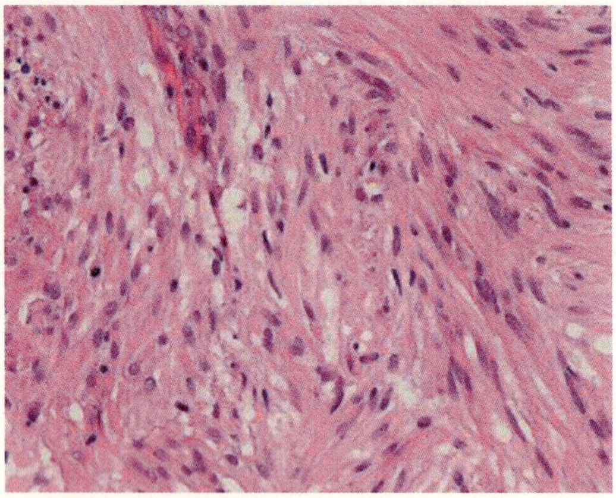

Fig. 17.6 High-magnification image (HE staining). The tumor was composed of spindle-shaped tumor cells. Immunohistochemical staining was positive for c-kit and CD34

17.2.2 GIST (Figs. 17.5 and 17.6)

- Next to the stomach, GIST occurs most frequently in the small intestine (20–30 %), and is more common in adults at 40–60 years old. Principal complaints include abdominal pain, black stool, and intestinal obstruction.
- Characteristic findings on endoscopy comprise submucosal elevations with a smooth surface and a gradual marginal rising appearance. The shape becomes more diverse as tumor diameter increases, with ulcer formation at the peak and a tendency for multiple nodules.
- Tumor diameter (>5 cm) and mitotic count (>5/50 high-power fields (HPF)) are generally used as indices of malignant potential. Biologically, small intestinal GIST is regarded as having higher malignant potential than gastric GIST, and a malignant potential classification has recently been proposed that takes account of the site of origin. This case was classified as low risk, with a tumor diameter of 20 mm and 4/50 HPF mitotic figures.

17.3 Case 3 [3]

17.3.1 Male, 70s (Fig. 17.7a–d)

Principal complaints: Black stool, malaise

- CE showed a friable mucosal abnormality in the lower small intestine. Although a large amount of residue resulted in poor observation, a non-epithelial tumor was suspected on the basis of the properties of the mucosal surface.
- Retrograde DBE revealed a circumferential tumor in the ileum approximately 110 cm on the proximal side of the ileocecal valve. The tumor had a comparatively steep marginal rising appearance, with auriculate protrusions at the margin.

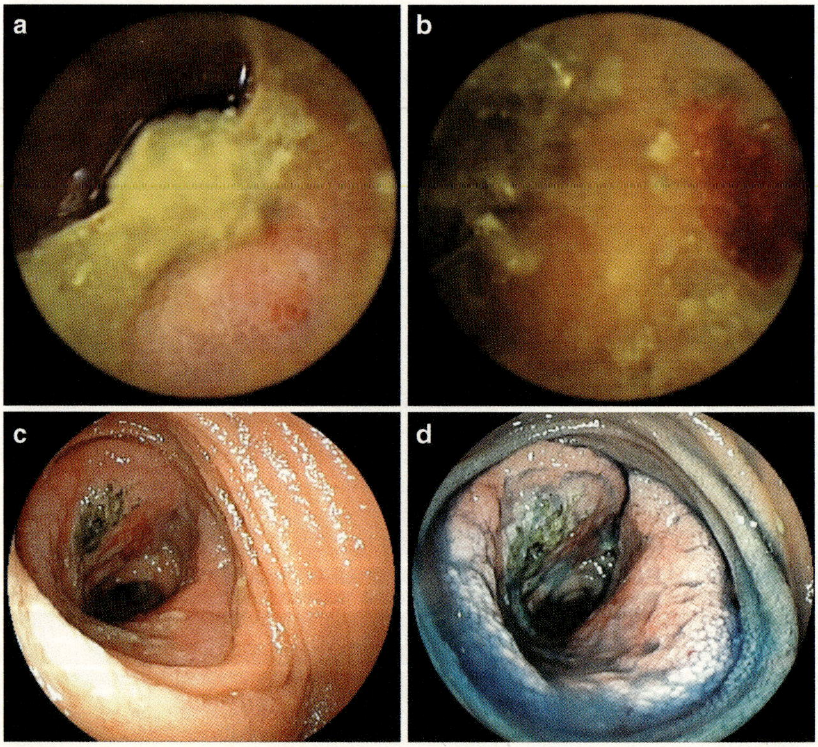

Fig. 17.7

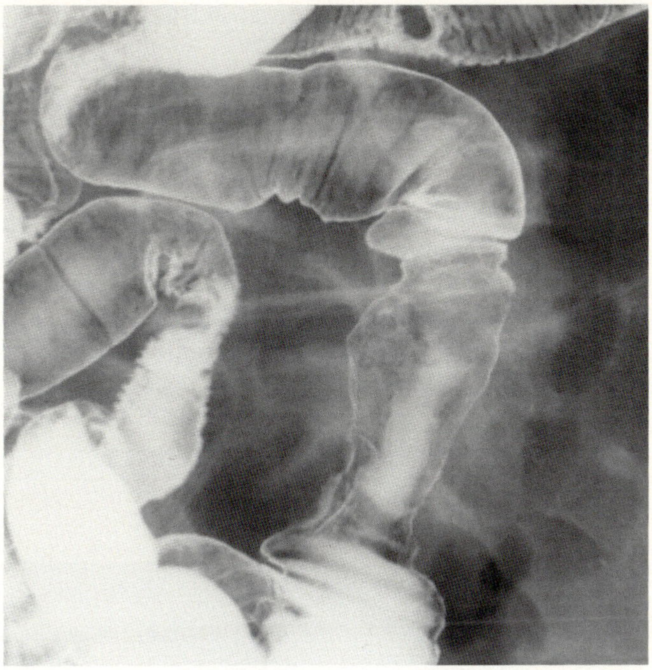

Fig. 17.8 Radiography showed an elevated lesion with gradual marginal rising appearance in the ileum, with luminal stenosis and ulceration inside. Distensibility of the lumen was comparatively good, with no rigidity

17.3.2 Malignant Lymphoma: Diffuse Large B-Cell Lymphoma (DLBCL) (Figs. 17.8 and 17.9a, b)

- Primary malignant lymphoma of the small intestine accounts for 30–40 % of all primary malignant small intestinal tumors. This lesion occurs more frequently in men, and can be found in all age groups from children to the elderly, with an average age of 55–59 years.
- Primary complaints frequently include abdominal pain, palpable abdominal tumor, ileus, weight loss, and melena.
- This pathology is divided into five categories in terms of macroscopic morphology: protrusive, ulcerated (stenotic, non-stenotic, or aneurysmal), multiple lymphomatous polyposis (MLP)-like, diffuse, and mixed/other. The ulcerated type is the most common. Histologically, the diagnosis of DLBCL is the most frequent.

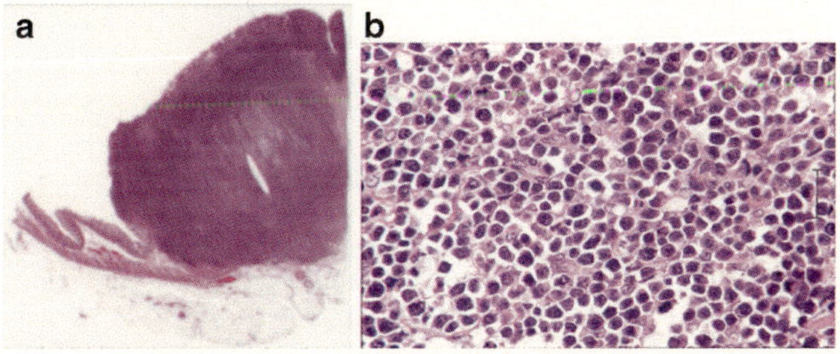

Fig. 17.9 (**a**, **b**) A magnified histopathological image of the surgical specimen showed a full-thickness tumor and diffuse proliferation of moderate-sized to large atypical lymphocytes on high-magnification images. Tumor cells were positive for CD20 in immunostaining

17.4 Case 4 [4]

17.4.1 Male, 80s (Fig. 17.10a–d)

Principal complaints: Lower abdominal pain, sensation of abdominal distension

- A large submucosal elevation of the terminal ileum escaped toward the cecum (a).
- Shallow ulceration had formed on the peak (b).
- An irregular submucosal elevation was evident in the duodenal bulb (c).
- After six courses of chemotherapy (R-CHOP), the lesion had disappeared, and an ulcer scar (arrow) believed to represent the base of the legion was visible (d).

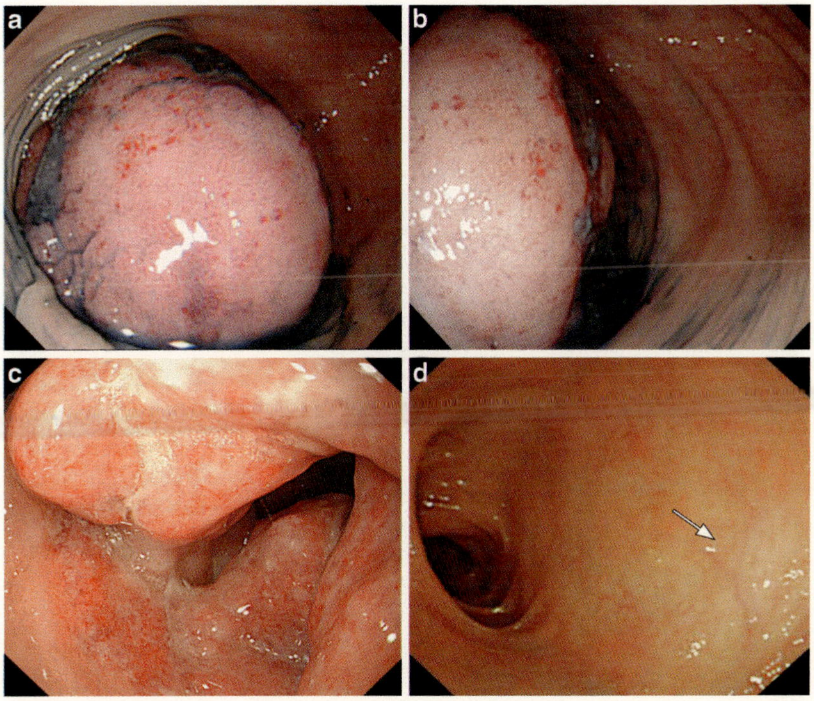

Fig. 17.10

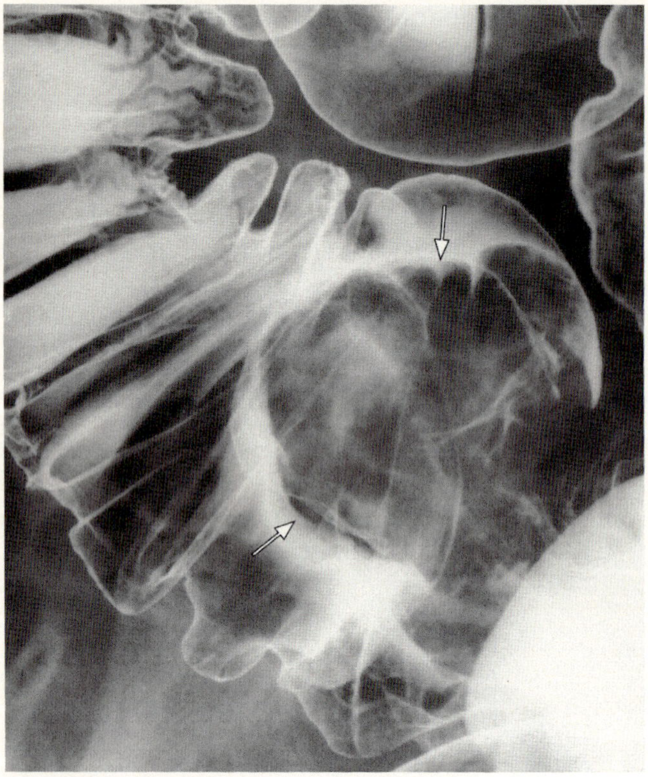

Fig. 17.11 Radiography showed a large submucusal elevation of the terminal ileum, sliding into the cecal side and measuring approximately 70 × 50 mm

17.4.2 Malignant Lymphoma: DLBCL (Figs. 17.11 and 17.12)

- Tumorous (protrusive) malignant lymphoma is classified as a localized small intestinal malignant lymphoma and is the next most common type after the ulcerated type. This lesion almost always occurs in the ileum.
- Most DLBCLs are sessile with smooth surfaces, and any ulceration that is present is often only a shallow erosion.
- Most cases are discovered due to abdominal pain, and as tumors enlarge they may become palpable and cause melena and intestinal intussusception.
- Histologically, most are derived from B cells, with DLBCL accounting for the majority of cases.

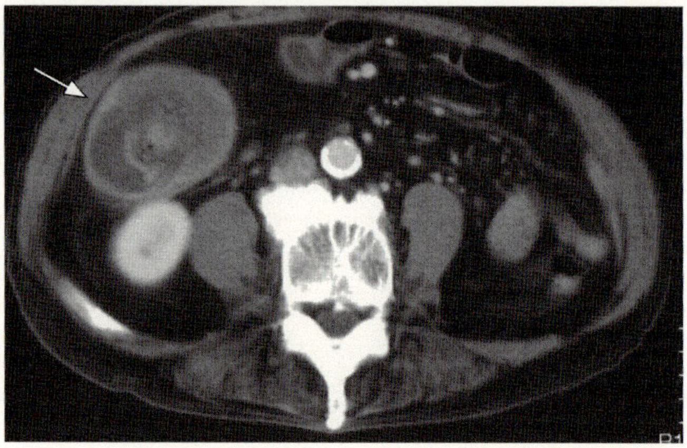

Fig. 17.12 Contrast-enhanced CT showed a stratified enhancing effect in the interior of the lesion, and the lesion in the terminal ileum had slid into an adjacent portion, causing intestinal intussusception at the cecum

17.5 Case 5 [5]

17.5.1 Female, 60s (Fig. 17.13a–d)

Principal complaints: Abdominal pain, melena, weight loss

- Upper gastronintestinal endoscopy revealed a saucer-like tumor in the third part of the duodenum, exhibiting a marginal rising appearance covered in normal mucosa (a, b).
- Antegrade DBE showed a saucer-like tumor in the upper jejunum similar to the duodenal lesion (c, d).
- An ulcer exposing the tumor had formed on the surface, with the margins forming a so-called "auriculate ulcer mound."

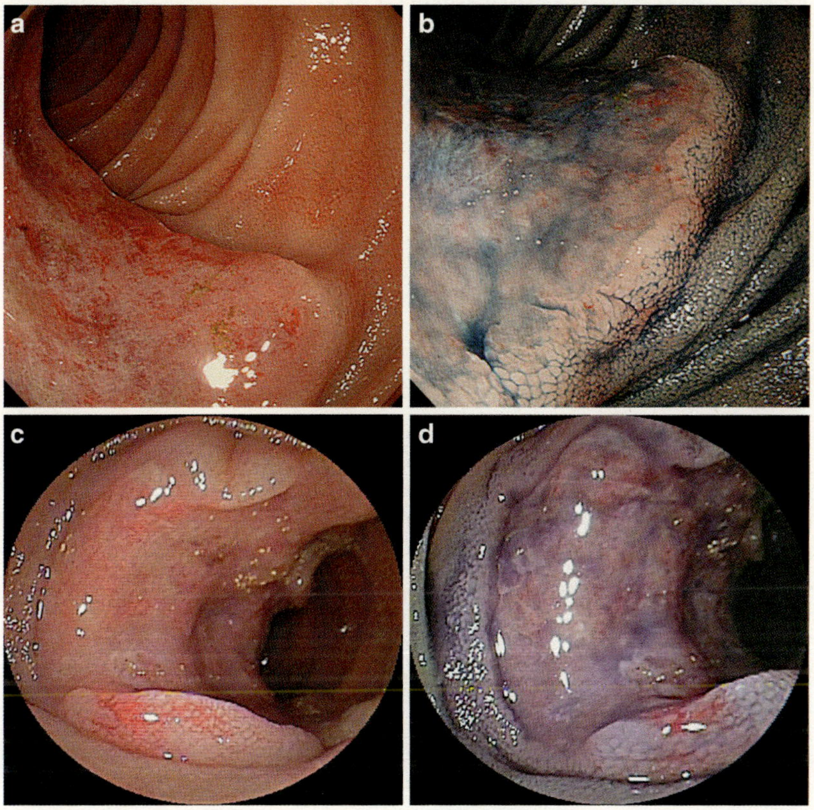

Fig. 17.13

17.5.2 Malignant Lymphoma: DLBCL (Fig. 17.14a, b)

- DLBCL is the most common lymphoma of the gastrointestinal tract, accounting for around 25–35 % of gastrointestinal malignant lymphomas and around 40 % of small intestinal lymphomas.
- The majority of small intestinal DLBCLs are ulcerated or protrusive. Depressions are frequently present on the surface of the protrusive type, as in this case.
- Lesions are frequently multiple. In this case, radiography revealed multiple protrusions and ulcerative lesions in the jejunum (a), in addition to a duodenal lesion (b).
- The points differentiating this condition from cancer were that the sides of the protrusions were covered in normal mucosa, and the ulcer margins took the form of an auriculate ulcer mound.

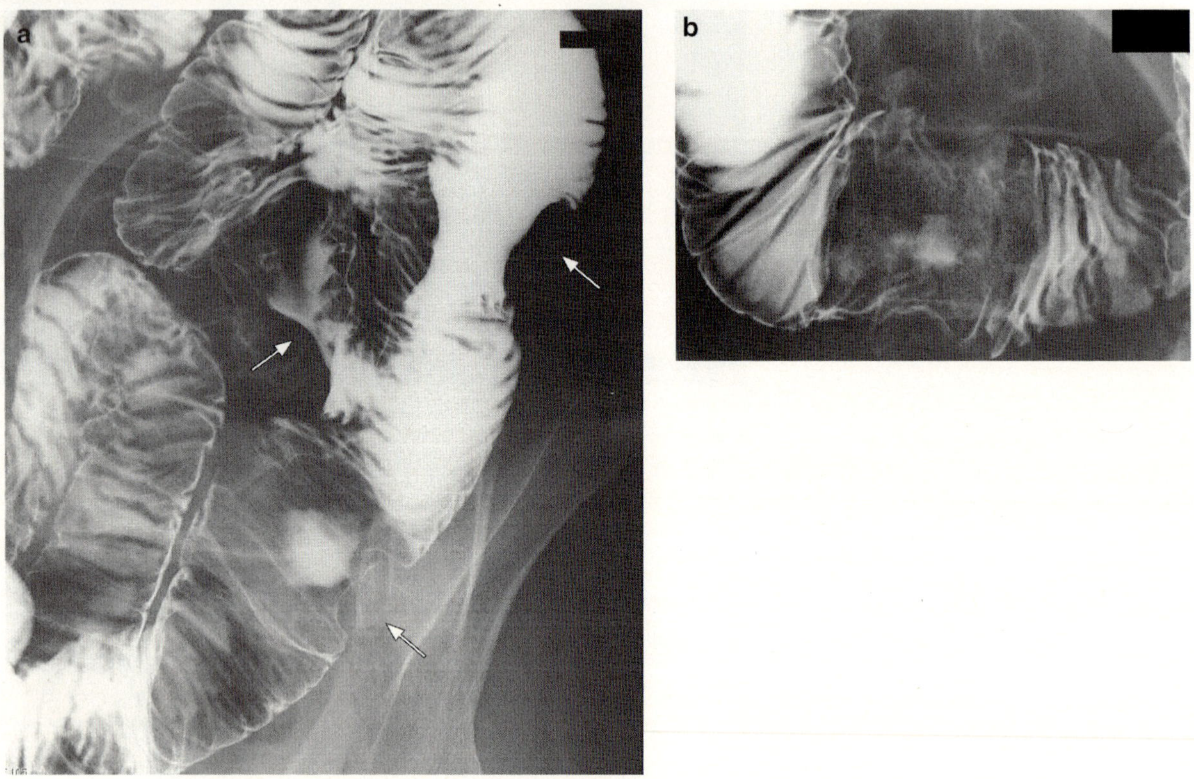

Fig. 17.14 (**a**, **b**) Radiography showed multiple protrusions and ulcerative lesions in the duodenum (*right*) and jejunum (*left*)

17.6 Case 6 [6]

17.6.1 Male, 50s (Fig. 17.15a–d)

Principal complaint: Abdominal pain

- Small intestinal examination under colonoscopy revealed an elevated lesion that had escaped to the large-intestinal side of the ileocecal valve (a, b), and which returned to the ileal side during examination (c, d).
- The surface of the protrusion was partly covered with normal ileal mucosa with villous structures, with shallow mucosal defects in places.
- The lesion was elastic-hard, and IFP, malignant lymphoma, and carcinoid were among the possible differential diagnoses.

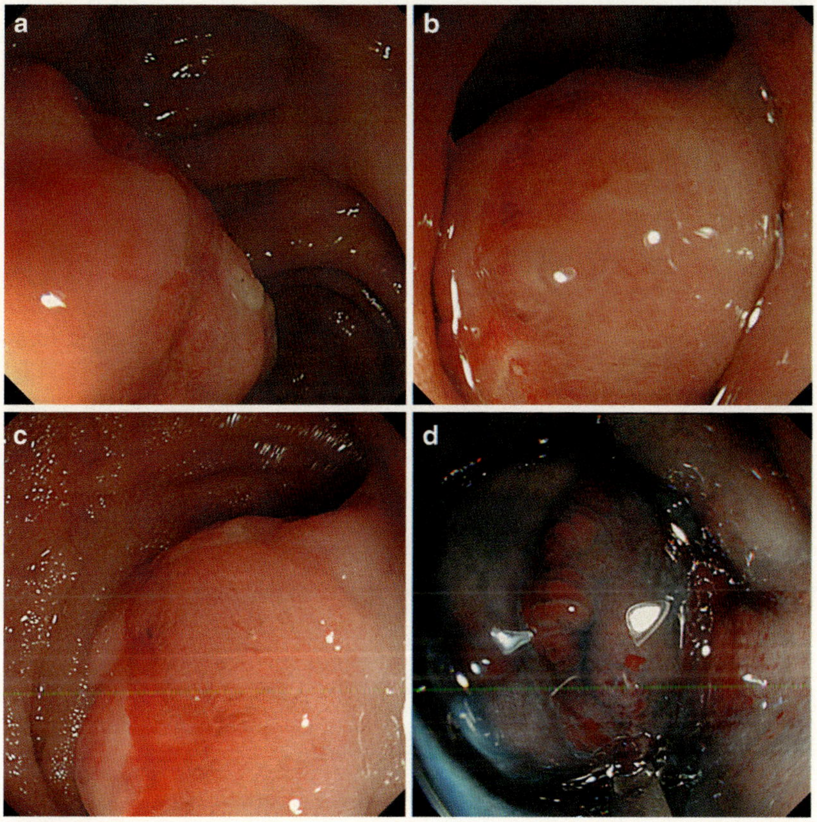

Fig. 17.15

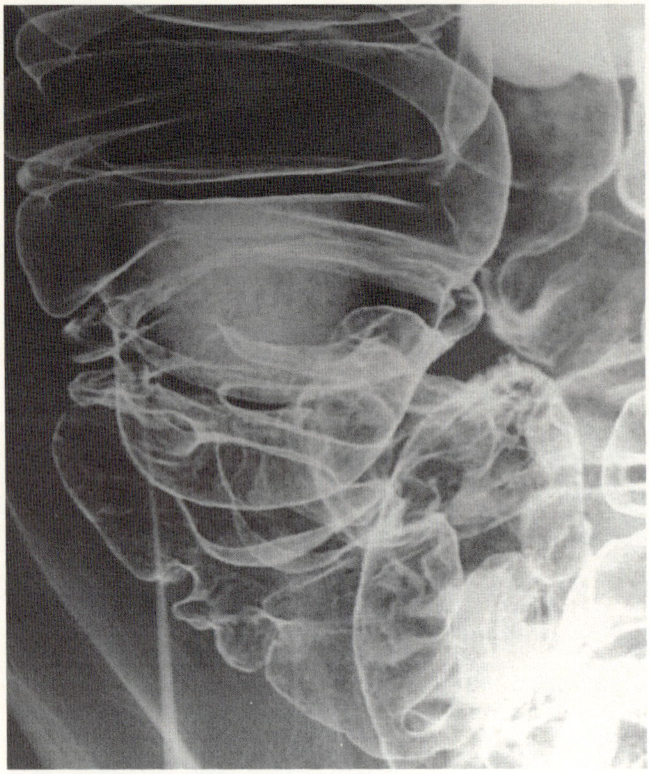

Fig. 17.16 Contrast enema showed an elevated lesion incarcerated in the ileocecal valve

17.6.2 Mucosa-Associated Lymphoid Tissue (MALT) Lymphoma (Figs. 17.16 and 17.17)

- MALT lymphoma is a form of lymphoma with low malignant potential, derived from marginal zone B-cells in MALT and forming in extranodal organs during chronic inflammation.
- In this case, a protrusive MALT lymphoma originating in the terminal ileum caused repeated intestinal intussusception into the large-intestinal side of the ileocecal valve (Fig. 17.16: contrast enema). In the resected specimen, the tumor was limited to the mucosa and submucosal surface layer, with a shallow mucosal defect in the area indicated by the arrow (Fig. 17.17).
- The terminal ileum is a region prone to lymphoma, with DLBCL accounting for the majority of ulcerative cases. In the case of protrusive lymphomas, however, the possibility of MALT lymphoma and follicular lymphoma must also be kept in mind.

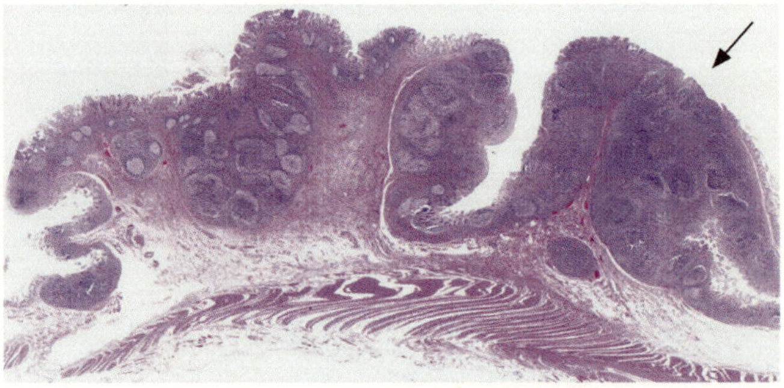

Fig. 17.17 In the resected specimen, the ileal tumor was limited to the mucosa and submucosal surface layer, with a shallow mucosal defect in the area indicated by the *arrow*

17.7 Case 7 [7]

17.7.1 Male, 60s (Fig. 17.18a–d)

Principal complaints: Anemia, black stool

- Lung cancer (non-small cell carcinoma) was identified.
- Antegrade DBE revealed a tumor with the rising marginal appearance of a submucosal tumor-like lesion in the jejunum (a).
- A well-demarcated ulcer was present in the center (b).
- An elevated lesion with a central depression of similar morphology was also evident on Kerckring's folds, separate from the lesion shown above. Multiple similar lesions were apparent nearby (c).
- CE revealed an ulcer with comparatively well-demarcated margins at the peak of the lesion (d).

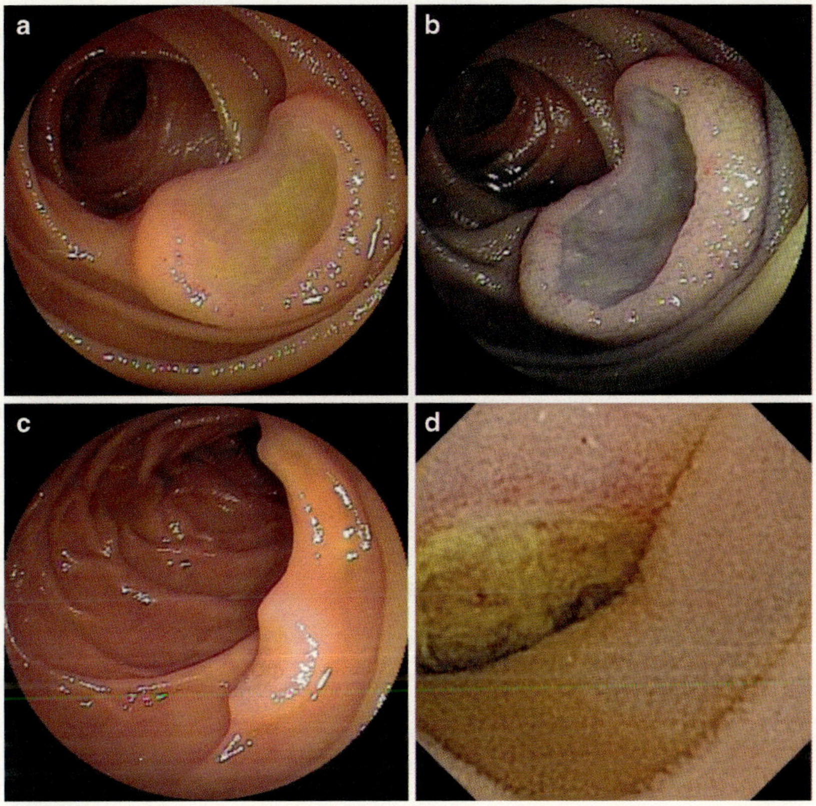

Fig. 17.18

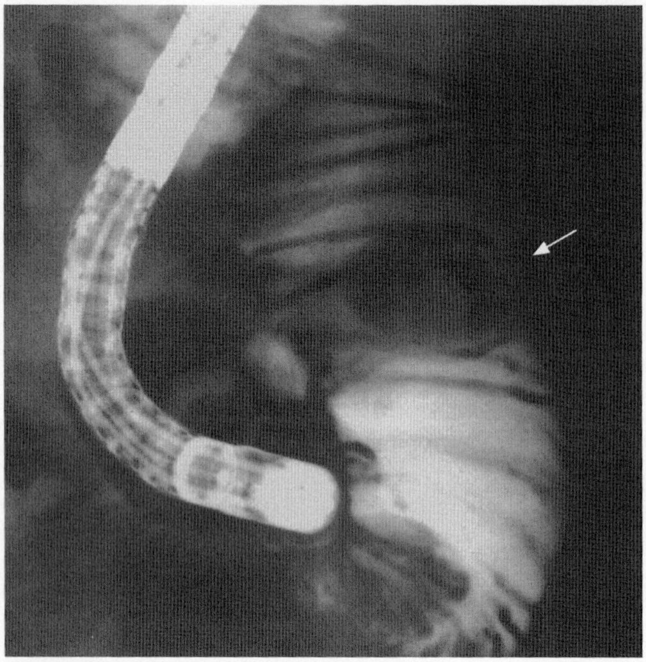

Fig. 17.19 Jejunal radiography revealed a filling defect with clear margins and a barium fleck in the center

17.7.2 Metastatic Intestinal Carcinoma (Primary Lung Cancer) (Figs. 17.19 and 17.20)

- Primary lesions that tend to cause small intestinal metastasis include lung cancer, malignant melanoma, breast cancer, gastric cancer, and pancreatic cancer.
- Clinical symptoms can be broadly categorized into melena, perforation, and stenosis.
- Metastatic intestinal carcinoma characteristically: (1) is common in the jejunum; (2) tends to occur as multiple lesions; and (3) frequently comprises large cell carcinoma.
- Macroscopically, metastatic intestinal carcinoma initially takes the form of a submucosal tumor, with ulcer formation as the lesion grows.

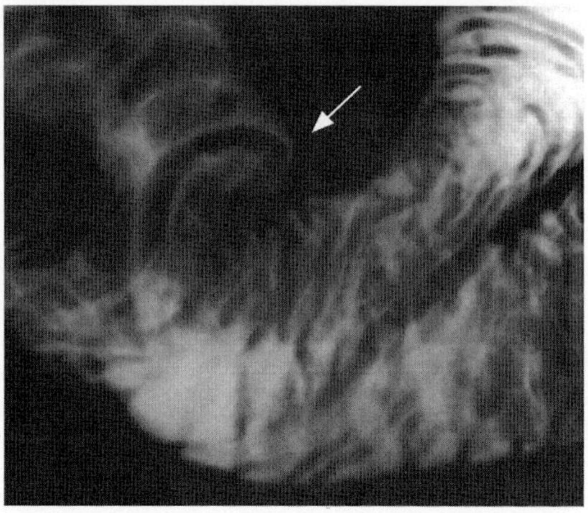

Fig. 17.20 The so-called "bull's-eye sign" was evident

17.8 Case 8 [8]

17.8.1 Female, 60s (Fig. 17.21a–d)

Principal complaints: Loss of appetite, weight loss, symptoms suggesting intestinal obstruction

- Upper gastrointestinal endoscopy showed stage III advanced carcinoma in the greater curvature of the gastric body. Histology showed poorly differentiated adenocarcinoma.
- Retrograde DBE revealed stenosis due to the formation of an almost circumferential tumor in the upper ileum, with the center of the legion comparatively depressed (a, b).
- Redness was present on the surface of the depression, but a flat-bottomed villous structure was also present, with preserved normal epithelium (c, d).
- The lesion was hard, and insertion of the endoscope through to the proximal side of the stenosis was not possible.
- Biopsy of the reddened surface exhibited poorly differentiated carcinoma on histological examination.

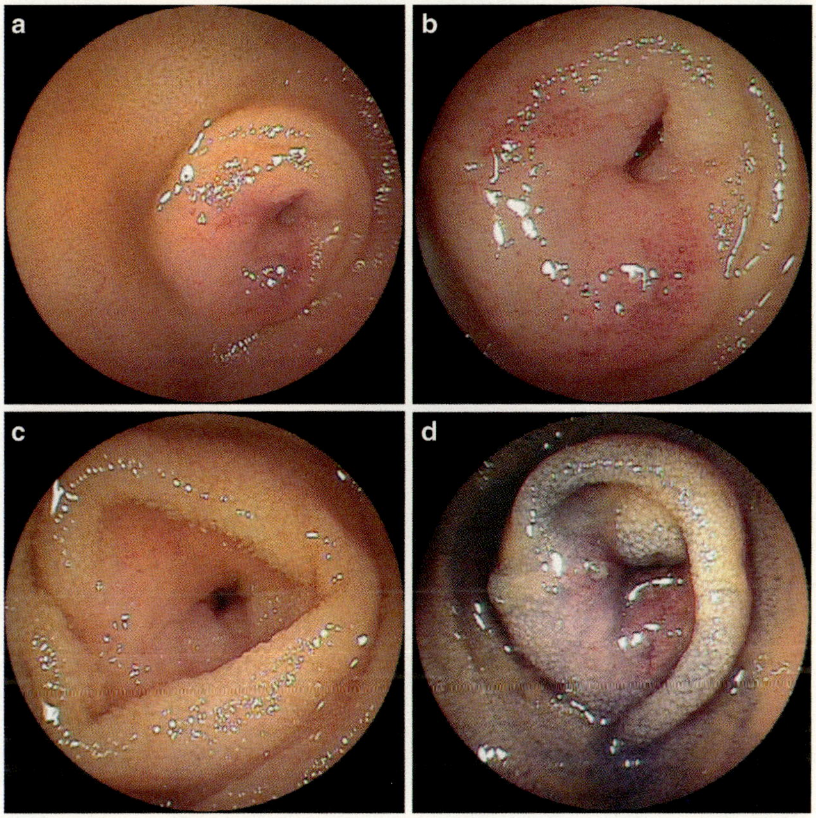

Fig. 17.21

17.8.2 Metastatic Intestinal Carcinoma (Primary Gastric Cancer) (Fig. 17.22a–c)

- Macroscopic findings of metastatic intestinal carcinoma vary according to tissue findings of the primary lesion and the type of metastasis. Blood-borne metastases to the small intestine tend to form as tiny metastatic foci in the shallow submucosal layers, followed by the development of (frequently multiple) lesions with a strong protrusive tendency into the mucosa. This type of metastasis occurs in lung and breast and cancer.
- Poorly differentiated carcinomas, including signet-ring cell carcinoma, may form a metastatic lesion on the small intestine via peritoneal dissemination. In this case, gastric cancer is frequently the primary tumor. Full-thickness invasion occurs from the serosa, and is visualized as tethered folds by radiography. As the tumor progresses, macroscopic findings may come to resemble those of ulcerative localized tumors (a).

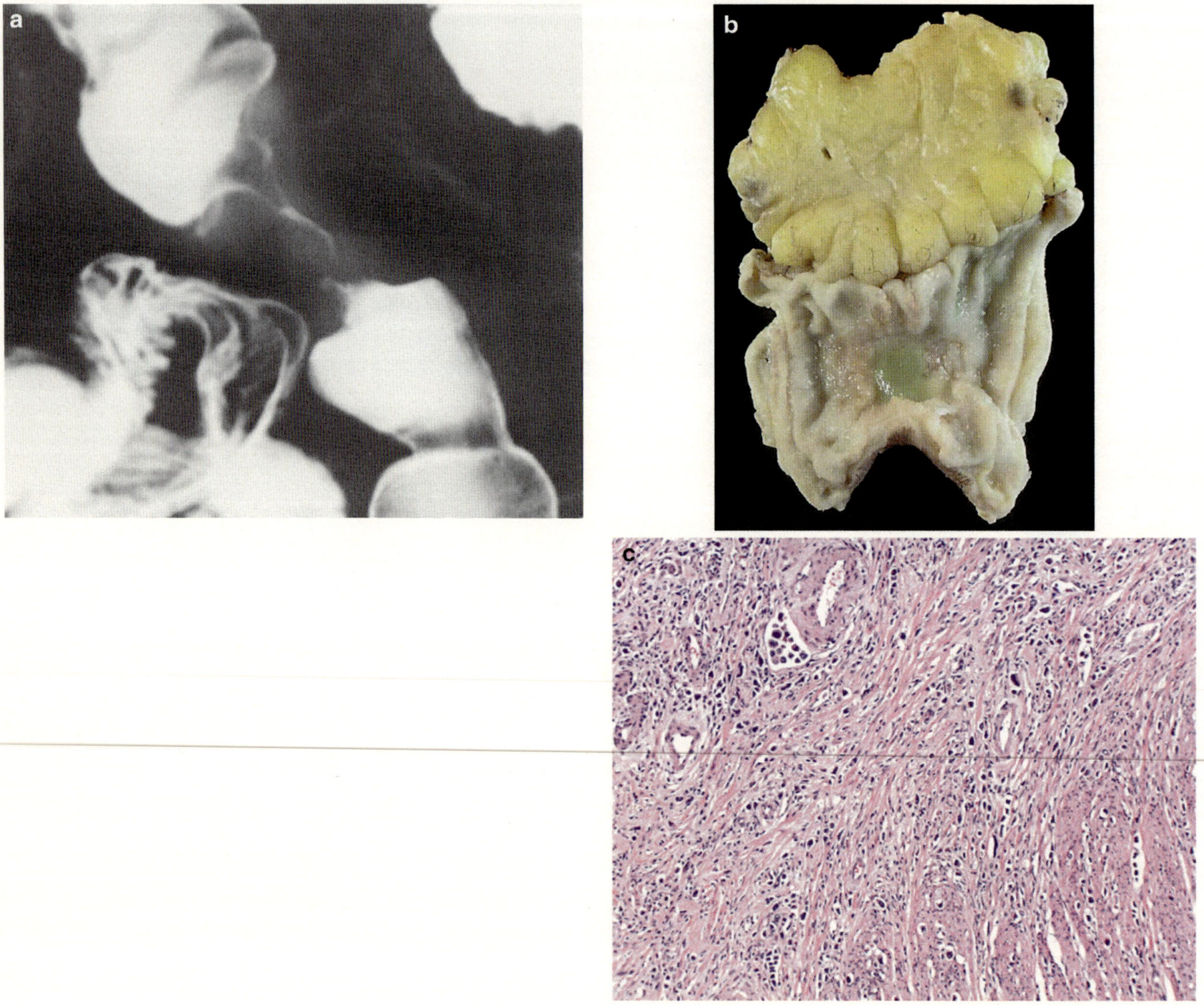

Fig. 17.22 (**a**) Tubular stenosis due to bilateral rigidity was evident. (**b**) Resected specimen showed an ulcerative localized tumor. (**c**) Histology showed poorly differentiated adenocarcinoma

17.9 Case 9 [9]

17.9.1 Male, 70s (Fig. 17.23a–d)

Principal complaint: Melena

- The patient had undergone surgery for right renal cell cancer 3 years previously.
- An elevated lesion occupying around one-quarter of the circumference of the lumen was evident approximately 130 cm distal to the ligament of Treitz.
- The peak was nodular, with erosion and adhering mucus (a, b).
- The tumor showed a gradual marginal rising appearance, and the base was covered in normal mucosa (c, d).

This case is quoted from Mulder CJJ (ed): Atlas of double balloon endoscopy. p.106, Medconnect, Munich, 2007.

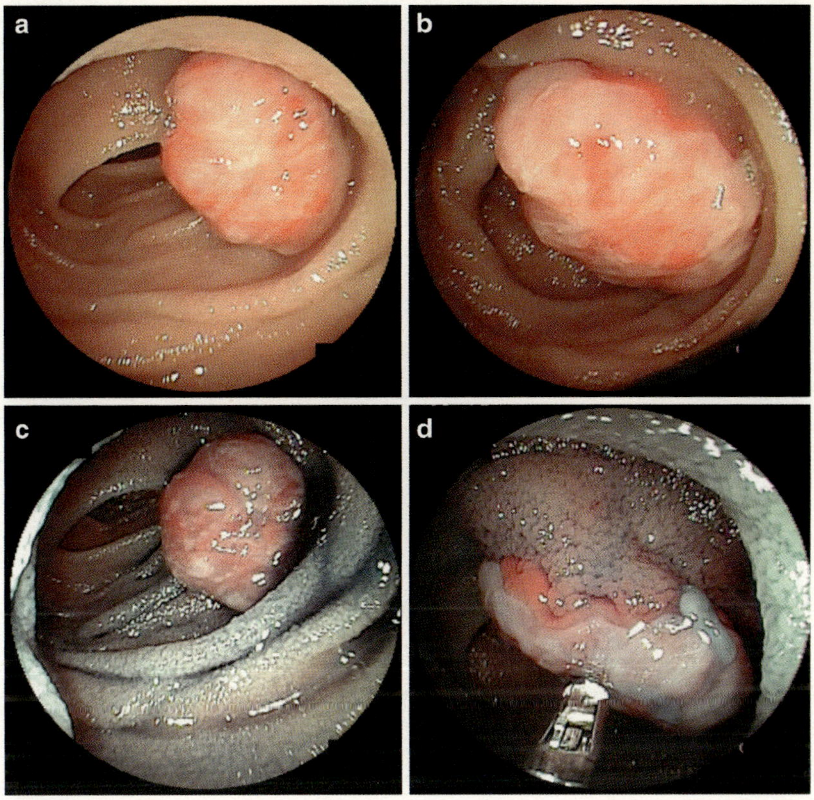

Fig. 17.23

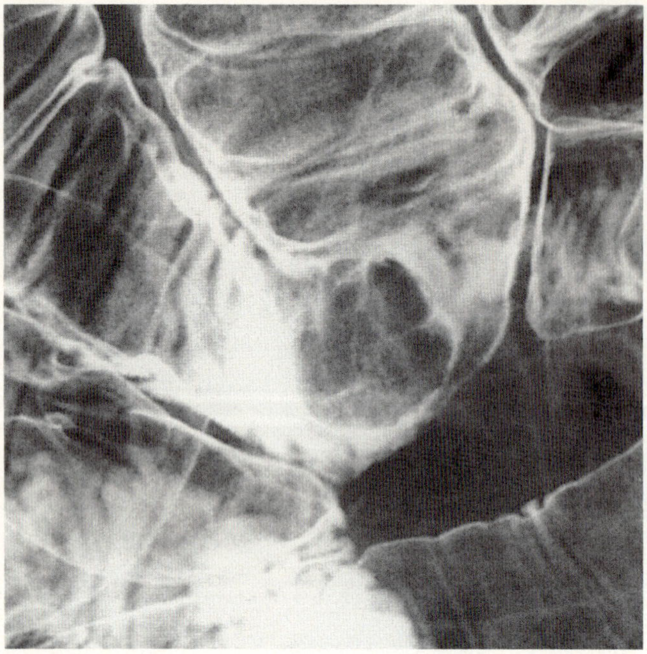

Fig. 17.24 Radiography revealed an elevated lesion around 2 cm in size with a nodular peak in the middle small intestine

17.9.2 Metastatic Intestinal Carcinoma (Primary Renal Cancer) (Figs. 17.24 and 17.25)

- Renal cell carcinoma metastasizes via the blood or lymph to organs including the lungs, bones, liver, and regional lymph nodes. Small intestinal metastasis is rare.
- Clinical symptoms include obstructive symptoms such as abdominal pain, vomiting, and loss of appetite, as well as gastrointestinal bleeding and anemia. Intestinal intussusception may also occur.
- Endoscopically, renal cell cancer metastasis is characterized by sides covered with normal mucosa, and may develop from a submucosal tumor into a pedunculated form. The peak may be ulcerated.

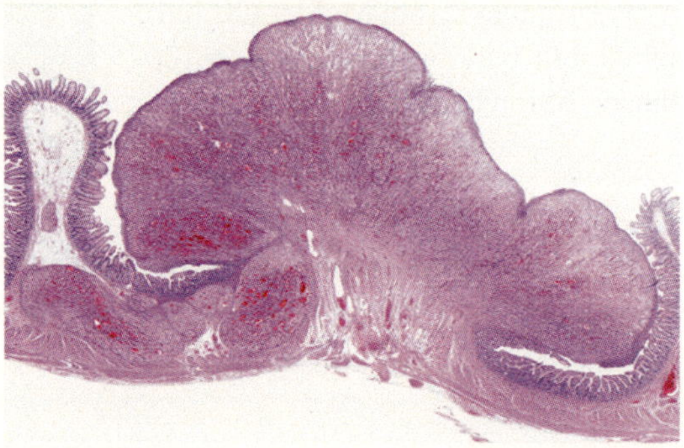

Fig. 17.25 Histopathology of the resected specimen showed solid proliferation of clear cell carcinoma, mainly in the submucosal layer

17.10 Case 10 [10]

17.10.1 Female, 60s (Fig. 17.26a–d)

Principal complaints: Persistent abdominal pain, nausea, high levels of carbohydrate antigen 19–9

- Antegrade DBE revealed a tumor covered with normal mucosa and converging folds from the surroundings (a, b).
- The lesion occupied almost the entire circumference of the central portion, with a suspected depression.
- A scope was unable to be passed through due to stenosis.
- Intraoperative endoscopic findings from the distal side of the lesion. A bumpy irregular ulcer with convergence of Kerckring's folds was evident at the site of stenosis (c, d).

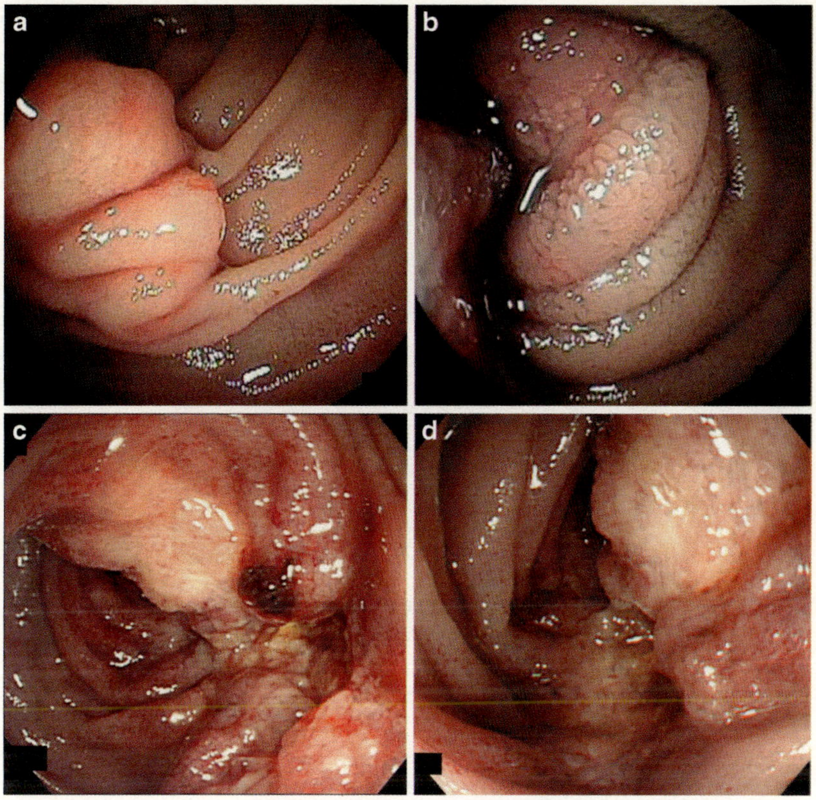

Fig. 17.26

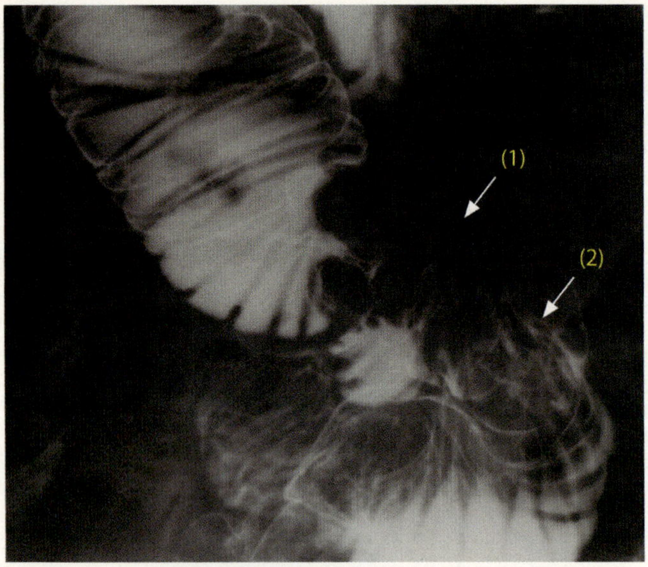

Fig. 17.27 Radiography revealed a smooth filling defect (*arrow 1*) and a faint barium fleck, together with convergence of the wall on the distal side (*arrow 2*)

17.10.2 Small Intestinal Carcinoma Arising from Heterotopic Pancreas (Figs. 17.27, 17.28 and 17.29)

- Gastrointestinal heterotopic pancreas may become cancerous, although this is comparatively rare.
- Around ten cases of small intestinal carcinoma arising from heterotopic pancreas have been reported in total from both Japan and overseas. This pathology tends to occur in the jejunum or Meckel's diverticulum, and frequently exhibits a form similar to that of an ulcerated submucosal tumor.
- If this disease concept is not kept in mind, preoperative diagnosis can be difficult.
- Radiographic and endoscopic findings in this case were characterized by an ulcerative tumor exhibiting different properties on the proximal and distal sides, corresponding on the proximal side to a submucosal tumor (Figs. 17.27 and 17.28).

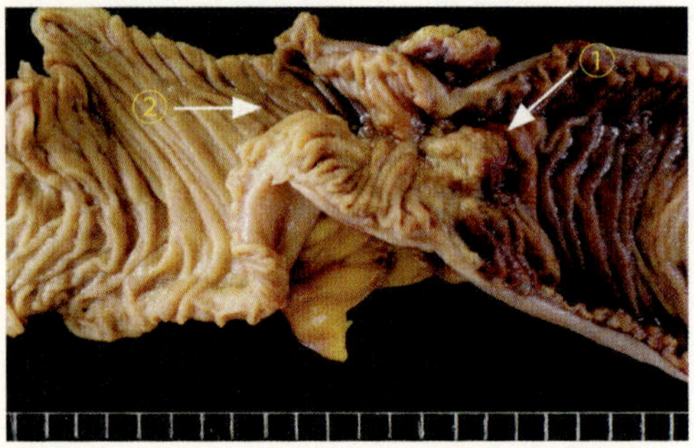

Fig. 17.28 A protrusion covered with normal mucosa was visible on the proximal side (*arrow 1*), and an ulcer was evident at the site of stenosis on the distal side (*arrow 2*)

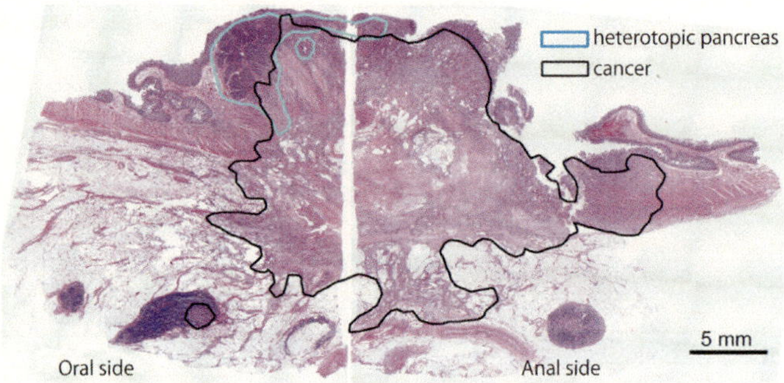

Fig. 17.29 The tumor was composed of heterotopic pancreatic tissue (*blue line*) and an adenocarcinomatous component (*black line*), with smooth transition between the two

References

1. Almeida N et al. Double-balloon enteroscopy and small bowel tumors: a South-European single-center experience. Dig Dis Sci. 2009;54:1520–4.
2. Grover S et al. Small intestine gastrointestinal stromal tumors. Curr Opin Gastroenterol. 2012;28:113–23.
3. Sopirjakova P et al. Small intestinal diffuse large B-cell lymphoma in a 58-year-old patient with coeliac disease. Acta Medica. 2011;54:25–8.
4. Weigand K et al. Chronic anemia masking a primary large B-cell lymphoma of the small intestine, finally diagnosed by double-balloon enteroscopy. Endoscopy. 2008;40 Suppl 2:E149.
5. Matsumoto T et al. Double-balloon endoscopy depicts diminutive small bowel lesions in gastrointestinal lymphoma. Dig Dis Sci. 2010;55:158–65.
6. Ohashi S et al. Education and imaging. Gastrointestinal: MALT lymphoma of the terminal ileum. J Gastroenterol Hepatol. 2006;21:1495.
7. Kobayashi N et al. Small intestinal metastasis from carcinoma of the lung. Clin Gastroenterol Hepatol. 2011;9:e103.
8. Mitsui T et al. Role of double-balloon endoscopy in the diagnosis of small-bowel tumors: the first Japanese multicenter study. Gastrointest Endosc. 2009;70:498–504.
9. Loualidi A et al. Duodenal metastasis: an uncommon cause of occult small intestinal bleeding. Neth J Med. 2004;62:201–5.
10. Arao J et al. A case of aberrant pancreatic cancer in the jejunum. Hepatogastroenterology. 1999;46:504–7.

18 Case Presentations: Multiple Protrusions

Shin Fujioka, Kunihiko Aoyagi, Yuji Maehata, Koichi Eguchi, Yutaka Yano, Shotaro Nakamura, Hiroshi Kawano, Yoshitaka Tomioka, Ritsuko Fujisawa, and Koichi Abe

18.1 Case 1, 2 [1]

18.1.1 Male, 70s (Fig. 18.1a, b)

Principal complaint: Black stool

- Three months after lung cancer surgery.
- Antegrade DBE showed dark-red semi-pedunculated elevated lesions scattered around the upper to middle small intestine.
- Tumor surfaces were markedly bumpy and friable, with adhesion of dirty material resembling necrotic tissue.

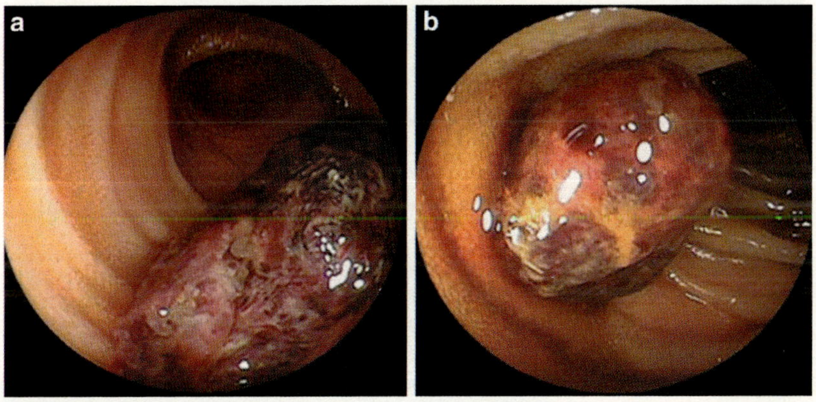

Fig. 18.1

18.1.2 Female, 70s (Fig. 18.2a, b)

Principal complaints: Black stool, anemia

- Lung cancer and metastatic adrenal tumor were present.
- Antegrade DBE revealed multiple submucosal elevations in the duodenum (b) and jejunum (a) with well-demarcated ulcers on the peaks.
- The margins of the ulcers were regular, with prominent vascular ectasia in the surrounding mucosa.
- The tumors were of varying sizes, with the duodenal lesion occupying about half the circumference of the lumen.

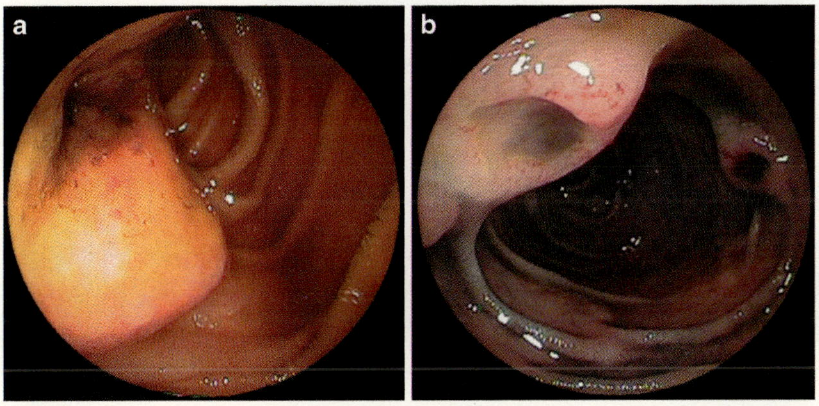

Fig. 18.2

S. Fujioka (✉) • Y. Maehata • S. Nakamura • R. Fujisawa
Department of Medicine and Clinical Science, Graduate School of Medical Sciences, Kyushu University, 3-1-1, Maidashi, Higashi-ku, Fukuoka City 812-8582, Japan
e-mail: sfujioka@intmed2.med.kyushu-u.ac.jp

K. Aoyagi • K. Eguchi • Y. Tomioka • K. Abe
Department of Gastroenterology and Medicine, Fukuoka University Faculty of Medicine, 7-45-1 Nanakuma, Jonan-ku, Fukuoka 814-0180, Japan

Y. Yano
Department of Gastroenterology, Fukuoka University Chikushi Hospital, 1-1-1 Zokumyoin, Chikushino 818-8502, Japan

H. Kawano
Division of Gastroenterology, Department of Medicine, Kurume University School of Medicine, 67 Asahi-machi, Kurume 830-0011, Japan

T. Matsui et al. (eds.), *Endoscopy in the Diagnosis of Small Intestine Diseases*, DOI 10.1007/978-4-431-54352-7_18, © Springer Japan 2014

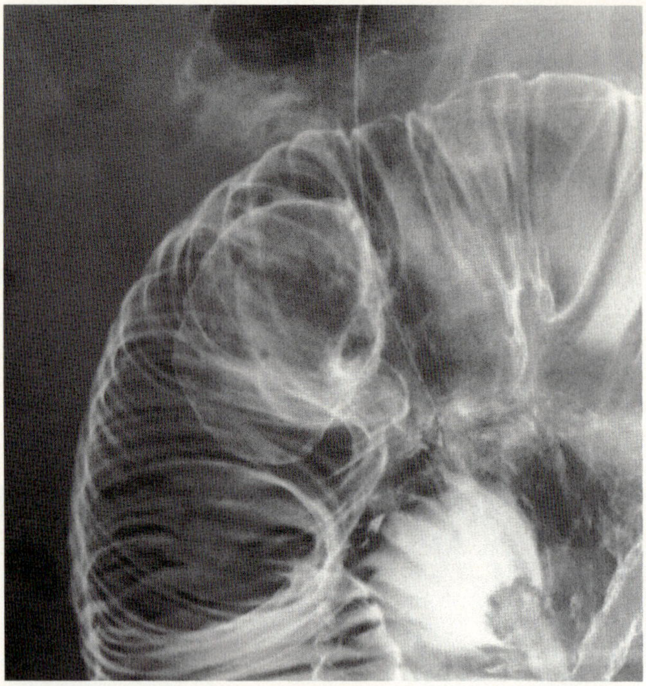

Fig. 18.3 Radiology for Case 1. A smooth, semi-pedunculated elevated lesion, 3 cm in diameter, was evident in the jejunum. At the start of the examination, intestinal intussusception was present on the presenting portion of the tumor, but this resolved during the examination

18.1.3 Metastatic Intestinal Carcinoma (Primary Lung Cancer) (Figs. 18.3 and 18.4)

- Other than direct invasion from abdominal organs, lung cancer metastasis is the most common form of secondary intestinal tumor, accounting for 60 % of metastatic intestinal carcinoma.
- In terms of histological type, large-cell carcinoma accounts for around half of cases and tends to occur in the jejunum, often as multiple tumors.
- It may be discovered as a result of intestinal obstruction, melena, perforation, or intestinal intussusception.
- Typically, they form submucosal tumor-like tumors with deep ulcers in the center, representing the so-called bull's-eye sign.
- Depending on the site of the primary lesion, histological type, site of metastatic focus, and level of development, cancers may take a range of forms, including sessile protrusion type, protrusive-depressed type, or ulcerated type in addition to tumor-like type.

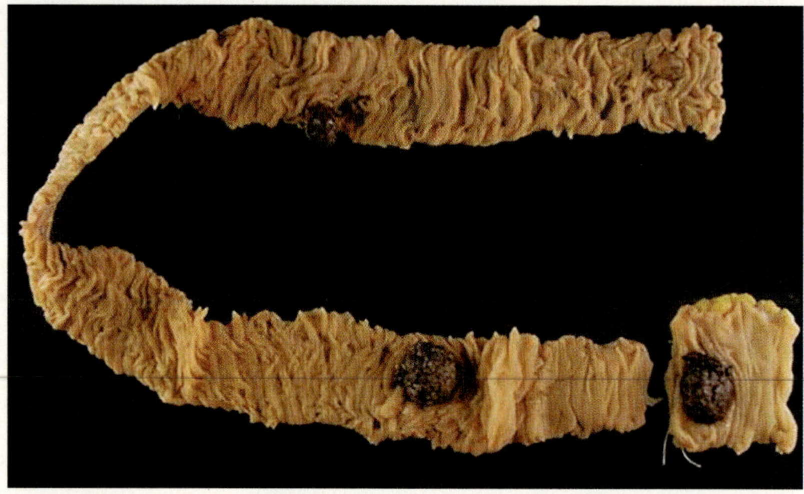

Fig. 18.4 Case 1 underwent partial small intestinal resection. Four nodular lesions were present in the resected small intestine

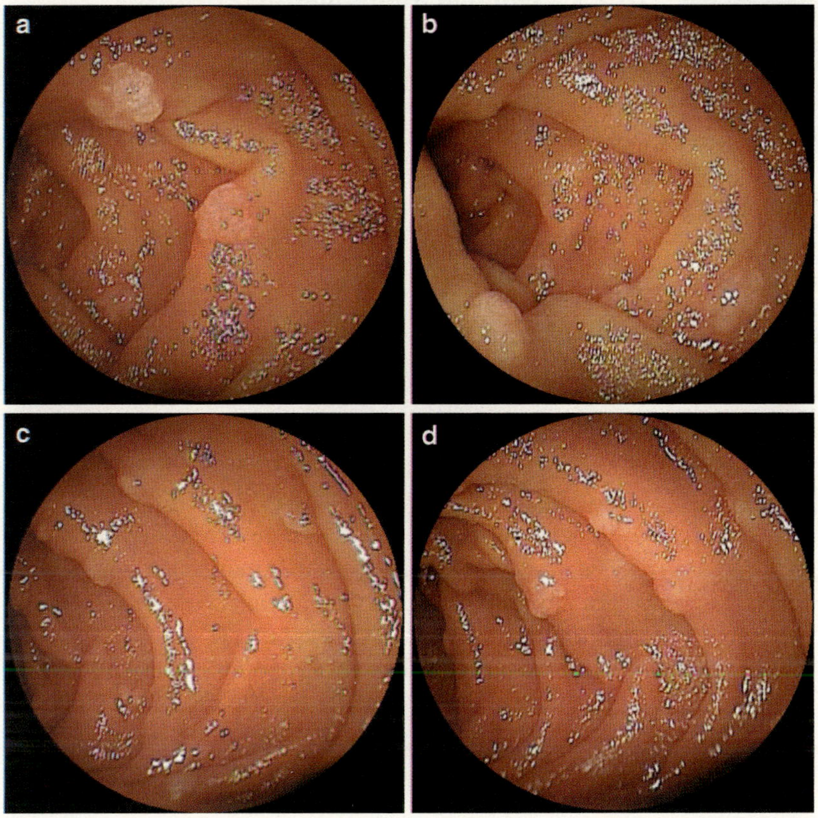

Fig. 18.5

18.2 Case 3 [2]

18.2.1 Male, 40s (Fig. 18.5a–d)

Principal complaint: Nothing in particular

- Multiple somewhat whitish, small elevated lesions were present in the jejunum (a, b).
- The multiple small protrusions in the jejunum were mainly located on top of folds. Their distribution became gradually sparser on the distal side (c, d).

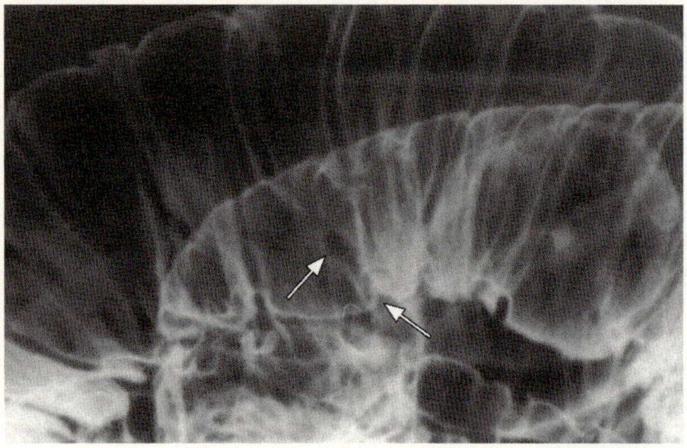

Fig. 18.6 Radiography (small intestinal double-contrast image) showed polyps as small filling defects

18.2.2 Familial Adenomatous Polyposis (FAP) (Fig. 18.6)

- This is a genetic disorder (dominant inheritance) in which a large number of adenomas develop in the large intestine and become cancerous. It is also seen in other parts of the gastrointestinal tract other than the large intestine, as fundic gland polyposis in the fundic gland region, and as adenoma in the pyloric region, duodenum, and small intestine.
- Small intestinal adenoma is more common in the jejunum than in the ileum. The rate of cancerous transformation is not as high as in the colon.
- Radiographically, FAP is characterized by multiple small filling defects, but adenoma of the terminal ileum is not easily distinguished from lymphoid polyps.
- Endoscopically, this pathology characteristically takes the form of small, white, sessile protrusions. In the terminal ileum, it must be distinguished from lymphoid polyp by the epithelial marginal rising appearance and comparatively well-demarcated white color.
- Other diseases from which this pathology must be distinguished include other types of gastrointestinal polyposis (Peutz-Jeghers syndrome, juvenile polyposis, Cowden disease, and Cronkhite-Canada syndrome).

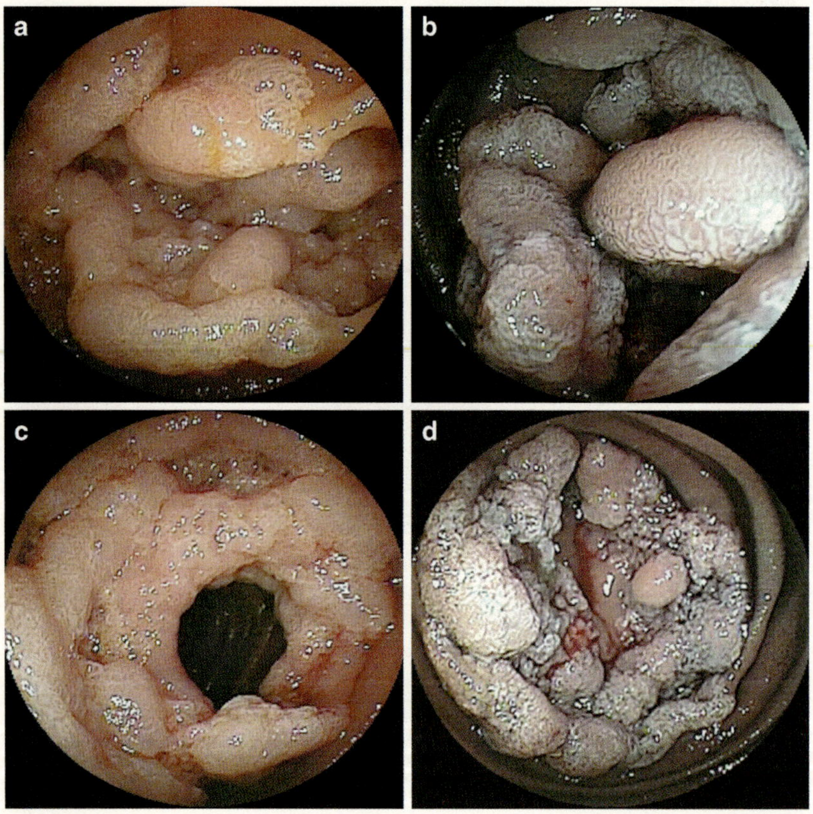

Fig. 18.7

18.3 Case 4 [3]

18.3.1 Female, 50s (Fig. 18.7a–d)

Principal complaint: Bloody stool

- The patient was diagnosed with colonic adenomatosis with advanced multiple carcinoma by a local physician, and underwent total colectomy. During this surgery, two nodule-aggregating lesions were identified in the jejunum (a, b).
- Antegrade DBE for monitoring purposes revealed a circumferential nodule- aggregating lesion in the upper jejunum, together with coarse nodules.
- A further circumferential nodule-aggregating lesion was also evident on the distal side. Nodules varied in size and the central area was unstructured, with pronounced redness (c, d).
- All lesions had increased in size compared with 3 years previously.

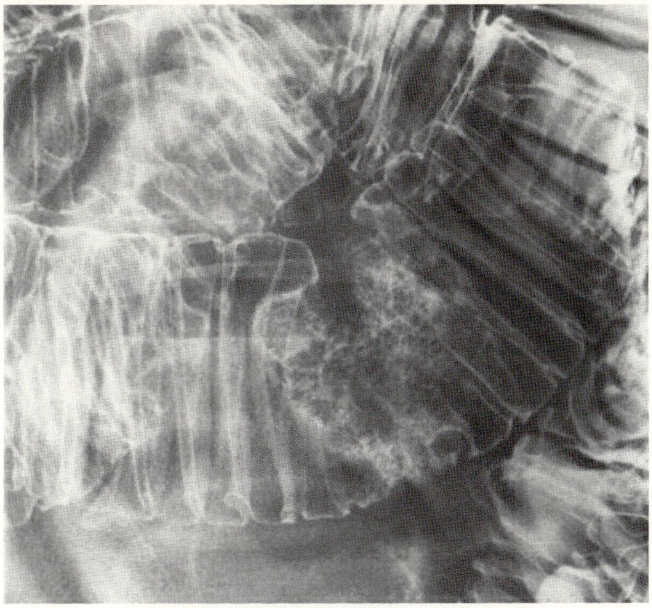

Fig. 18.8 Radiology revealed a circumferential nodule-aggregating lesion in the upper jejunum

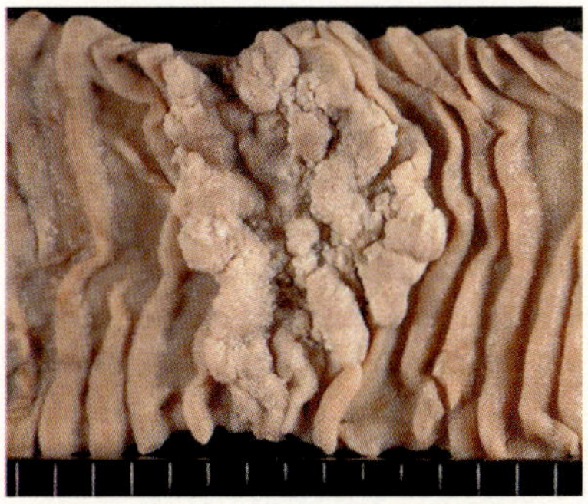

Fig. 18.9 A protrusion with a maximum diameter of around 5 cm was seen in the specimen after partial small intestinal resection

18.3.2 Familial Adenomatous Polyposis (FAP) (Figs. 18.8, 18.9 and 18.10)

- Colonic adenomatosis is a genetic disease in which multiple adenomas develop in the large intestine, and which has a high rate of complication with colorectal carcinoma from a young age. Adenomas also occur at a high rate in the duodenum and upper small intestine.
- Intestinal adenoma occurs in approximately 60 % of cases, but many points regarding the long-term course remain unclear.
- Although cancerous transformation is believed to occur in around 2 % of cases, the number of reported cases of complication with intestinal carcinoma has been increasing in recent years in line with the increase in long-term survival.
- Although the cases we have treated have comprised nodule-aggregating lesions, there have also been a few reports of other advanced cancers.

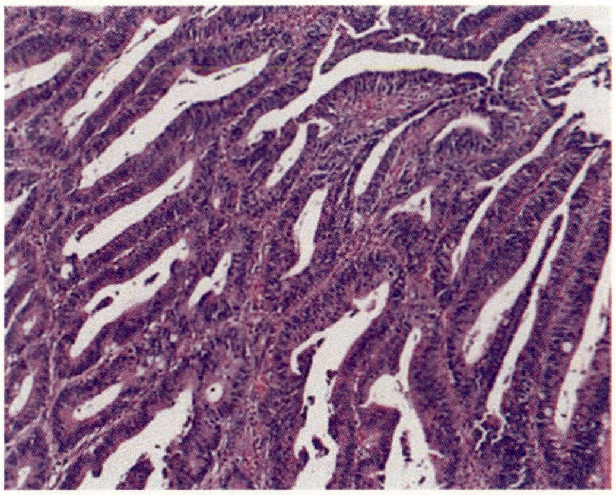

Fig. 18.10 Histopathology showed signs of highly differentiated adenocarcinoma mixed with tubulo-villous adenoma

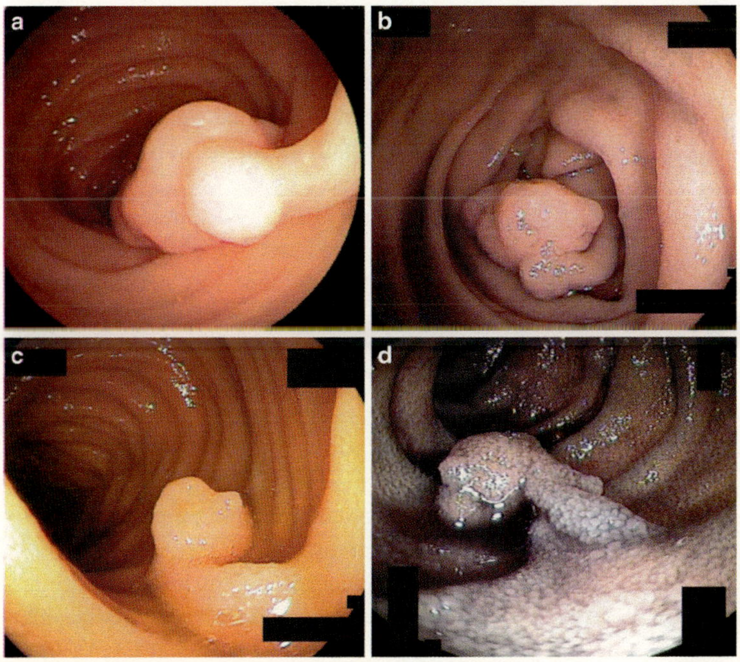

Fig. 18.11

18.4 Case 5 [4]

18.4.1 Female, 20s (Fig. 18.11a–d)

- The patient was diagnosed with Peutz-Jeghers syndrome as an elementary school student.
- A pedunculated polyp around 10 mm in size with a nodular peak of the same color as the surrounding mucosa was evident in the third part of the duodenum (a, b).
- A 7-mm pedunculated polyp of the same color with a lobulated peak was also evident in the upper small intestine of the same patient (c, d).

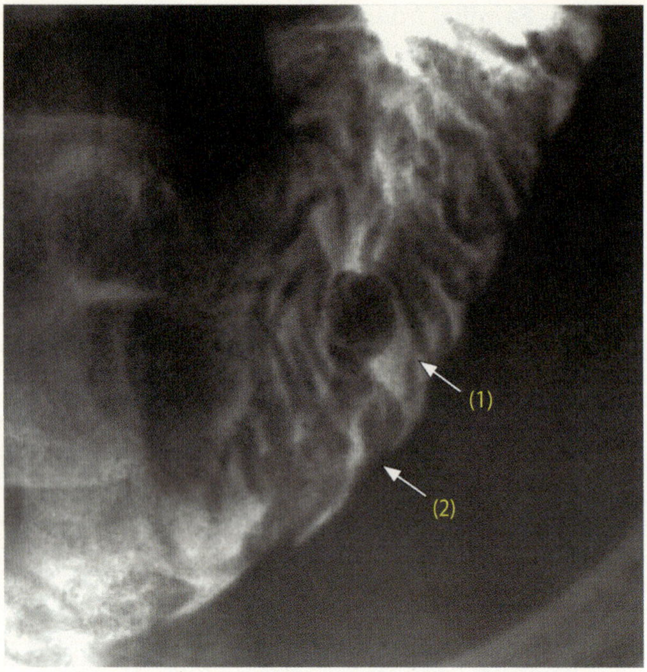

Fig. 18.12 Radiography of the polyp showed a nodular peak (*arrow 1*) and a long peduncle (*arrow 2*)

18.4.2 Peutz-Jeghers Syndrome (PJS) (Figs. 18.12 and 18.13)

- PJS is an autosomal dominant genetic condition characterized by pigmented patches on the lips, oral mucosa, and distal portions of the extremities, as well as gastrointestinal polyposis.
- Polyps arise sporadically, but may be densely concentrated. They vary in size, with most being 5–20 mm in diameter, but some may exceed 40 mm, and these frequently cause intestinal intussusception.
- Polyps are often pedunculated, with nodular or lobulated surfaces.
- Histologically, they mainly comprise glandular hyperplasia and dendritic growth of the muscularis mucosae.

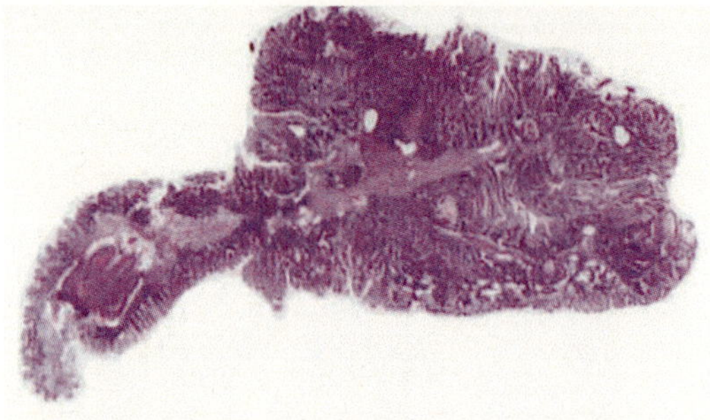

Fig. 18.13 Histopathology of the polypectomy specimen is diagnosed as Peutz-Jeghers polyp because this tumor is composed with a hamartomatous polyp with extensive smooth muscle arborization

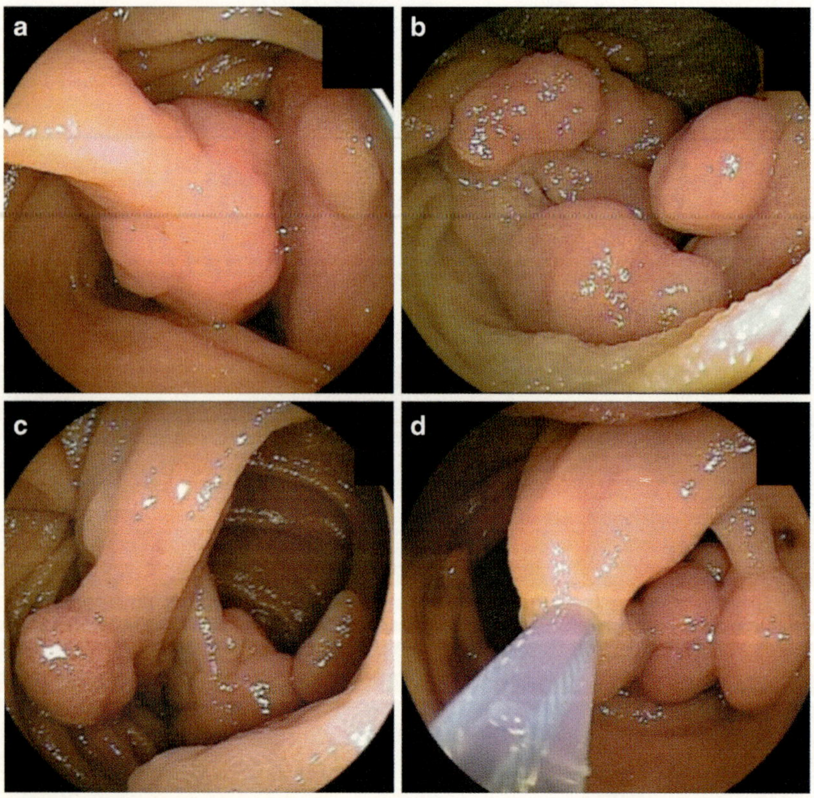

Fig. 18.14

18.5 Case 6 [5]

18.5.1 Female, 30s (Fig. 18.14a–d)

Principal complaint: Intermittent abdominal pain

- The patient was diagnosed with PJS at 2 years old. She had undergone laparotomic small intestinal polypectomies at both 15 and 24 years old.
- Antegrade DBE showed numerous polyps in the second part of the duodenum.
- The upper jejunum was densely packed with pedunculated or semi-pedunculated polyps around 2–3 cm in diameter (a, b, c).
- The surface of the polyps was lobulated with a coarse nodular or convoluted appearance.
- Polyps varied in color from whitish or normal to reddish.
- Pedunculated polyps were removed by polypectomy (d).
- Densely packed polyps had caused intestinal intussusception, resulting in intermittent abdominal pain, but this resolved after polyp removal.

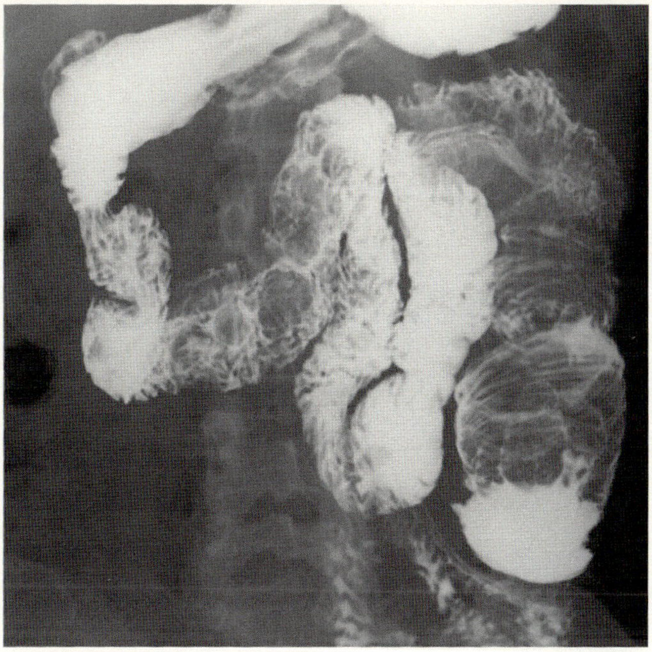

Fig. 18.15 Multiple filling defects ranging in size from 2 cm to a maximum of 4 cm were evident from the third part of the duodenum to the jejunum. Numerous polyps were particularly densely concentrated in the upper jejunum in the upper left abdomen, and intestinal intussusception was evident on the presenting portion of the polyps

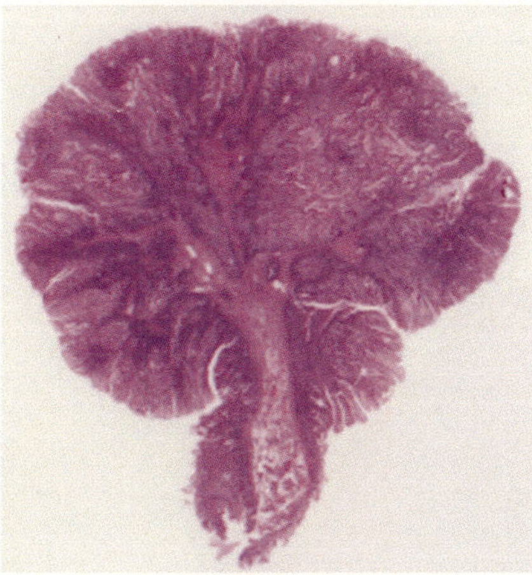

Fig. 18.16 Histopathology of the resected specimen. There was dentritic growth of the branches of the muscularis mucosae, and non-atypical hyperplastic mucosa

18.5.2 PJS (Figs. 18.15 and 18.16)

- PJS is an autosomal-dominant genetic disease that causes pigmentation in the oral cavity and on the lips, fingers, and toes, together with multiple gastrointestinal polyps.
- This syndrome occurs in 1 in 10,000–12,000 people. About 50 % of patients show a family history of the disease. In terms of distribution, polyps are found in the stomach, small intestine, and large intestine, excluding the esophagus. Polyps occur equally in the stomach, small intestine, and large intestine in Japan, but are more common in the jejunum in Europe and the United States. The number of polyps ranges from a few to several hundred in some cases.
- Polyps may be pedunculated, semi-pedunculated, or non-pedunculated, with a lobular surface that is coarse nodular or convoluted. Coloration varies from white to red.
- Histopathologically, these lesions are regarded as hamartomas, and polyps in the stomach, duodenum, small intestine, or large intestine may turn cancerous. Adenoma is also present in 10 % of polyps. Carcinoma is also present in 1–3.8 %. The rate of complication with gastrointestinal cancer is 20–25 %, with cancer of the large intestine being most common.

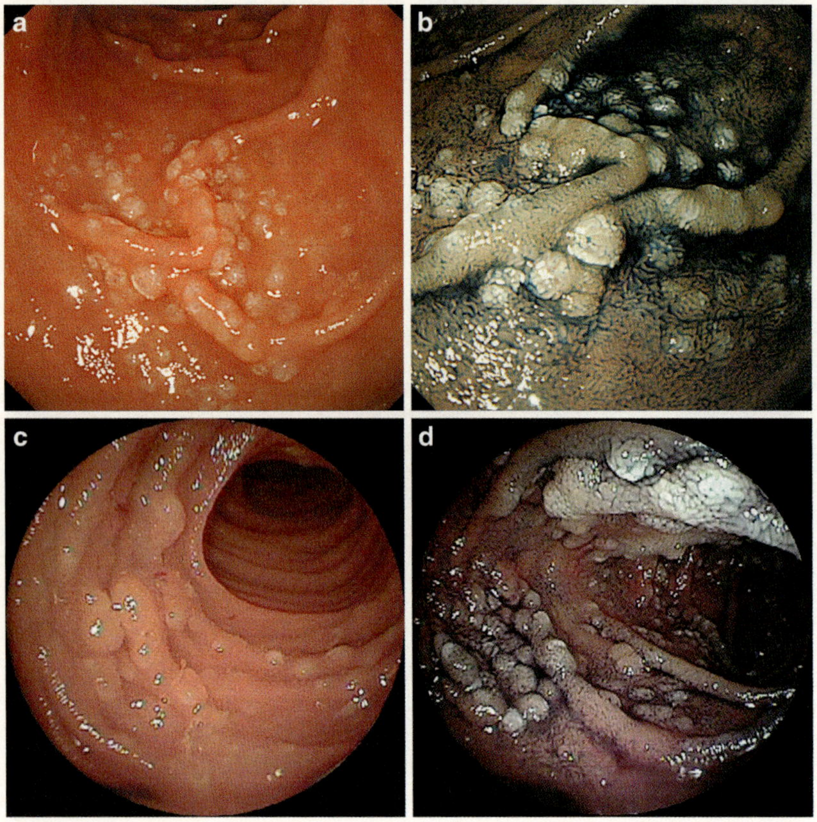

Fig. 18.17

18.6 Case 7 [6]

18.6.1 Female, 50s (Fig. 18.17a–d)

- Although the patient was asymptomatic, upper gastrointestinal endoscopy was performed as part of a health checkup.
- Multiple small white protrusions, some of which were nodular, were clustered in the second part of the duodenum on the opposite side to the papilla (a, b).
- Antegrade DBE revealed numerous small, smooth-surfaced protrusions in the jejunum (c, d).

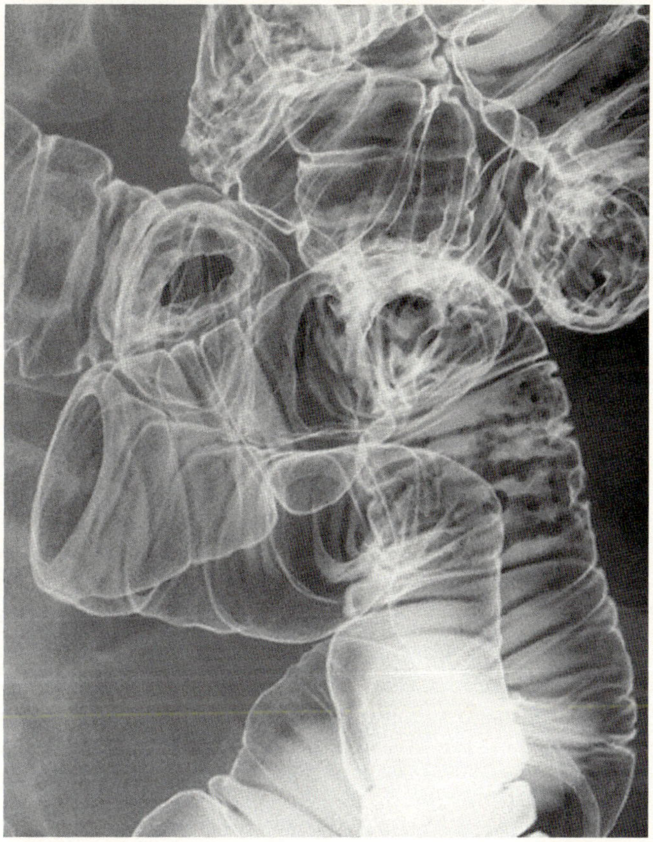

Fig. 18.18 Radiography visualized clusters of small protrusions. Small lesions may be difficult to distinguish from air bubbles

18.6.2 Follicular Lymphoma (Figs. 18.18 and 18.19a, b)

- The spread of small intestinal endoscopy has increased the number of reported cases of small intestinal follicular lymphoma.
- This pathology is most commonly identified in the second part of the duodenum, but lesions are also frequently found in the jejunum and ileum.
- Macroscopically, it tends to appear as MLP, in the form of widespread multiple small protrusions. Radiographically, it is visualized as clusters of small protrusions, but in the small intestine these may be difficult to distinguish from air bubbles (Fig. 18.18).
- Reaching a definitive diagnosis from HE specimens alone is difficult. Confirmation requires positive immunostaining for both CD10 and Bcl2 (Fig. 18.19).

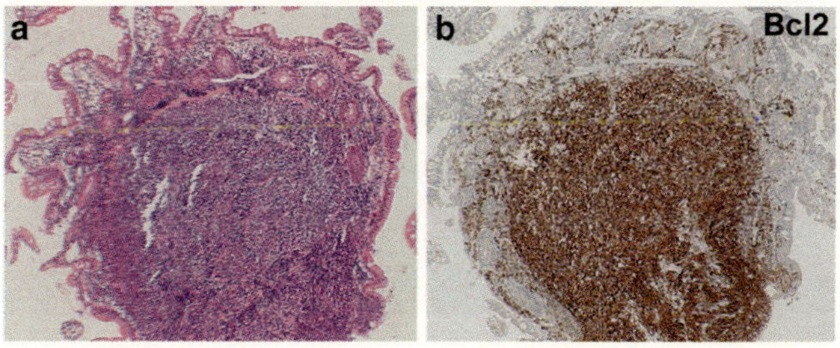

Fig. 18.19

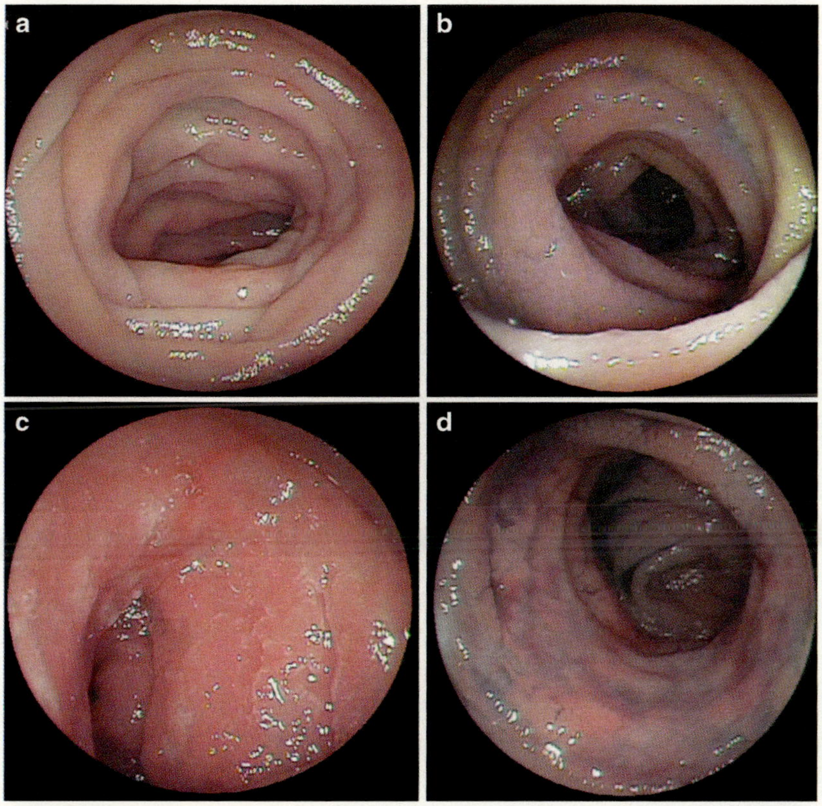

Fig. 18.20

18.7 Case 8 [7]

18.7.1 Female, 40s (Fig. 18.20a–d)

Principal complaint: Diarrhea

- Widespread irregular swelling of the folds was evident in the small intestine, with scattered small areas of redness. The intestine was somewhat distensible with air (a, b).
- Swelling of the folds was pronounced in part of the jejunum, which was indistensible, and narrowing of the intestinal tract was seen. Reddening and erosion were evident (c, d).

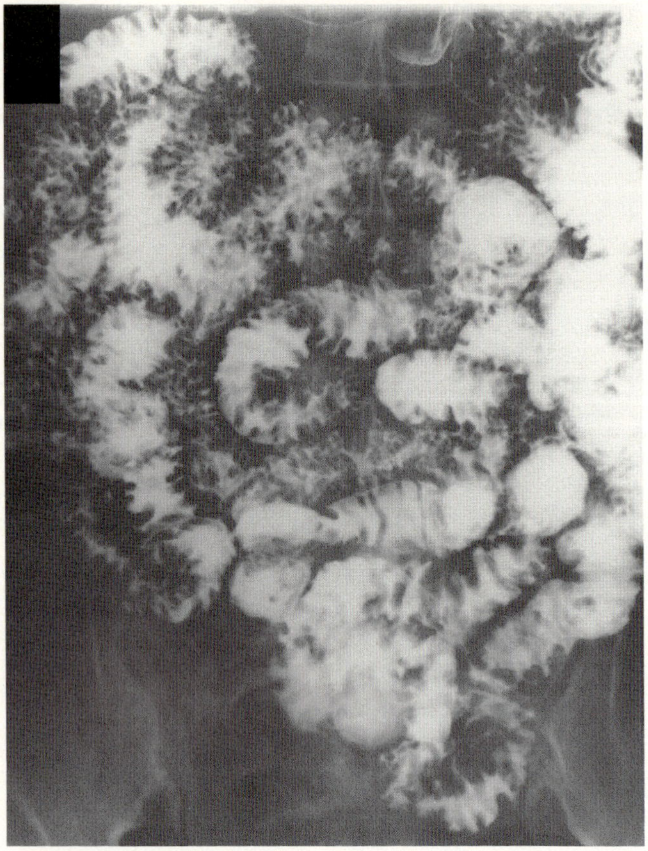

Fig. 18.21 Radiography showed widespread irregular swelling of the folds in the small intestine

18.7.2 Malignant Lymphoma: T-Cell Lymphoma (Fig. 18.21)

- Main complaints include diarrhea, abdominal pain, and general malaise, and hypoproteinemia, perforation/fistula, ileus, and abdominal tumor are frequently evident. T-cell lymphoma has also been reported as a complication of celiac disease.
- On small intestinal barium-contrast radiography, this pathology is characterized by swelling of the folds due to tumor cell infiltration, accompanied by ulceration or luminal narrowing.
- Endoscopically, although T-cell lymphoma is characteristically edematous lesions, somewhat hardened swelling of the folds, fine granular mucosa, redness, erosion, and ulceration are also present.
- Histologically, villous atrophy and intraepithelial lymphocyte infiltration are evident.
- In this case, immunostaining of small intestinal mucosa biopsy was positive for CD3, CD45RO, CD8, and bcl-2, and negative for CD4, CD20, CD56, CD79, MPO, TIA-1, κ, λ, and EMA. Serum HTLV-1 also yielded negative results.

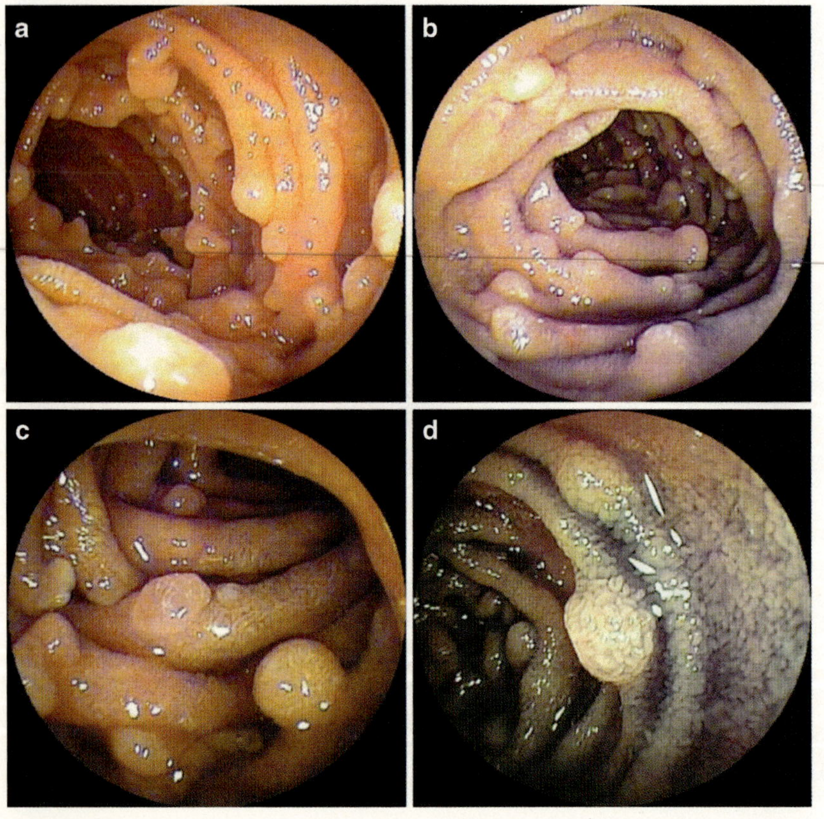

Fig. 18.22

18.8 Case 9 [8]

18.8.1 Male, 40s (Fig. 18.22a–d)

Principal complaint: Positive test for fecal occult bleeding

- DBE showed that the entire small intestine was densely packed with small, wide-based elevated lesions that were around 2–3 mm in diameter and almost the same color as the surrounding mucosa. No abnormality of the intervening mucosa was seen.
- After spraying with indigo carmine, elevated lesions were clearly demarcated (a, b).
- Indigo carmine spraying showed lesions with a variety of macroscopic forms, including some with prominent protrusions and others that were flat elevations. The lesions were covered in villous epithelium that was either similar to the surrounding normal intestinal mucosa or somewhat coarse (c, d).

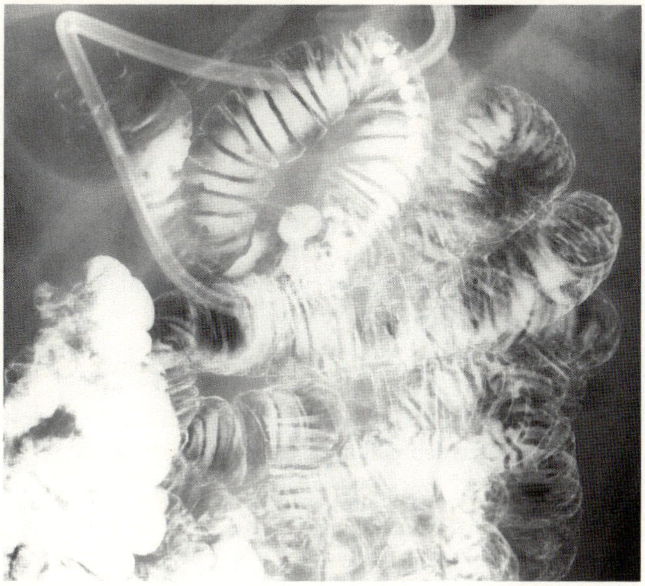

Fig. 18.23 The multiple small, well-demarcated filling defects visible in this radiographic image, mainly in the jejunum, can be interpreted as a sign of multiple lesions.

18.8.2 Cowden Disease (Figs. 18.23 and 18.24a, b)

- Cowden disease is a form of PTEN hamartoma tumor syndrome characterized by mutation of the PTEN gene and hamartoma. It is an autosomal-dominant genetic disease that causes facial trichilemmoma, cutaneous and mucosal lesions including keratotic papules on the limbs and small papules in the oral mucosa, and papilloma, as well as the simultaneous appearance of hamartoma-like hyperplasias and malignant tumors in multiple organs.
- In terms of gastrointestinal lesions, polyposis is frequently present from the esophagus to the large intestine. Esophageal polyposis in particular is a finding not encountered in other forms of polyposis. Polyposis of the small intestine occurs in around 50–60 % of cases, in the form of multiple sessile elevated lesions a few millimeters in size.
- Histopathologically, it takes the form of hyperplasia or hamartoma.
- As Cowden disease has a high risk of complication with malignant tumors of other organs such as the breast, thyroid, or uterus, careful monitoring is required.

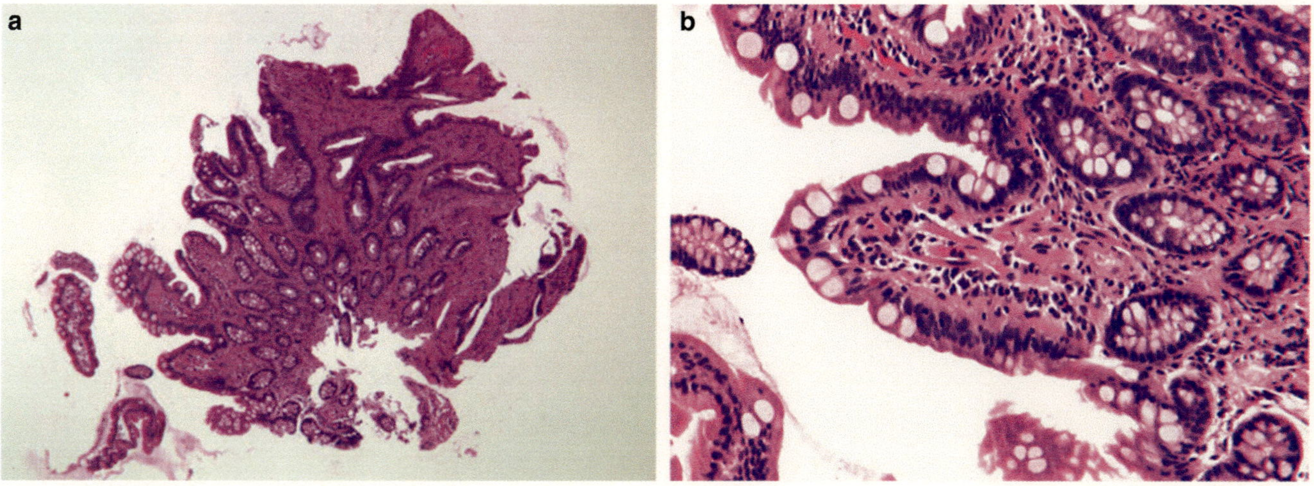

Fig. 18.24 Histopathology of a biopsy sample showed hyperplasic changes of small intestinal villous epithelium

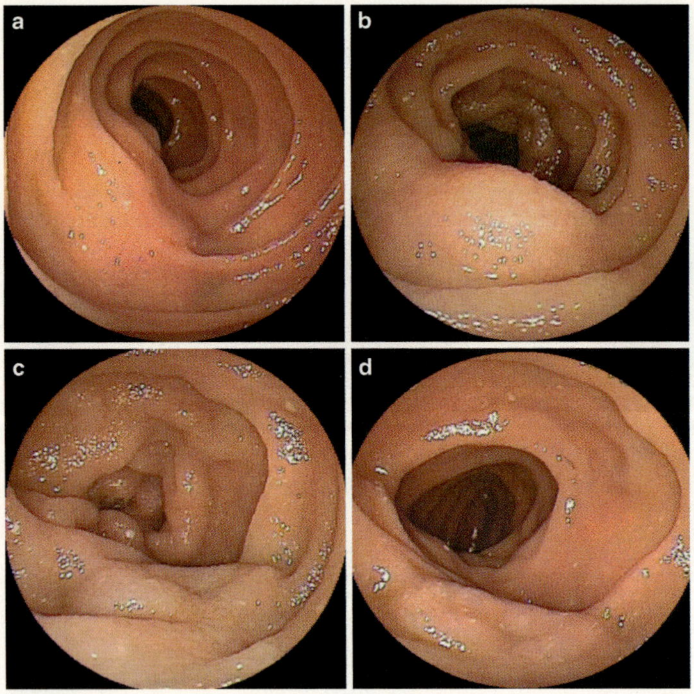

Fig. 18.25

18.9 Case 10 [9]

18.9.1 Male, 50s (Fig. 18.25a–d)

- Peritoneal tumors were identified by abdominal ultrasonography during a health checkup.
- Submucosal tumors with a comparatively gradual marginal rising appearance were evident in the jejunum (a, b).
- Submucosal elevations were also present in the same vicinity.
- A submucosal elevation with comparatively low height and depressions at the peak was apparent (c, d).

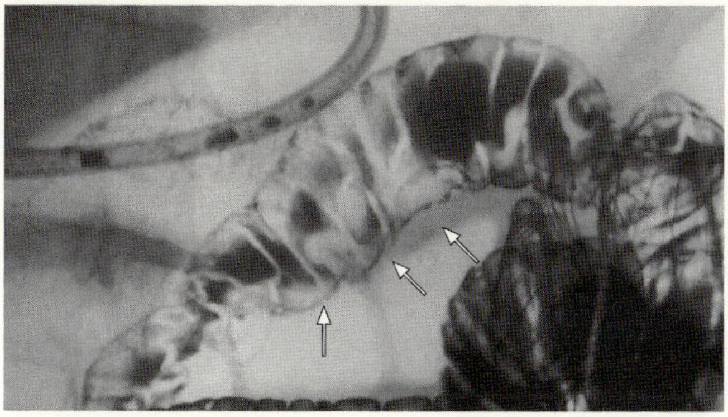

Fig. 18.26 Contrast enhancement with a small amount of air showed multiple submucosal elevations in the jejunum. The surface was comparatively smooth, with no obvious ulceration or erosion (*arrows*)

18.9.2 Recklinghausen's Disease (VRD) (Figs. 18.26, 18.27 and 18.28)

- VRD is a genetic disease that affects 30–40 people per 100,000, causing café-au-lait pigmentation and fibroma in the skin or peripheral nerves.
- Gastrointestinal tumors occur in around 25 % of cases of VRD, with GIST seen as a frequent complication.
- Endoscopically, GIST as a complication of VRD appears as a submucosal elevation in the same way as ordinary GIST, but with a tendency for multiple extraluminal growths.

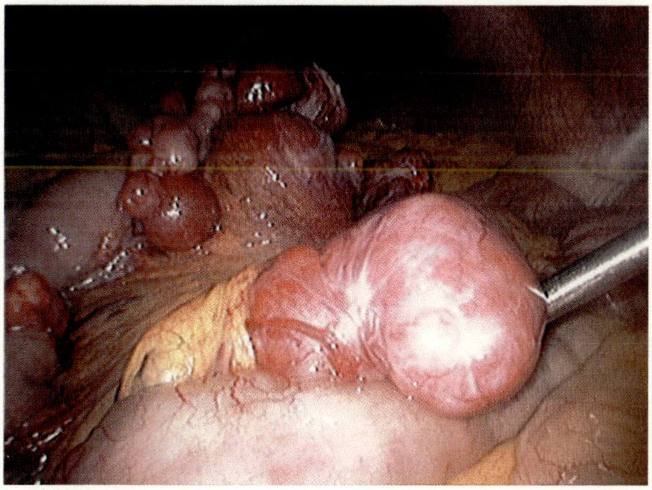

Fig. 18.27 Multiple tumors were present outside the gastrointestinal wall on the antimesenteric side of the small intestine

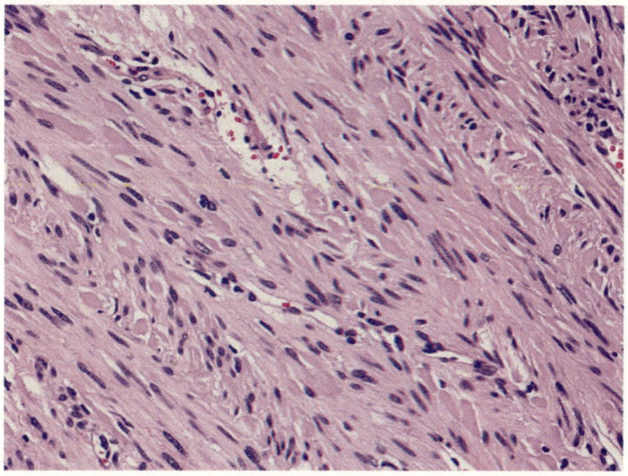

Fig. 18.28 Chromatin-rich spindle-shaped cells had proliferated in bundles

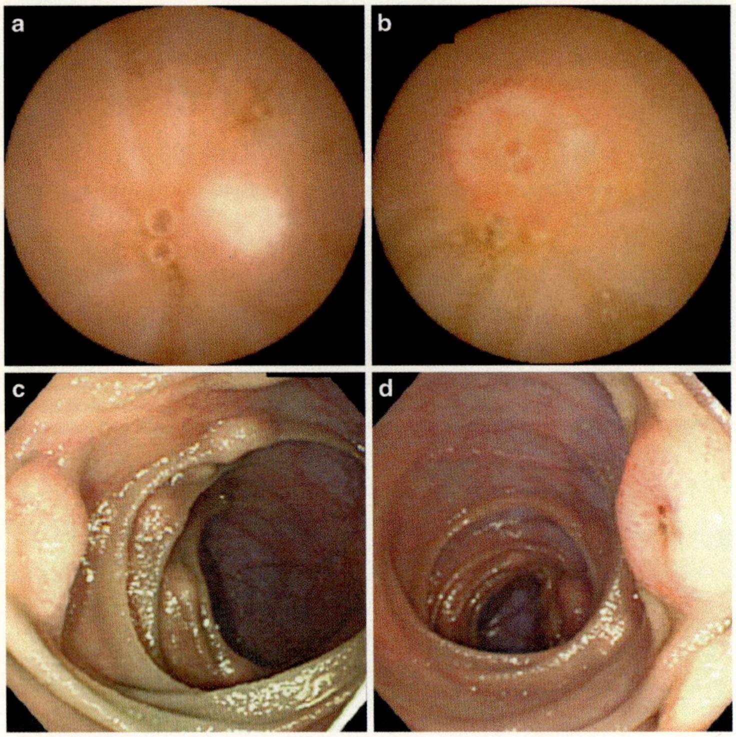

Fig. 18.29

18.10 Case 11 [10]

18.10.1 Male, 50s (Fig. 18.29a–d)

Principal complaint: Black stool, anemia

- CE revealed numerous yellowish-white submucosal elevations of varying sizes.
- In some places, reddish submucosal elevations with depressions at the peaks were also evident (a, b).

- Intraoperative endoscopy showed multiple elastic-hard submucosal elevations with a gradual marginal rising appearance (c, d).
- Protrusions were of varying sizes, with the larger lesions exhibiting indentation or erosion at the peak.

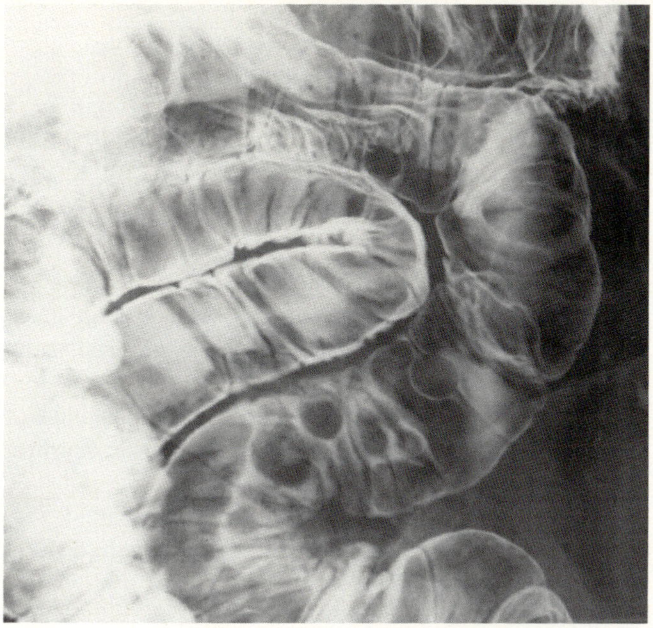

Fig. 18.30 Radiography revealed multiple oval or round filling defects in the central and lower small intestine, some of which displayed barium flecks in the center

18.10.2 Carcinoid (Figs. 18.30 and 18.31)

- Carcinoid tumors are malignant epithelial tumors derived from neuroendocrine cells, and account for 1.3–1.7 % of malignant small intestinal tumors. Venous infiltration is frequent, and the prognosis is poor.
- Although small intestinal carcinoid tumor is believed to arise multicentrically in 20–40 % of cases, cases of multiple small intestinal carcinoid tumor are rare in Japan. The number of tumors is usually less than 10.
- Endoscopically, these lesions take the form of yellowish-white submucosal elevations, some of which show an indentation or erosion at the peak. They must be differentiated from metastatic intestinal tumor and lymphoproliferative disease.

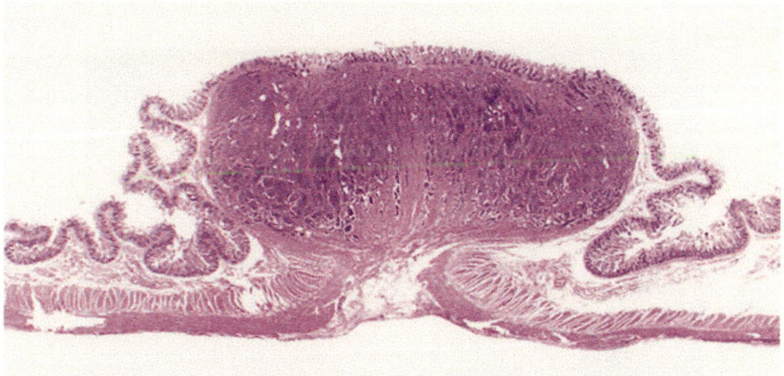

Fig. 18.31 For large-diameter tumors, cellular infiltration had reached the muscularis propria

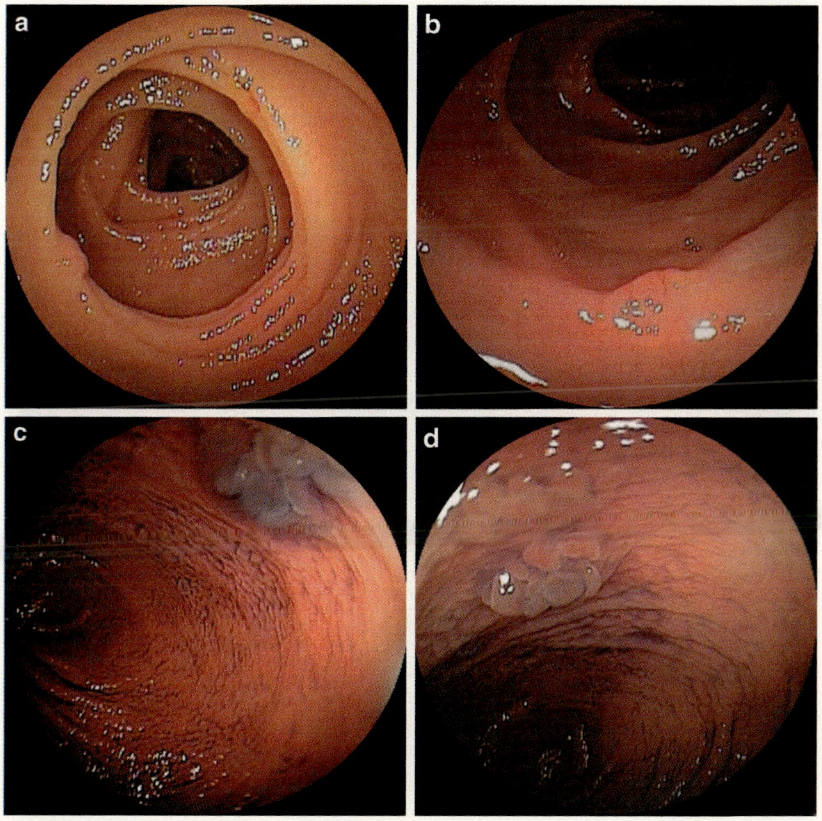

Fig. 18.32

18.11 Case 12 [11]

18.11.1 Female, 70s (Fig. 18.32a–d)

Principal complaints: diarrhea, alopecia, pigmentation of fingers

- Small, slightly reddish protrusions were evident in the jejunum (a, b).
- Dye spraying revealed that the polyps were somewhat papillary in form, with widespread granular mucosa (c, d).

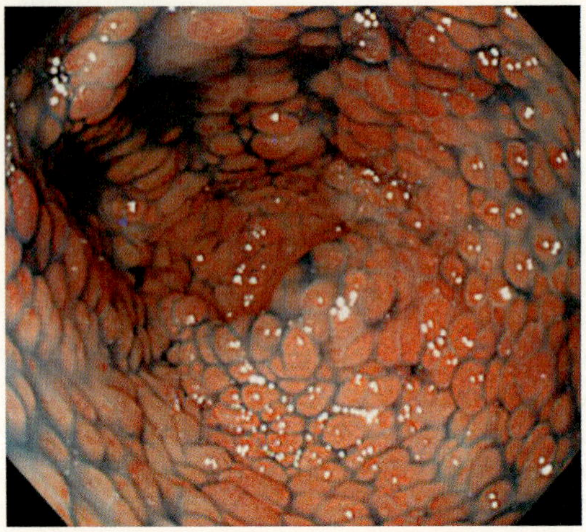

Fig. 18.33 The gastric antrum was densely packed with reddish protrusions

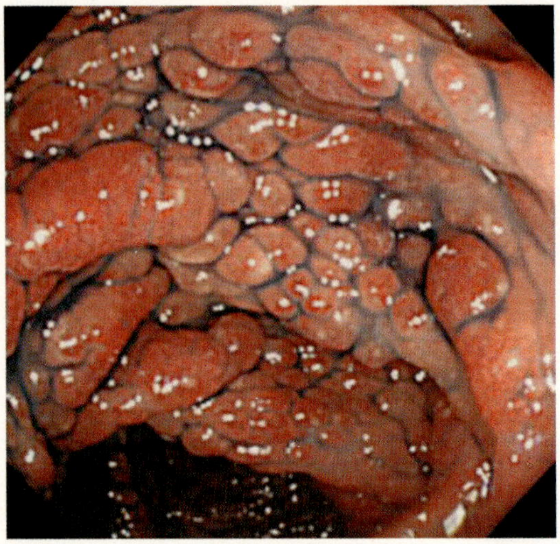

Fig. 18.34 Lesions of the large intestine. Multiple reddish protrusions with a "salmon roe" appearance were also present in the ascending colon

18.11.2 Cronkhite-Canada Syndrome (Figs. 18.33 and 18.34)

- This cryptogenic non-genetic syndrome comprises gastrointestinal polyposis together with other symptoms including alopecia, pigmentation of the skin, and atrophy of the nails.
- It is more common from middle age.
- Polyps frequently occur in the stomach and large intestine, and less commonly in the esophagus and small intestine.
- Clinical symptoms comprise alopecia, pigmentation of the skin, atrophy of the nails, taste disturbance, diarrhea, and weight loss.
- Endoscopically, it appears as numerous edematous, sessile or semi-pedunculated protrusions that may be densely or non-densely distributed.

References

1. Yoshimoto A et al. Gastrointestinal metastases from primary lung cancer. Eur J Cancer. 2006;42:3157–60.
2. Matsumoto T et al. Small-intestinal involvement in familial adenomatous polyposis: evaluation by double-balloon endoscopy and intraoperative enteroscopy. Gastrointest Endosc. 2008;68:911–9.
3. Ruys AT et al. Jejunal cancer in patients with familial adenomatous polyposis. Clin Gastroenterol Hepatol. 2010;8:731–3.
4. Ohmiya N et al. Management of small-bowel polyps in Peutz-Jeghers syndrome by using enteroclysis, double-balloon enteroscopy, and videocapsule endoscopy. Gastrointest Endosc. 2010;72:1209–16.
5. Sakamoto H et al. Nonsurgical management of small-bowel polyps in Peutz-Jeghers syndrome with extensive polypectomy by using double-balloon endoscopy. Gastrointest Endosc. 2011;74:328–33.
6. Nakamura S et al. Endoscopic features of intestinal follicular lymphoma: the value of double-balloon enteroscopy. Endoscopy. 2007; 39:E26–7.
7. Yanai S et al. Endoscopic findings of enteropathy-type T-cell lymphoma. Endoscopy. 2007;39 Suppl 1:E339–40.
8. Thomson M et al. Double balloon enteroscopy in children: diagnosis, treatment, and safety. World J Gastroenterol. 2010;16: 56–62.
9. Hirashima K et al. Multiple gastrointestinal stromal tumors in neurofibromatosis type 1: report of a case. Surg Today. 2009; 39:979–83.
10. Ramage JK et al. Guidelines for the management of gastroenteropancreatic neuroendocrine (including carcinoid) tumours (NETs). Gut. 2012;61:6–32.
11. Watanabe T et al. Cronkhite-Canada syndrome. Gastroenterology. 2008;135:e7–8.

Case Presentations: Ulcers

19

Takahiro Beppu, Masashi Yamaguchi, Shotaro Nakamura, Kozue Tsurumi, Yoichiro Ono, Mitsue Sogawa, Kenji Watanabe, Takashi Watanabe, Motohiro Esaki, Naoya Kubokura, Fumihito Hirai, Hideki Ishibashi, Satoshi Ishikawa, Tomoko Nawata, and Yoshitaka Tomioka

19.1 Case 1 [1]

19.1.1 Female, 70s (Fig. 19.1a–d)

- Presented with abdominal pain, vomiting, and ileus.
- A circumferential stenotic lesion was present in the jejunum, as a slightly discolored tumor with a gradual marginal rising appearance (a, b).
- Half of the circumference of the tumor was covered with a thin white coat, and the lumen showed extremely poor distensibility, even with a large amount of insufflation.
- Dye spraying clearly demarcated the boundary between the tumor and surrounding normal mucosa.
- Partly nodular changes were also visible at the site of stenosis (c, d).

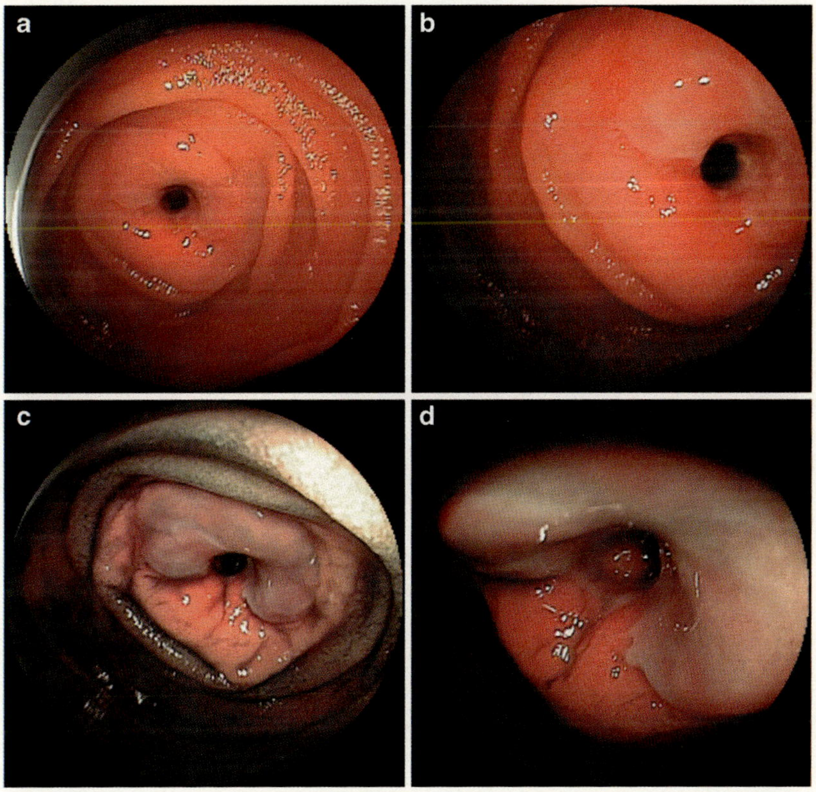

Fig. 19.1

T. Beppu (✉) • M. Yamaguchi • T. Watanabe • T. Nawata • Y. Tomioka
Department of Gastroenterology and Medicine, Fukuoka University Faculty of Medicine, 7-45-1 Nanakuma, Jonan-ku, Fukuoka 814-0180, Japan
e-mail: bouzutb@yahoo.co.jp

S. Nakamura • M. Esaki • N. Kubokura
Department of Medicine and Clinical Science, Graduate School of Medical Sciences, Kyushu University, 3-1-1 Maidashi, Higashi-ku, Fukuoka 812-8582, Japan

K. Tsurumi • Y. Ono • F. Hirai • H. Ishibashi • S. Ishikawa
Department of Gastroenterology, Fukuoka University Chikushi Hospital, 1-1-1 Zokumyoin, Chikushino 818-8502, Japan

M. Sogawa • K. Watanabe
Department of Gastroenterology, Osaka City University Graduate School of Medicine, 1-4-3 Asahi-machi, Abeno-ku, Osaka 545-8585, Japan

T. Matsui et al. (eds.), *Endoscopy in the Diagnosis of Small Intestine Diseases*, DOI 10.1007/978-4-431-54352-7_19, © Springer Japan 2014

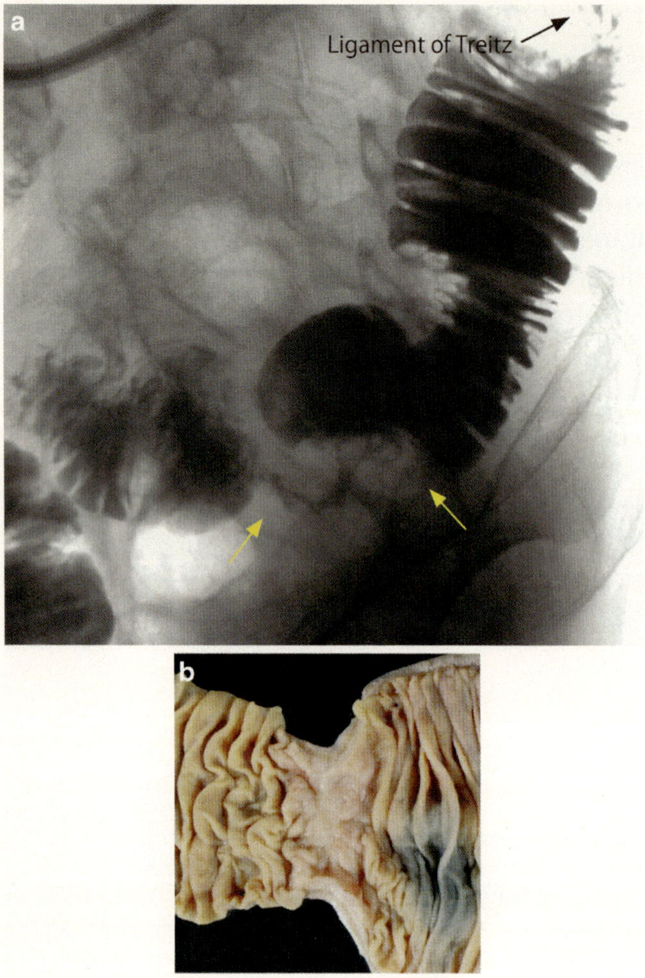

Fig. 19.2 (**a**, **b**) After fixation in formalin, a depression containing shallow ulceration was evident in the resected specimen

19.1.2 Small Intestinal Carcinoma (Primary) (Figs. 19.2a, b and 19.3)

- Primary small intestinal malignant tumors are rare, accounting for 1 % of all gastrointestinal malignant tumors. Of these, around 30 % are carcinoma. The 5-year survival rate is 30 %, and average survival is poor, at around 20 months.
- This pathology is frequently discovered due to symptoms such as abdominal pain, melena, and ileus.
- In the jejunum, it more commonly occurs within 60 cm of the ligament of Treitz (black arrow), and in the ileum around 80 % of cases occur within 60 cm of the ileocecal valve.
- On this radiographic image, a severely stenotic lesion 2 cm in length was evident in the upper jejunum, 15 cm from the ligament of Treitz (yellow arrow). Granular epithelial changes of varying sizes were evident at the margin on the proximal side. Contrast agent was pooled in the intestine on the proximal side, which was dilated. The lesion showed poor distensibility for the size of the tumor.

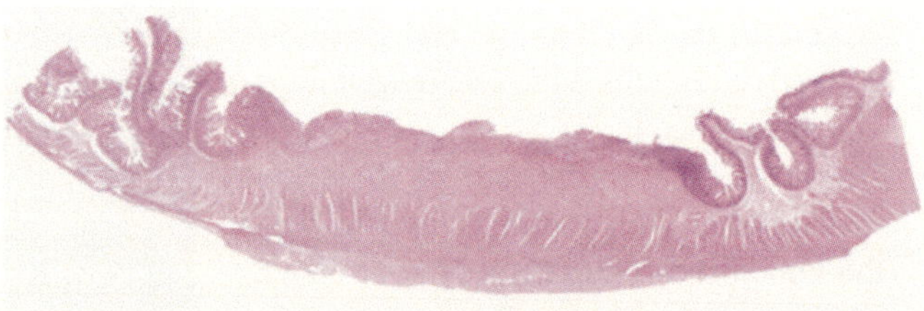

Fig. 19.3 Histopathological findings from the resected specimen showed poorly differentiated adenocarcinoma with signet-ring cells. Metastasis to regional lymph nodes was evident

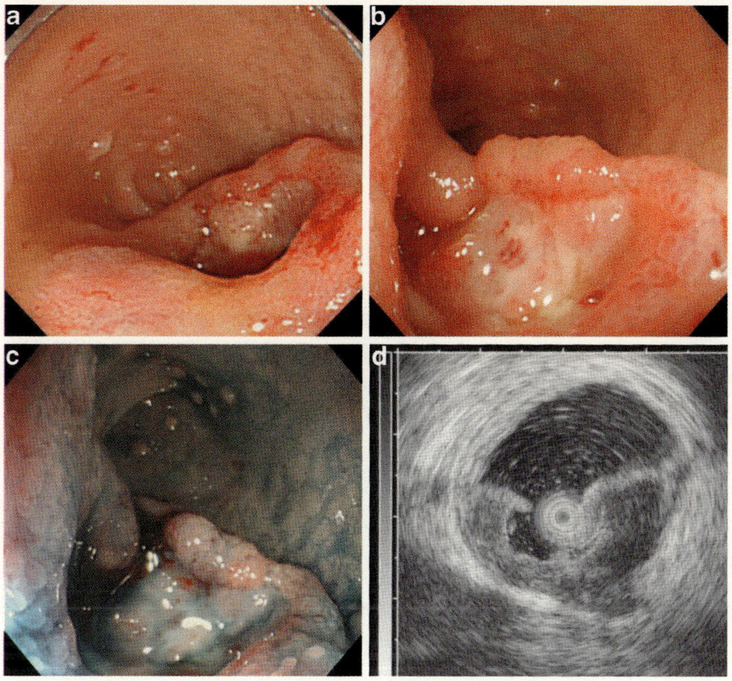

Fig. 19.4

19.2 Case 2 [2]

19.2.1 Male, 40s (Fig. 19.4a–d)

Principal complaint: Melena. Interleukin-2 receptor (IL-2R) 281 U/mL

- A submucosal elevation with an irregularly shaped ulcer deep in the central area was evident in the terminal ileum (a).
- Close-up image showing formation of deep ulcers (b).
- The lesion after dye-spraying (c).
- Ultrasound endoscopy (d). The lesion was visualized as a hypoechoic tumor extending across 2–4 layers.

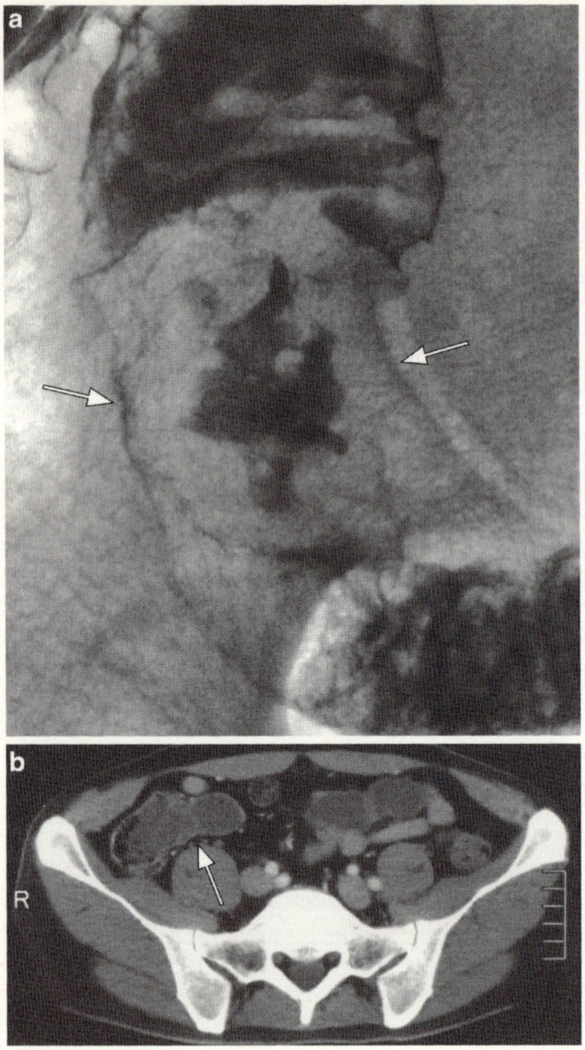

Fig. 19.5 Radiography showed formation of an irregularly shaped ulcer with a deep central area (**a**). Contrast-enhanced CT showed thickening of the ileal wall with mild dilation of the intestine on the proximal side (**b**)

19.2.2 Malignant Lymphoma: DLBCL (Figs. 19.5a, b and 19.6)

- The ulcerative type, classified as localized small intestinal malignant lymphoma, is the most common.
- Localized lesions may be difficult to differentiate from type 2 advanced carcinoma, with the presence of submucosal tumor-like findings in the protrusive portion being key to distinguishing these pathologies.
- Malignant lymphoma causes stenosis of the intestine as it progresses, and may be discovered due to intestinal obstruction. However, obstructive symptoms are not common, because malignant lymphoma is softer than carcinoma. Radiographically, the lesion does not exhibit rigidity, with little dilation of the intestine on the proximal side.

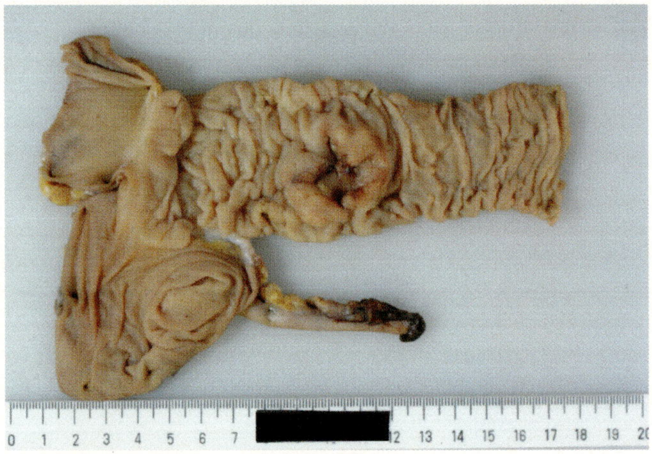

Fig. 19.6 The lesion was localized, and was treated surgically (with postoperative adjuvant chemotherapy). The specimen was fixed postoperatively. The tumor measured 30×35 mm. The lesion represented ulcerative-type DLBCL with a deep irregularly shaped ulcer in the central area

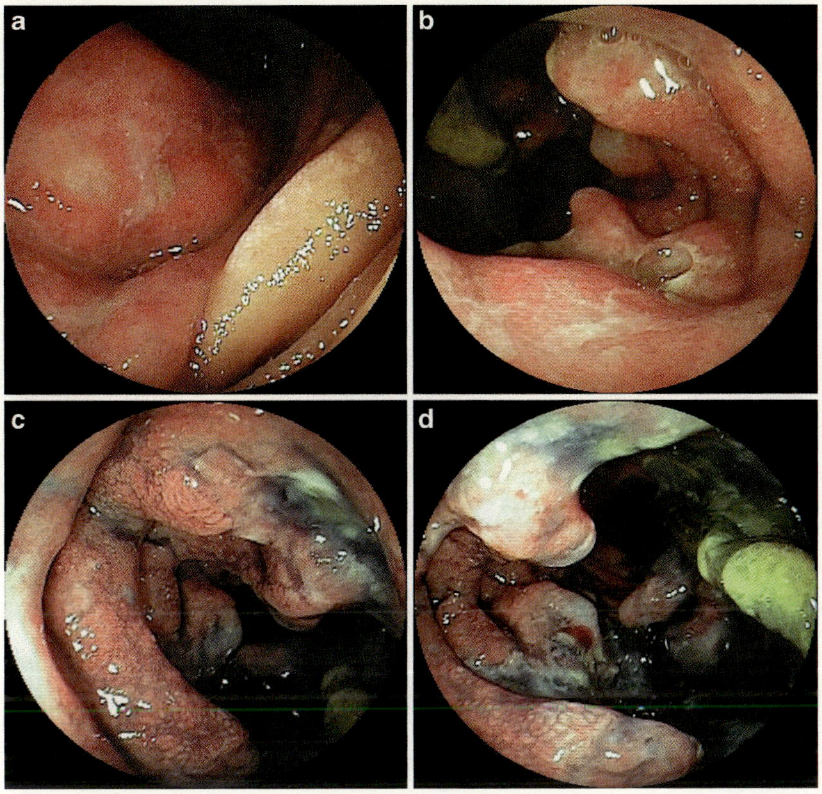

Fig. 19.7

19.3 Case 3 [3]

19.3.1 Female, 70s (Fig. 19.7a–d)

- Admitted to hospital with principal complaints of abdominal pain, weight loss, and abdominal tumor.
- Antegrade DBE revealed a circumferential ulcerative lesion that was longer in the longitudinal direction in the jejunum, with reddish swollen folds on the proximal side (a, b).
- Internally, mixed protrusions and ulcers with a submucosal tumor-like marginal rising appearance were also evident, and the lumen was comparatively wide, permitting easy passage of the scope (c, d).

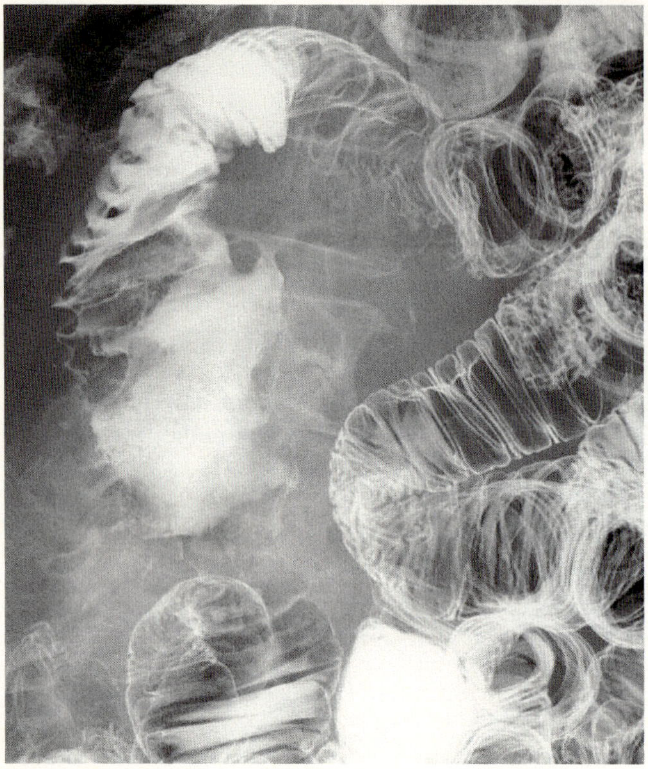

Fig. 19.8 In this case, radiography showed an aneurysmal-type tumor

19.3.2 Malignant Lymphoma: DLBCL (Figs. 19.8 and 19.9)

- DLBCL is the most frequent histological type of small intestinal malignant lymphoma.
- Macroscopically, around 60 % of small intestinal DLBCLs are of the ulcerative type.
- The ulcerative type is subcategorized as stricturing, non-stricturing, or aneurysmal on the basis of radiographic findings.
- The non-stenotic type exhibits no obvious stenosis or dilation of the intestine at the site of the lesion, whereas the aneurysmal type shows clear dilation of the intestine at the lesion site. Both are typical forms of small intestinal lymphoma.

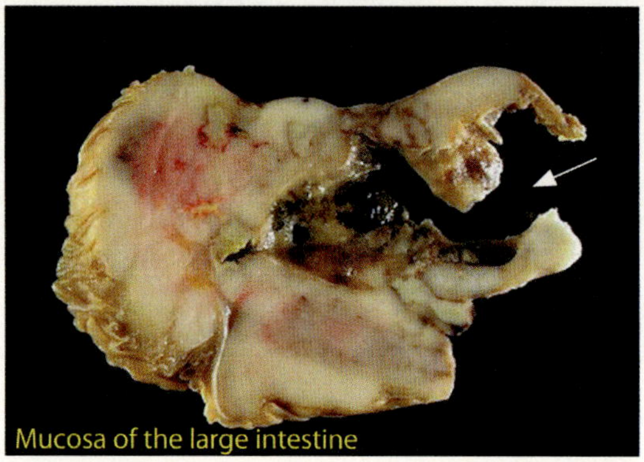

Fig. 19.9 In the resected specimen, the lumen was dilated on the small intestinal side of the tumor (*arrow*), which had infiltrated the wall of the large intestine

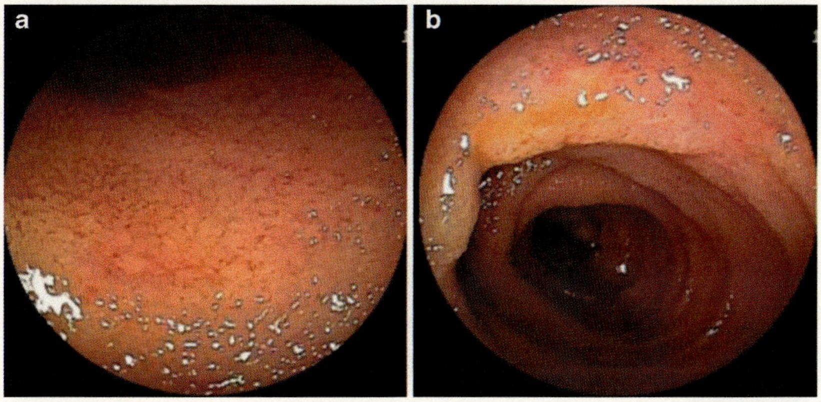

Fig. 19.10

19.4 Case 4, 5 [4]

19.4.1 Male, Teens (Fig. 19.10a, b)

Principal complaints: Lower abdominal pain, diarrhea, fever

- Scattered aphthae with a white coat and surrounded by a scarlet halo were evident.
- Circular erosion was also apparent.

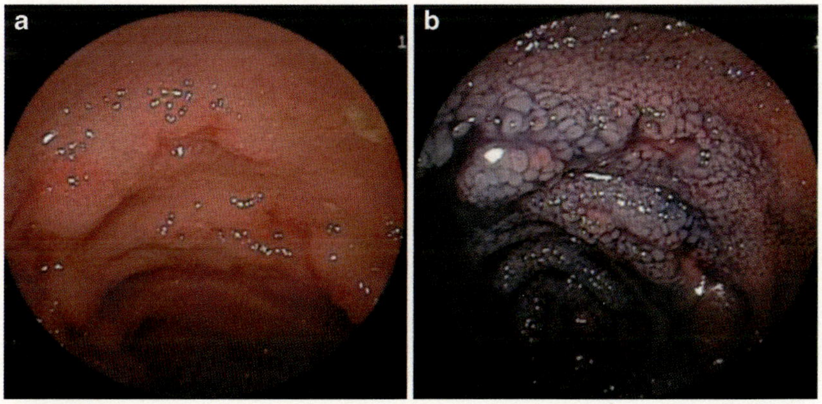

Fig. 19.11

19.4.2 Male, Teens (Fig. 19.11a, b)

Principal complaints: Sore throat, lower abdominal pain, diarrhea, fever

- Longitudinal/circular erosion was evident in the ileum.

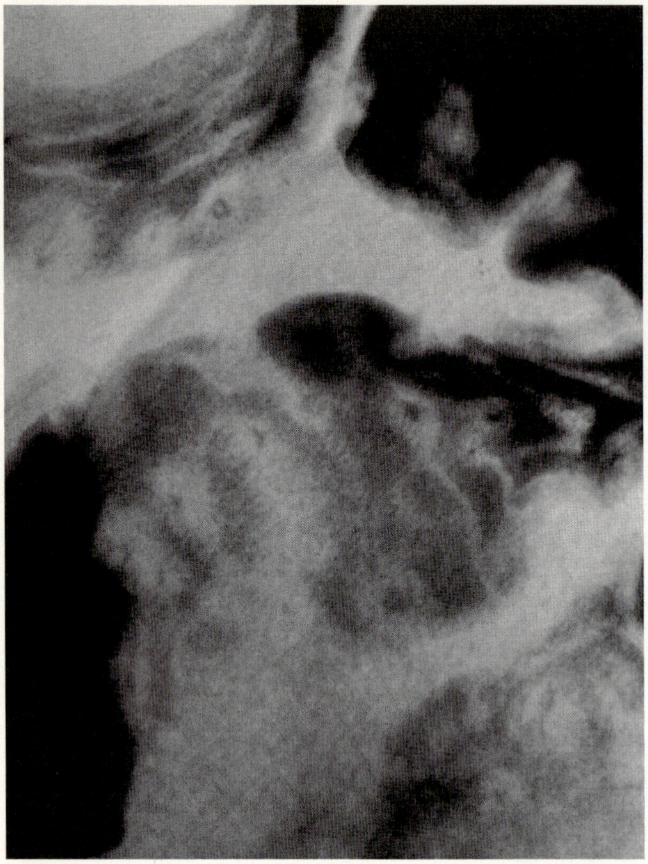

Fig. 19.12 Case 4: Endoscopy and radiography performed at around the same time revealed multiple aphthae allined longitudinally from the middle small intestine to the terminal ileum

19.4.3 Aphthous-Type Crohn's Disease (Fig. 19.12)

- The aphthous type is believed to account for around 5 % of cases of Crohn's disease.
- When only aphthous lesions are present in Crohn's disease, without the typical longitudinal ulceration or cobblestone appearance, they are regarded as constituting early-stage Crohn's disease lesions, and a biopsy test for non-caseating epithelioid cell granuloma is indispensible to the confirmation of this diagnosis.

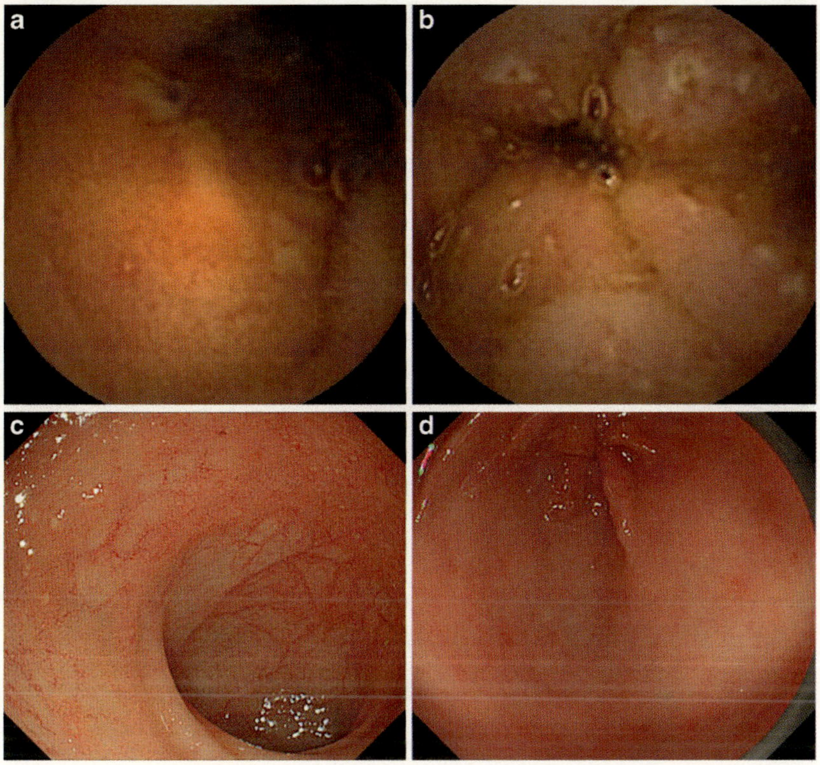

Fig. 19.13

19.5 Case 6 [5]

19.5.1 Female, Late 20s (Fig. 19.13a–d)

Principal complaints: Abdominal pain, diarrhea, melena, fever

- CE revealed aphthae and redness in the middle small intestine (a) and multiple erosions and aphthae with a white coating in the terminal ileum (b).
- Small intestinal examination by colonoscopy during the same time period showed multiple aphthae with a tendency to run longitudinally, as well as redness in the terminal ileum (c).
- Upper gastrointestinal endoscopy of the same patient during the same time period revealed multiple aphthae in the gastric antrum (d).

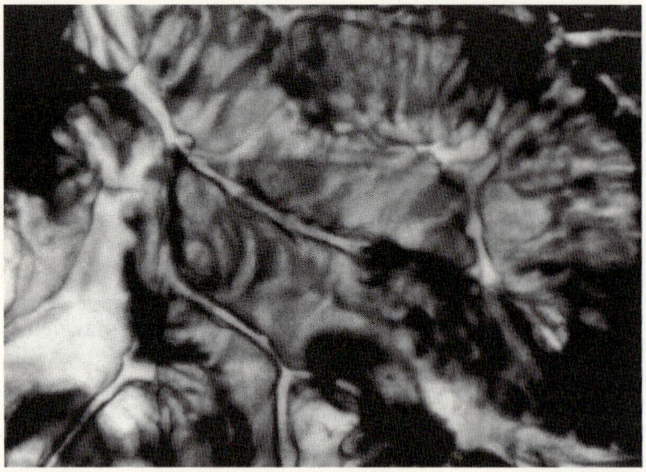

Fig. 19.14 Small intestinal radiography of a different case. Multiple aphthae were evident

19.5.2 Aphthous-Type Crohn's Disease (Figs. 19.14 and 19.15a, b)

- Non-caseating epithelioid cell granuloma may be detected not only from aphtha biopsy, but also from biopsies of upper gastrointestinal lesions or intervening normal mucosa.
- In some cases, progression to typical lesions may occur.
- Anal lesions are also frequently present.

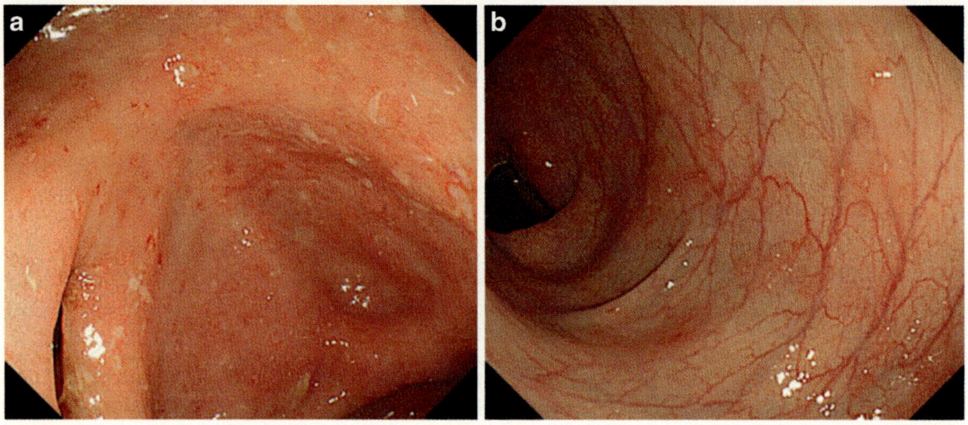

Fig. 19.15 Endoscopy of the lower region in the same case at around the same time revealed scattered aphthae skipping the entire colon, some of which tended to run longitudinally (**a**). Epithelioid cell granuloma was detected in the large intestine and confirmed the diagnosis (**b**)

19.6 Case 7, 8 [6]

19.6.1 Male, 20s (Fig. 19.16a, b)

- A comparatively wide longitudinal ulcer was evident at the mesenteric side in the ileum, surrounded by pronounced mucosal convergence.
- Ulcer margins were somewhat irregular and edematous. The ulcer bed showed a thick white coat.

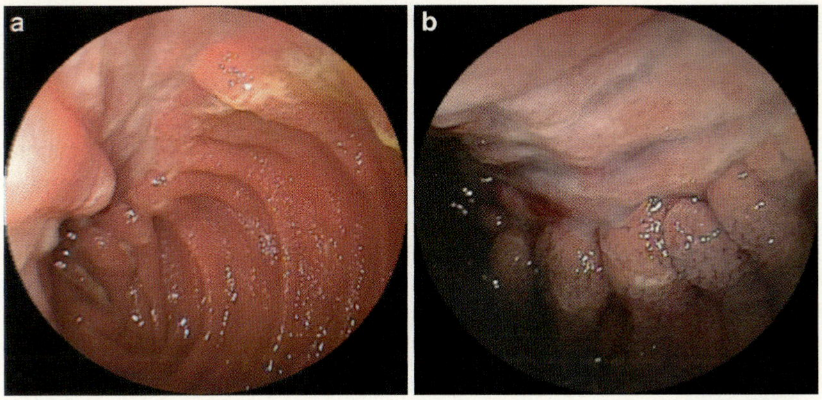

Fig. 19.16

19.6.2 Female, 50s (Fig. 19.17a, b)

- Shallow longitudinal ulceration of the ileum was evident.
- Unilateral deformity of the intestine and longitudinal ulceration with a white coating was present on the mesenteric side.

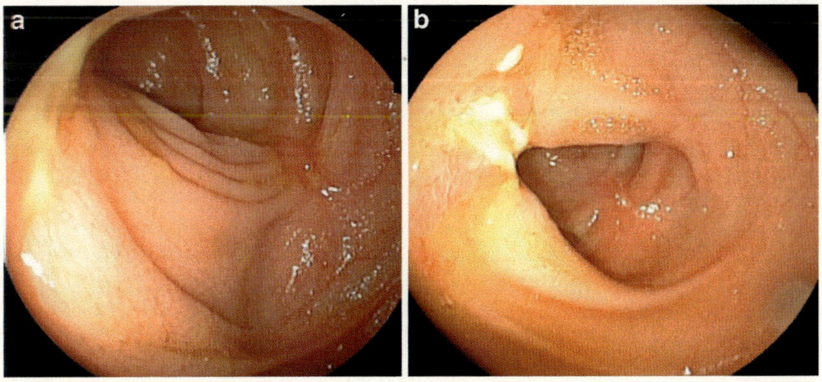

Fig. 19.17

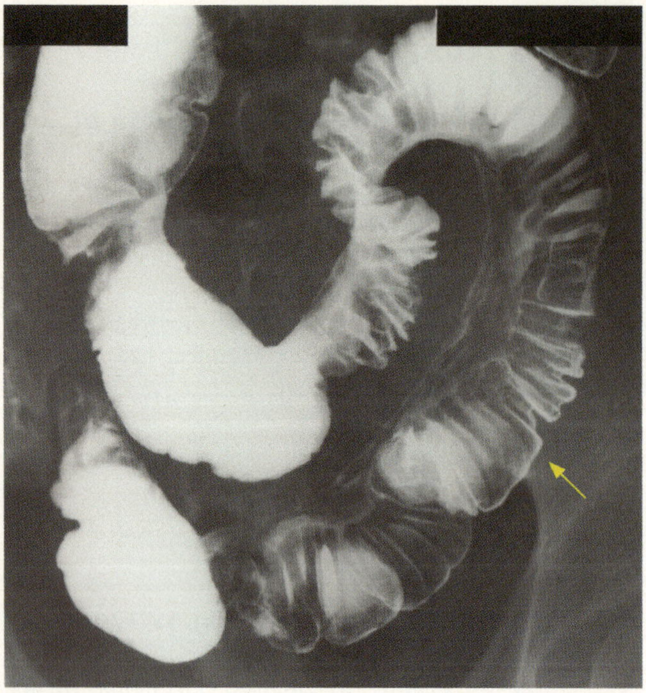

Fig. 19.18 Case 7: Radiography showed multiple longitudinal ulcers causing lateral deformation of the intestine and pronounced mucosal convergence, together with irregular open ulcers on the mesenteric side. The *arrow* indicates the site of endoscopic observation

19.6.3 Crohn's Disease (Fig. 19.18)

- Longitudinal ulcers and a cobblestone appearance form the characteristic signs of Crohn's disease.
- Active longitudinal ulcers are evident in the great majority of small intestinal lesions, and represent an important finding of Crohn's disease small intestinal lesions.
- Solitary or sporadic irregularly shaped ulcers frequently merge to become longitudinal, and are regarded as taking on a longitudinal form after healing.
- Longitudinal ulcers with a length of several centimeters along the axis of the intestine may take a variety of forms, including broad or girdle-like ulcers and narrow, linear ulcers. They occur more commonly on the mesenteric side, causing contraction of the mesentery, and thus tend to be visualized as lateral rigidity during radiography.

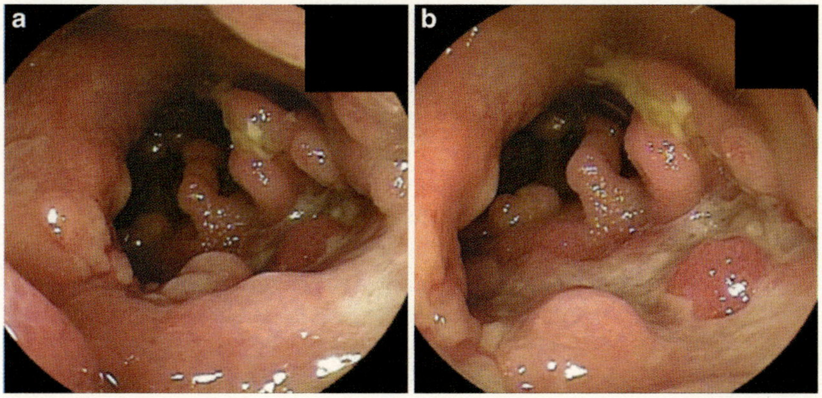

Fig. 19.19

19.7 Case 9, 10 [7]

19.7.1 Male, 50s (Fig. 19.19a, b)

- Irregularly shaped ulcer was evident in the terminal ileum, with edematous swelling of the surrounding mucosa and remaining mucosa surrounded by ulceration, producing a cobblestone-like external appearance.

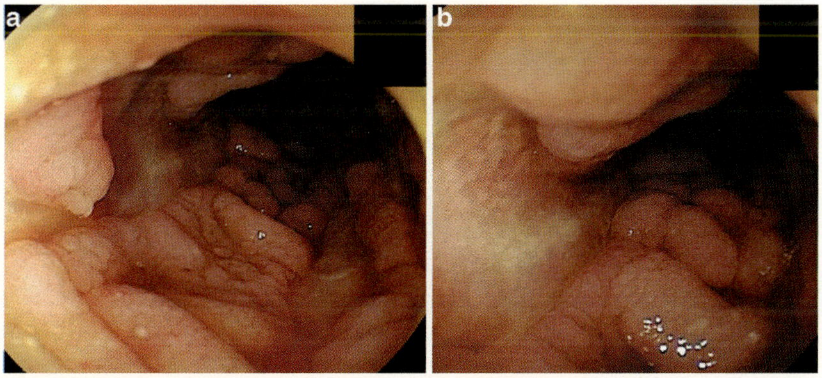

Fig. 19.20

19.7.2 Male, 60s (Fig. 19.20a, b)

- Two or three longitudinal ulcers were shown surrounded by a pronounced cobblestone appearance.

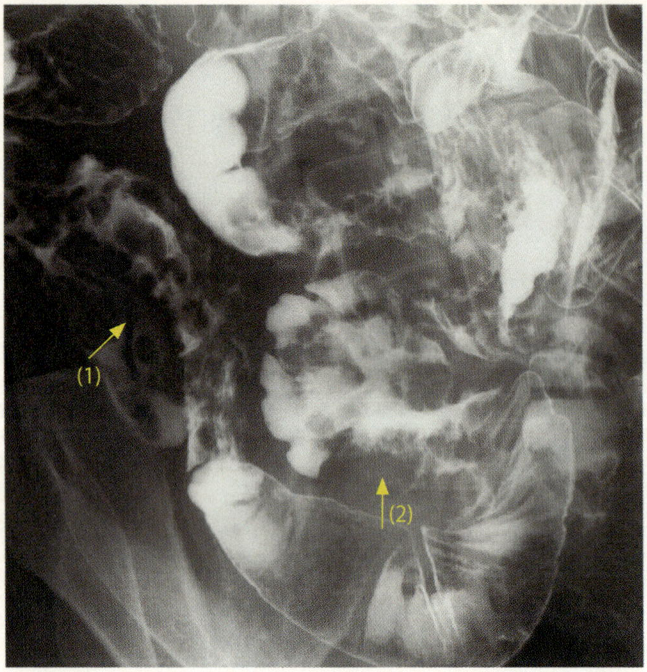

Fig. 19.21 Case 9: Radiography showed irregular barium flecks in the terminal ileum, surrounded by scattered small filling defects, forming a cobblestone appearance (*arrow 1*, site of endoscopic observation). Non-continuous deep ulcers with a cobblestone appearance were present (*arrow 2*)

19.7.3 Crohn's Disease (Fig. 19.21)

- Histologically, Crohn's disease is a chronic inflammatory disease characterized by non-caseating epithelial granuloma.
- In Japan, occurrence tends to be seen in young people aged from their late teens to their 20s, with a male:female ratio of around 2:1.
- Imaging findings comprise aphthous ulcers/lesions and irregular ulcers that become longitudinal and progress to form longitudinal ulcers and a cobblestone appearance, with complications including stenosis, fistula, and abscess.
- Cobblestone appearance ranks alongside longitudinal ulcers as a characteristic sign of Crohn's disease. This appearance results when mucosa surrounded by a mesh of ulceration forms swellings or polyps due to contraction of the muscularis mucosae, edema of the submucosa, or fibrosis or cellular infiltration.
- Cobblestone appearance is often evident in the neighborhood of longitudinal ulcers, and may be difficult to distinguish from inflammatory polyps in mild cases.

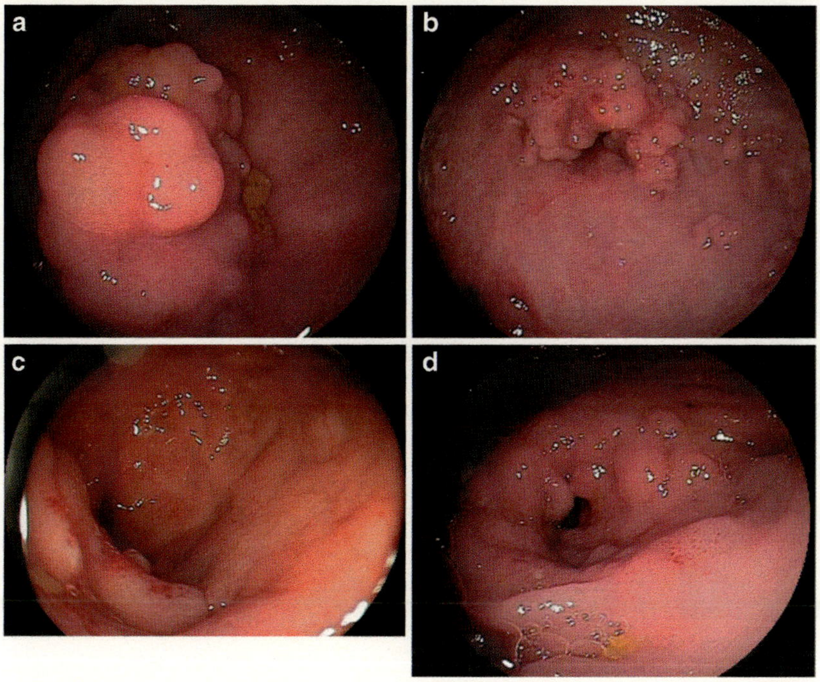

Fig. 19.22

19.8 Case 11, 12 [8]

19.8.1 Male, 40s (Fig. 19.22a–d)

- The patient had developed a refractory anal fistula 15 years earlier, and had been monitored for the previous 3 years for ileocolic Crohn's disease. As radiography showed stenosis in the neighborhood of the jejuno-ileal junction and in the lower ileum, and the patient reported an increasing sensation of abdominal distension, antegrade DBE was performed with the objective of balloon dilation.
- Stenosis associated with papillary protrusion was evident in the upper ileum, surrounded by inflammatory mucosal tags and mucosal scar (a, b).
- Tightly twisted stenosis was evident in the middle ileum. Cobblestone-like changes were evident on the proximal side of the stenosis (c, d).

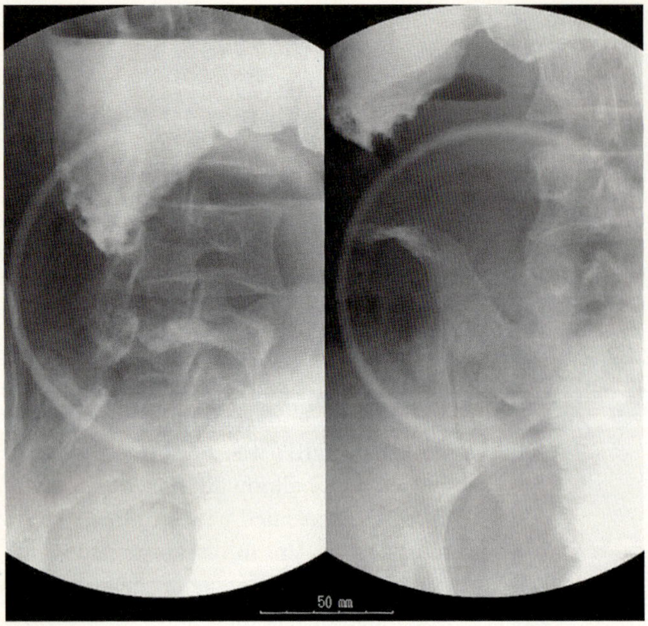

Fig. 19.23 Radiography revealed stenosis in the neighborhood of the ileo-jejunal junction. The mucosa in front of the site of stenosis was irregular, with prestenotic dilation

19.8.2 Crohn's Disease with Intestinal Carcinoma (Figs. 19.23, 19.24 and 19.25)

- Small intestinal cancer occurring together with Crohn's disease has rarely been reported in Japan.
- According to statistics from 154 cases in the United States and Europe collected by Dossett et al., this pathology occurs more often in men (male:female ratio, 2.4:1), and at a younger average age of 24.5 years compared with that of 51.3 years for sporadic small intestinal cancer, with more cases undergoing long-term monitoring.
- As detection is anatomically difficult and tumor formation is difficult to recognize as a result of intestinal deformation due to Crohn's disease, the preoperative rate of diagnosis is a low 3.1 %, compared with 35.4 % during surgery and 61.5 % after surgery.
- Prognosis is poor due to the difficulty of early detection, with low 1- and 2-year survival rates of 49.6 % and 27.0 %, respectively.

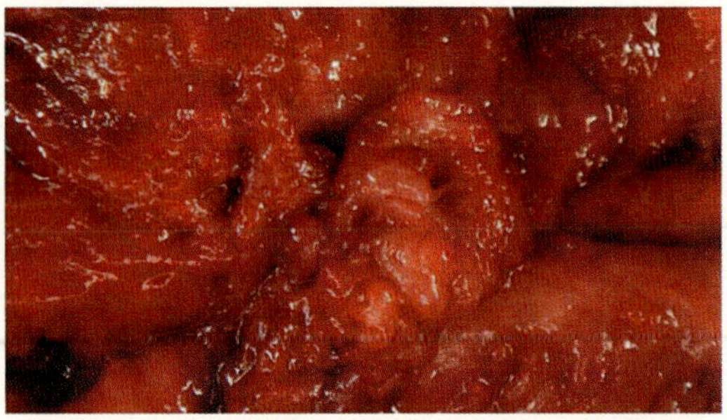

Fig. 19.24 Macroscopic image of the surgically resected specimen. Cancer and surrounding inflammatory polyps were evident

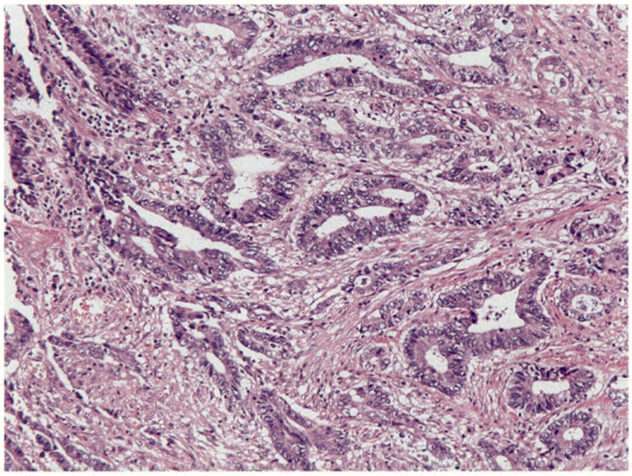

Fig. 19.25 Histopathologically, the stenotic site in the middle ileum constituted moderately differentiated adenocarcinoma (pSS), and the stenotic site in the upper ileum represented highly differentiated adenocarcinoma (pMP)

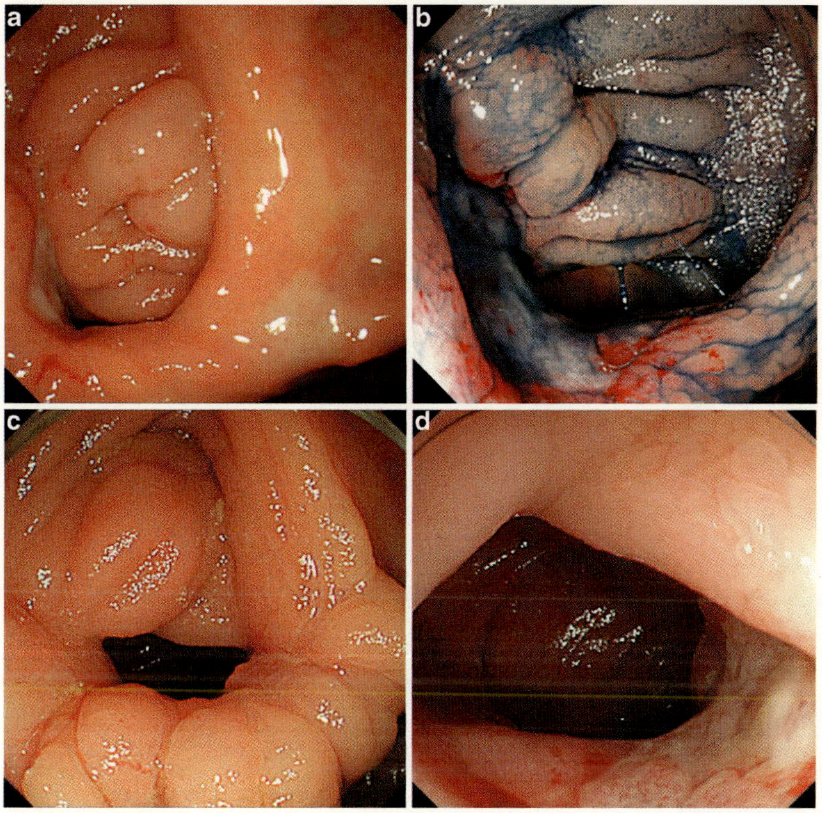

Fig. 19.26

19.9 Case 13 [9]

19.9.1 Female, 50s (Fig. 19.26a–d)

Principal complaints: Abdominal pain, bloody stool

- The ileocecal valve was dilated, with an oval or round-shaped ulcer on the valve.
- There was no irregularity of the ulcer margins (a, b).
- The intervening mucosa was normal.
- Endoscopic images were obtained 1.5 years after those shown in the top row.
- Convergence of the mucosal folds due to ulcer scarring was evident on the ileocecal valve, which was narrowed (c, d).
- The scope was able to pass through.
- Geographic ulcers were present in the deeper area.
- Ulcer borders were clearly demarcated.
- The intervening mucosa was normal.

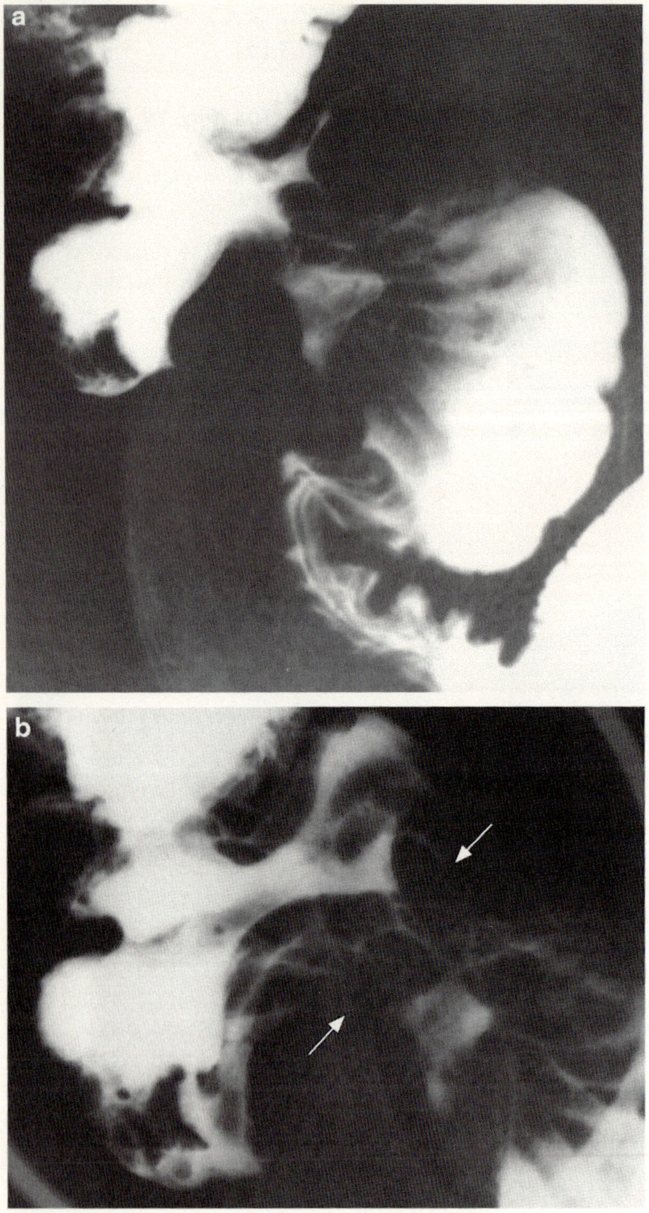

Fig. 19.27 (a) Radiography (at the same period as Fig. 19.26 c, d) showed clearly demarcated pools of barium and convergence of intestinal folds in the ileocecal area. (b) Radiography (Fig. 19.26 c, d) revealed narrowing of the ileocecal area due to ulcer scarring

19.9.2 Behçet Disease (Fig. 19.27a, b)

- Gastrointestinal lesions, most commonly ileocecal ulcers, are listed as accessory lesions in the diagnostic criteria for intestinal Behçet disease. They typically constitute deep ulcers covered with a thick white coat with clear margins in the ileocecal area.
- The patient shown here exhibited ileocecal ulcers, oral aphthae, genital ulcers, and arthritis, and was diagnosed with incomplete Behçet disease.

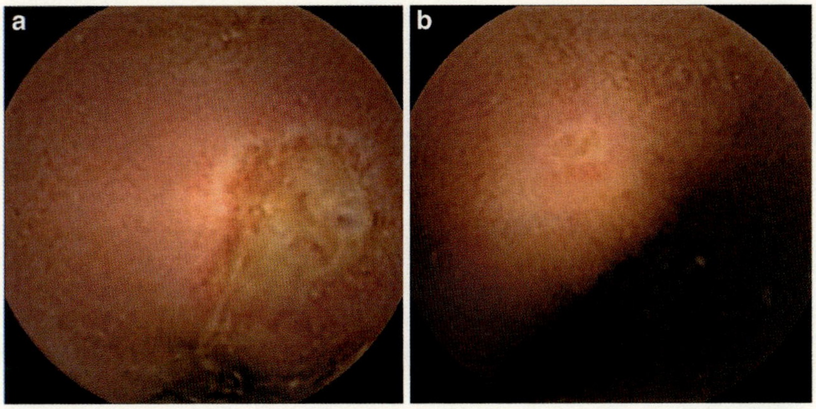

Fig. 19.28

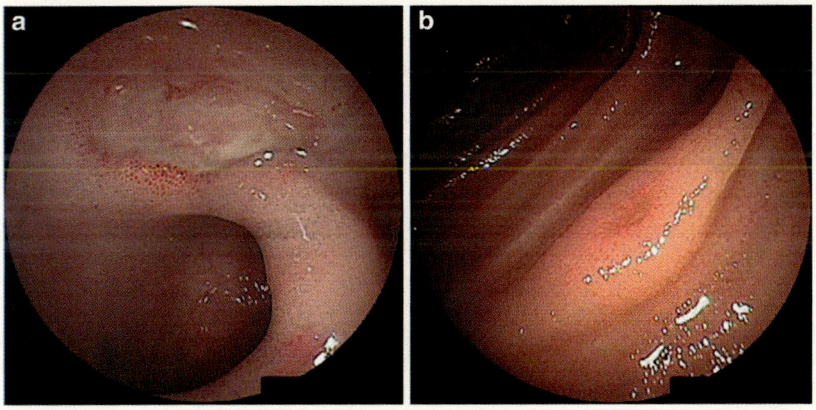

Fig. 19.29

19.10 Case 14 [10]

19.10.1 Male, 70s (Fig. 19.28a, b)

- Principal complaints were fever ≥38°C, recurrent oral aphthae, and pain in both knees.
- Colonoscopy showed a large open ulcer on the lip of the ileocecal valve and scattered small ulcers in the terminal ileum.
- CE showed multiple oval or round ulcerative lesions, and erosions with halo in the ileum.

19.10.2 Male, 60s (Fig. 19.29a, b)

- The principal complaint was repeated gastrointestinal bleeding. The patient also had a history of recurrent oral aphthous ulcers and genital ulcers.
- Retrograde DBE showed multiple erosive and ulcerative lesions extending throughout almost the entire region from the middle to lower small intestine.
- Ulcer scarring was also observed, suggesting a chronic/recurrent course.

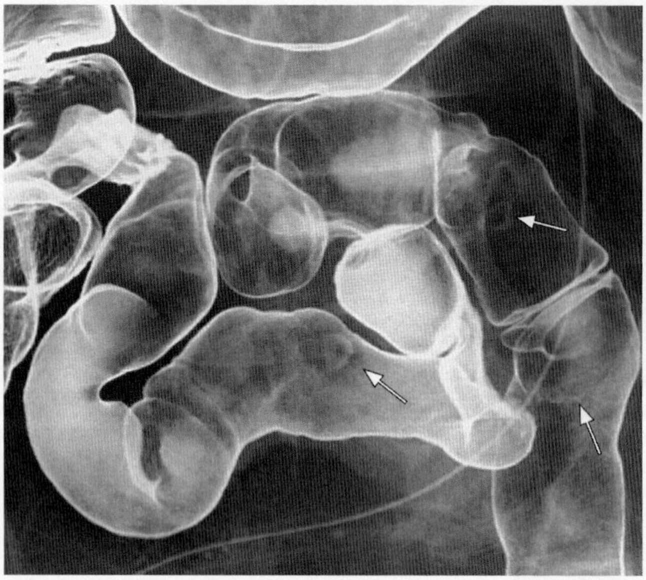

Fig. 19.30 Radiography revealed sharply demarcated barium flecks with filling defects at the borders in the terminal ileum (*arrows*)

19.10.3 Behçet's Disease (Fig. 19.30)

- Behçet's disease is a disorder characterized by repeated and protracted inflammatory lesions of the oral mucosa, skin, eyes, and genital area.
- The prevalence of intestinal lesions in this disorder is around 1 %.
- Gastrointestinal lesions in Behçet's disease may occur in any part of the gastrointestinal tract from the esophagus to the anus. However, in around 70 % of cases, punched-out like ulcers form in the ileocecal area; these are considered to represent typical lesions.
- Aphthae, erosions, small ulcers, and other lesions occurring outside the ileocecal area are known as atypical lesions. They mainly occur on the antimesenteric side, but with no obvious longitudinal pattern.

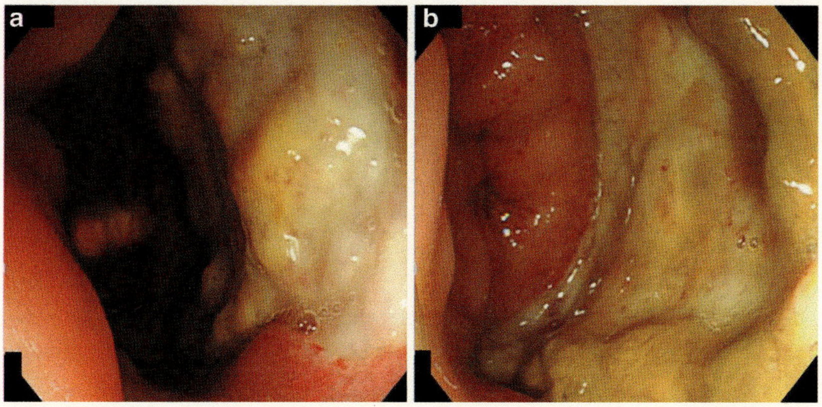

Fig. 19.31

19.11 Case 15, 16 [11]

19.11.1 Male, 30s (Fig. 19.31a, b)

- The principal complaint was abdominal pain and fever persisting for about 3 months.
- Although repeated oral aphthae were present, no ophthalmologic, cutaneous, or joint symptoms or genital ulcers were identified.
- Colonoscopy revealed a large, deep ulcer covered in a thick, dirty white coat in the terminal ileum.
- Ulcer margins were clearly demarcated.

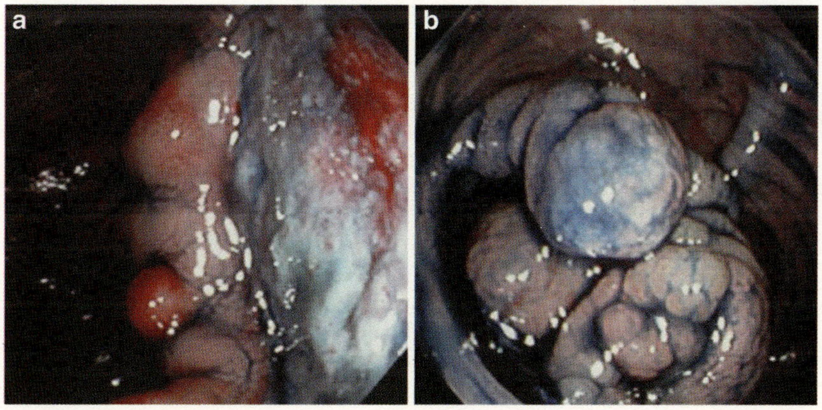

Fig. 19.32

19.11.2 Male, 60s (Fig. 19.32a, b)

- The principal complaint was abdominal pain persisting for about 6 months.
- No symptoms of Behçet disease were evident.
- Colonoscopy revealed an undermining ulcer covered with a thick white coat in the terminal ileum, with protruding surroundings (a).
- The ileocecal valve was enlarged and deformed (b).

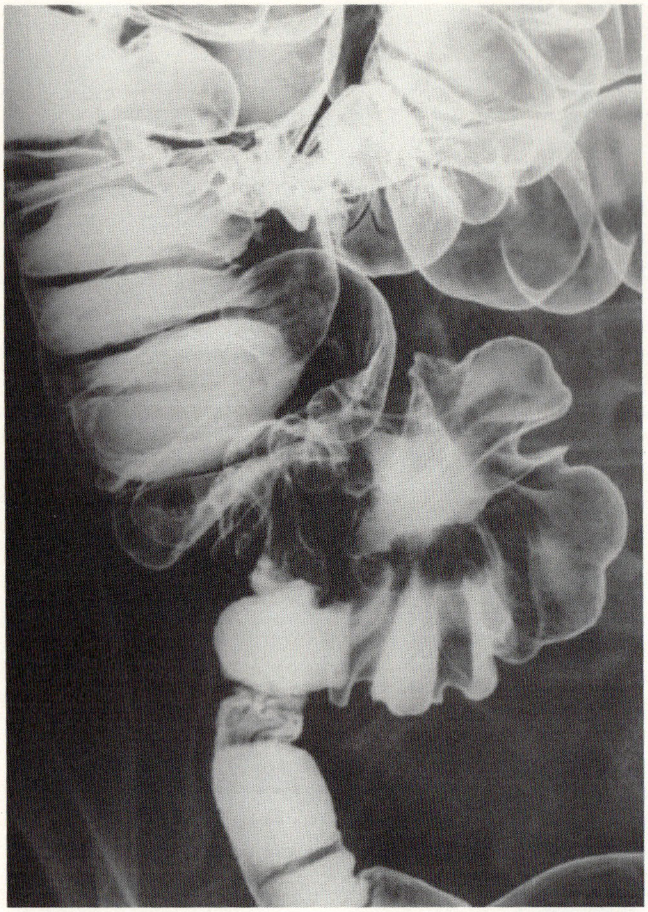

Fig. 19.33 Radiography showed a deep barium fleck in the terminal ileum. The borders of the ulcer were clearly demarcated, and surrounding enlarged mucosal folds were evident

19.11.3 Simple Ulcers (Fig. 19.33)

- Round or egg-shaped punched-out like refractory ulcers very similar to the typical lesions of intestinal Behçet disease that are present in the ileocecal area are called simple ulcers if any suspicion remains that they may not meet the diagnostic criteria for Behçet disease.
- The differences between simple ulcers and Behçet's disease remain unclear.
- Ulcers tend to be undermining, and histologically comprise Ul-IV ulcers with chronic active nonspecific inflammatory findings.
- They are visualized radiographically as deep, clearly demarcated barium flecks surrounded by mound-like filling defects.
- Endoscopically, they appear as clearly demarcated ulcers covered with a thick white coat, with nodular protrusions surrounding large lesions. Even if multiple ulcers are present, the intervening mucosa is normal.

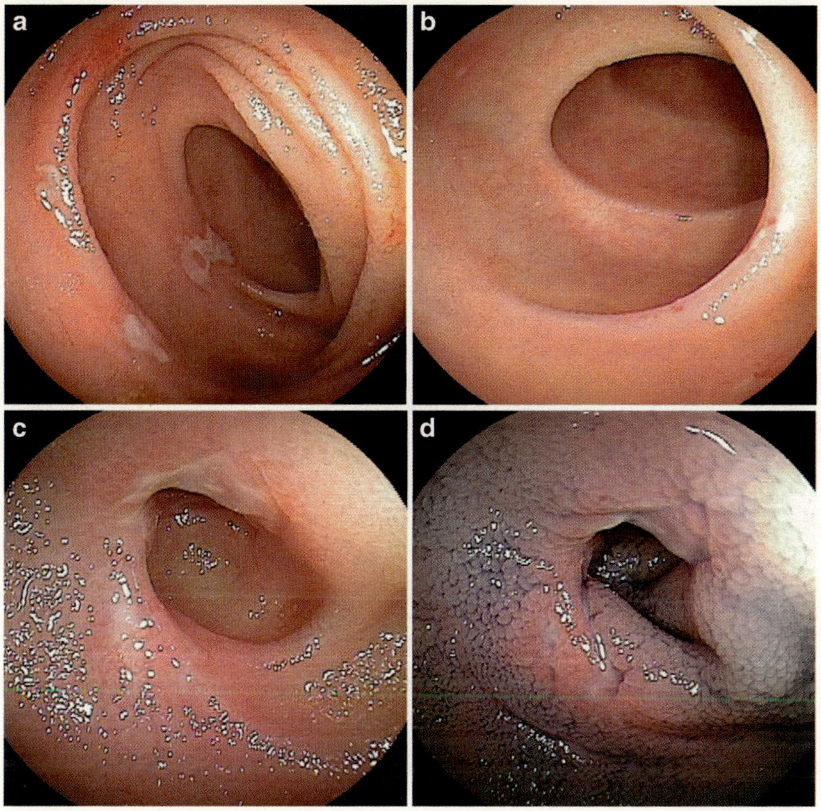

Fig. 19.34

19.12 Case 17 [12]

19.12.1 Female, 50s (Fig. 19.34a–d)

- The patient had previously undergone two partial resections of the small intestine for intestinal obstruction.
- Iron-deficiency anemia persisted after surgery, and the patient was monitored by endoscopy.
- Abnormal course of Kerckring's folds and shallow ulcers were evident (a), as was an oblique line of ulcer scarring (b).
- Endoscopy at the site of stenosis. In this disease, sites of stenosis often exhibit a spiral form, frequently showing shallow ulcers running in a circumferential or oblique direction to the intestinal axis (c, d).

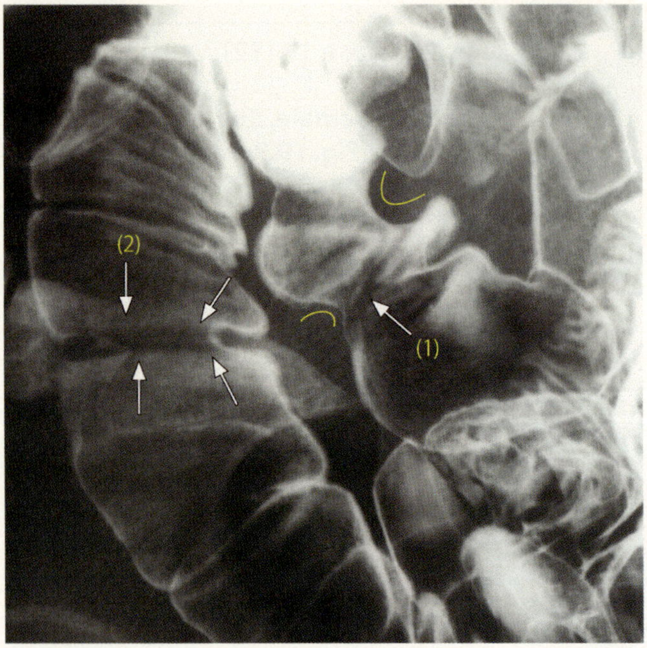

Fig. 19.35 Indentations in the ileum were evident, with the intestine asymmetrically deformed. A shallow, linear ulcer was present in the area of the deformity (*arrow 1*). A shallow, linear ulcer running obliquely to the axis of the intestine was also visualized (*arrows 2*). Both are characteristic radiological signs of this condition

19.12.2 Chronic Non-specific Multiple Ulcers of the Small Intestine (Fig. 19.35)

- This disease concept was first described in the late 1960s by Japanese doctors Okabe and Sakimura.
- This condition mainly affects young people. Clinically, the main symptoms are long-term occult or overt bleeding and severe persistent anemia, with hypoproteinemia, growth retardation, and varying degrees of abdominal pain.
- The cause remains unknown, although a genetic component has been suggested.
- Morphologically, the pathology appears as multiple ulcerative lesions in a comparatively narrow region of the ileum (excluding the terminal ileum), causing varying degrees of deformation and stenosis.
- The characteristic ulcer morphology is that of narrow tape-shaped ulcers running in a circumferential or oblique fashion. Histopathologically, they comprise shallow Ul-I or II ulcers that are clearly demarcated from their surroundings.
- This condition possesses defined sets of clinical and histopathological characteristics, and care must be taken not to mistakenly allocate small intestinal ulcers without a confirmed diagnosis to this disorder.
- Response to nutritional and other therapies is seen with improvement of ulcers, but the condition is refractory over the long term, and surgery is frequently required to treat stenosis.

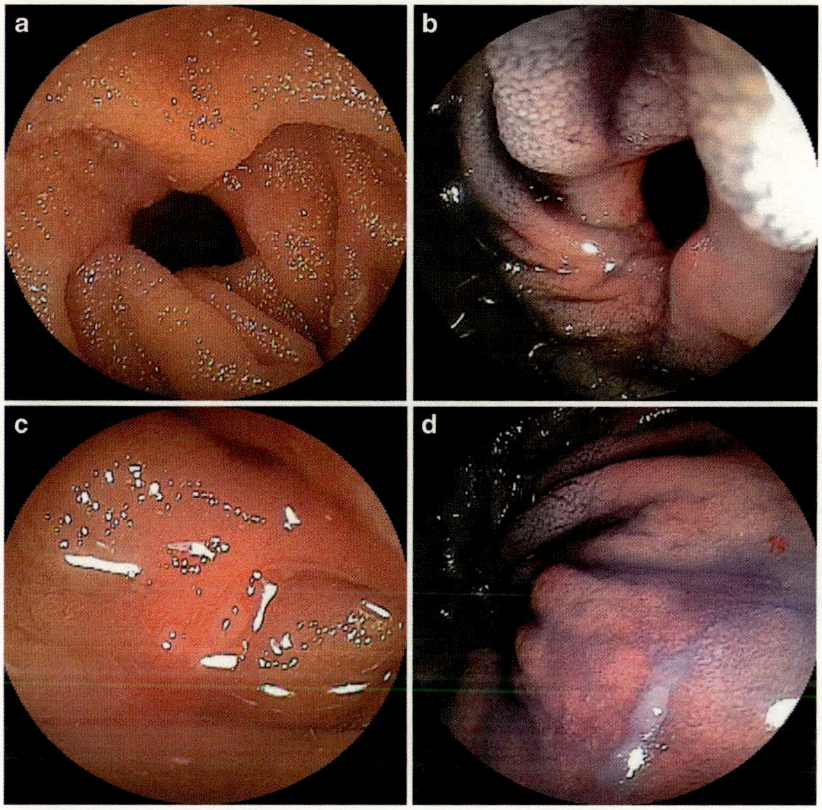

Fig. 19.36

19.13 Case 18 [13]

19.13.1 Male, 60s (Fig. 19.36a–d)

- The patient had a history of small intestinal resection for intestinal obstruction.
- Although symptoms resolved after surgery, testing for fecal occult blood yielded positive results every year.
- As shown on the left, moderate stenosis was seen in the anastomotic area, although the patient remained asymptomatic (a, b).
- Endoscopic view of the distal side of the site of stenosis. Small ulcers and erosions were present (c, d).

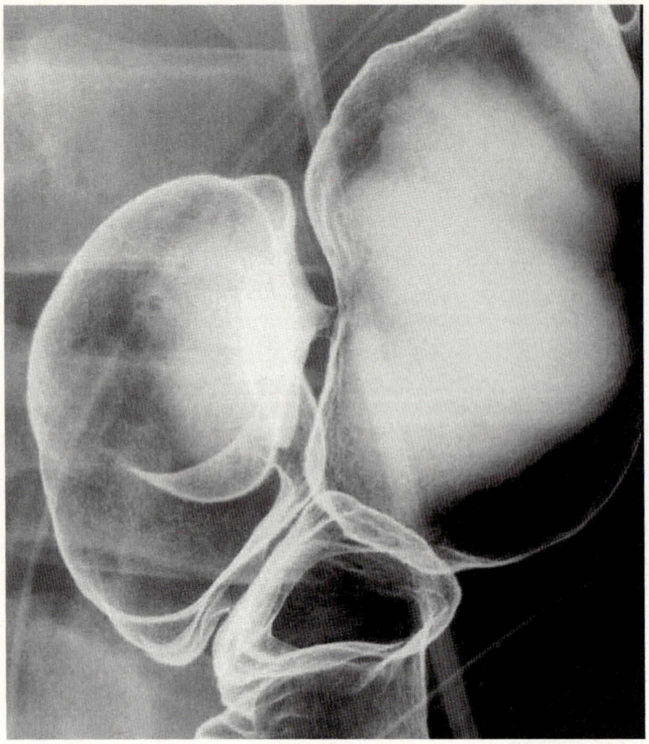

Fig. 19.37 Radiographic findings of the site of stenosis revealed by endoscopy. EBD was performed at a later date, after the endoscope was unable to be passed through. After EBD, the endoscope did pass through, enabling endoscopic observation of the proximal side

19.13.2 Chronic Non-specific Multiple Ulcers of the Small Intestine (Figs. 19.37 and 19.38a, b)

- This condition causes multiple stenoses, and intestinal resection is frequently required as a result. Stenosis also tends to occur at the site of anastomosis.
- Endoscopic balloon dilation (EBD) by DBE is effective for avoiding frequent surgery.
- In this condition, ulcers are shallow, and the fistula formation and transfer of inflammation outside the intestine seen in conditions such as Crohn's disease do not occur. This makes the pathology a good candidate for EBD.

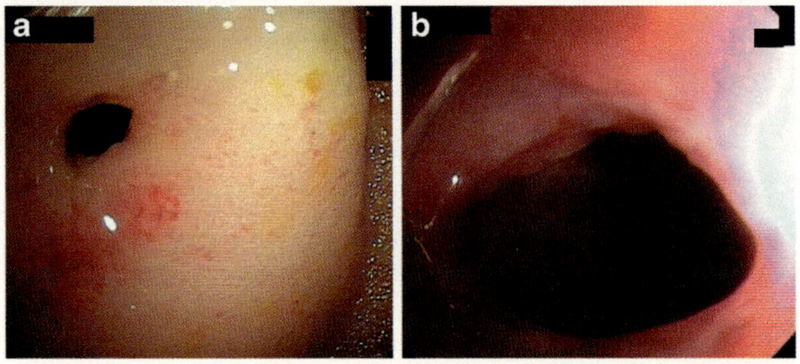

Fig. 19.38 (**a**, **b**) Endoscopic views before and after EBD (different patient to the image on the left). A 12- to 15-mm TTS balloon was dilated to relieve severe stenosis at the anastomosis site. After EBD, the scope was able to be passed through the site of stenosis to the proximal side. Surgery was thus avoided for the long-term future

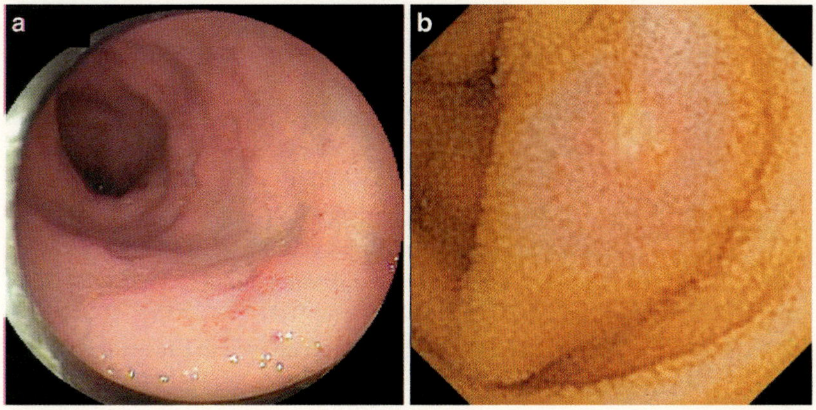

Fig. 19.39

19.14 Case 19, 20 [13]

19.14.1 Female, 70s (Fig. 19.39a, b)

Principal complaint: Melena. The patient was taking loxoprofen for elbow pain.

- Retrograde DBE revealed small, irregularly distributed ulcers in the ileum.
- CE showed aphthae in the ileum.

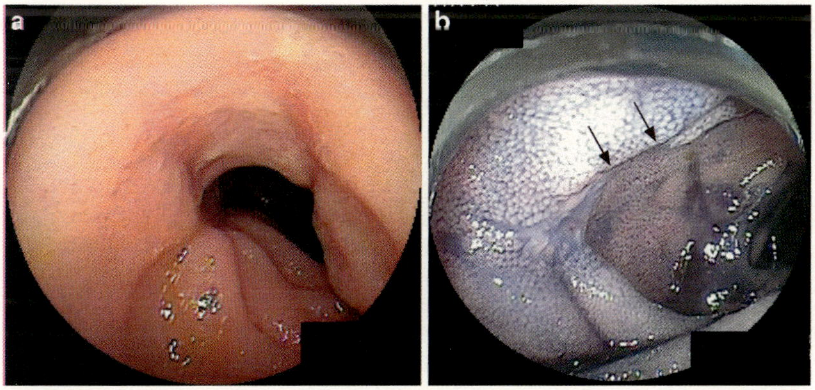

Fig. 19.40

19.14.2 Female, 70s (Fig. 19.40a, b)

Principal complaint: Tarry stools. The patient was taking lornoxicam for mandibular osteomyelitis.

- Retrograde DBE revealed a shallow open oval or round-shaped ulcer with fold convergence in the ileum (a). The irregularly shaped ulcers on the distal side (b) included partial linear outgrowth on the top of the fold (arrows).

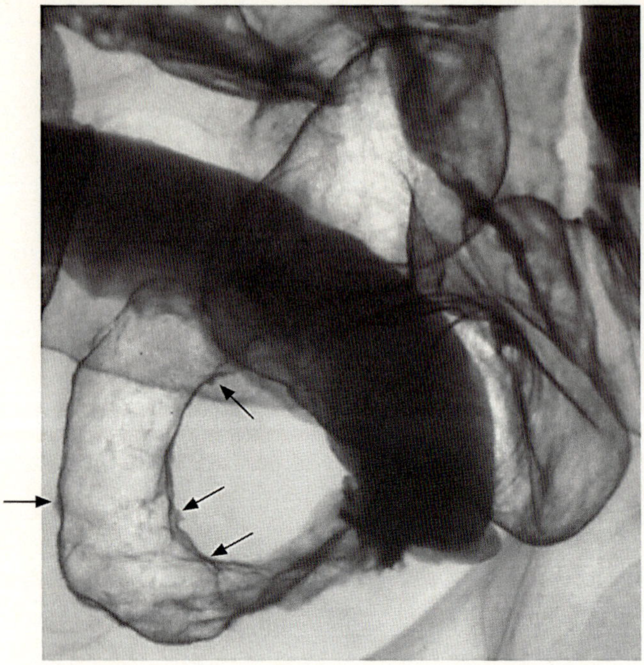

Fig. 19.41 Case 19: Radiography undertaken during the same period as endoscopy revealed numerous small barium flecks (*arrows*) in the ileum

19.14.3 NSAID-Induced Enteropathy (Fig. 19.41)

- In NSAID-induced enteropathy, lesions may take on diverse forms, including round, geographical, irregular, circular, longitudinal, or oblique ulcers.
- Small lesions characteristically comprise irregularly distributed aphthous lesions of varying sizes and small ulcers.
- Lesion distribution is considered unrelated to the position of the mesentery.
- Long-term use of NSAIDs is believed to cause diaphragm-like stenosis when a circular ulcer becomes scarred.

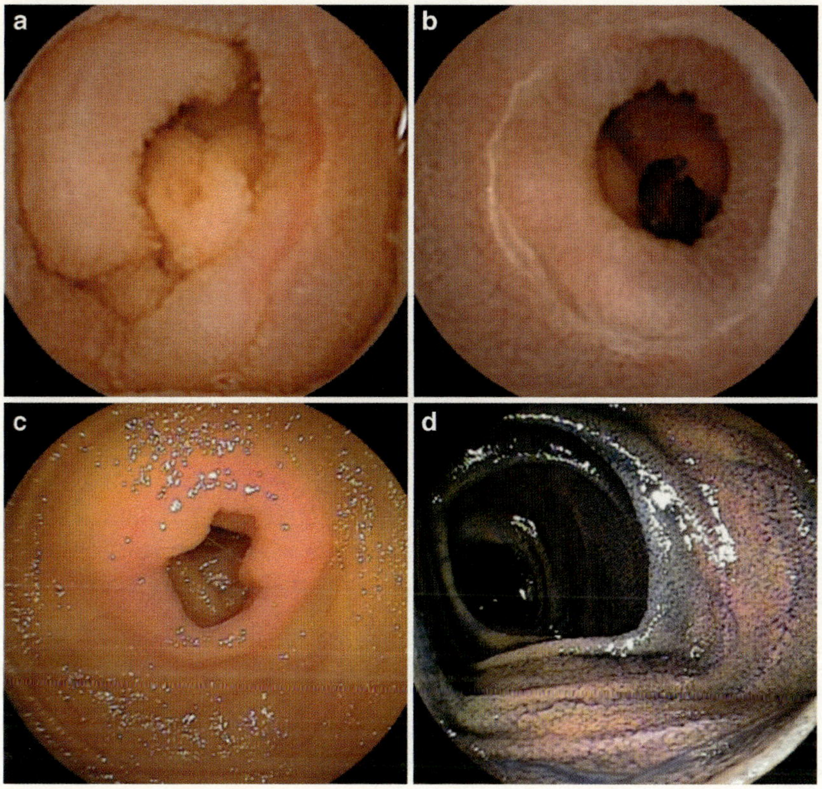

Fig. 19.42

19.15 Case 21 [14]

19.15.1 Male, 60s (Fig. 19.42a–d)

- Lower abdominal pain had persisted for over 3 months. The patient was taking low-dose aspirin and a non-steroidal anti-inflammatory drug (NSAID).
- CE revealed circumferential circular ulcers, ulcer scarring, and small erosions throughout the small intestine (a, b).
- Retrograde DBE 2 weeks after CE. Low-dose aspirin and NSAID had been discontinued after CE.
- Circular ulceration causing stenosis (c), ulcer scarring (d), redness, and erosions were evident in the ileum, but had healed somewhat compared with when CE was performed.

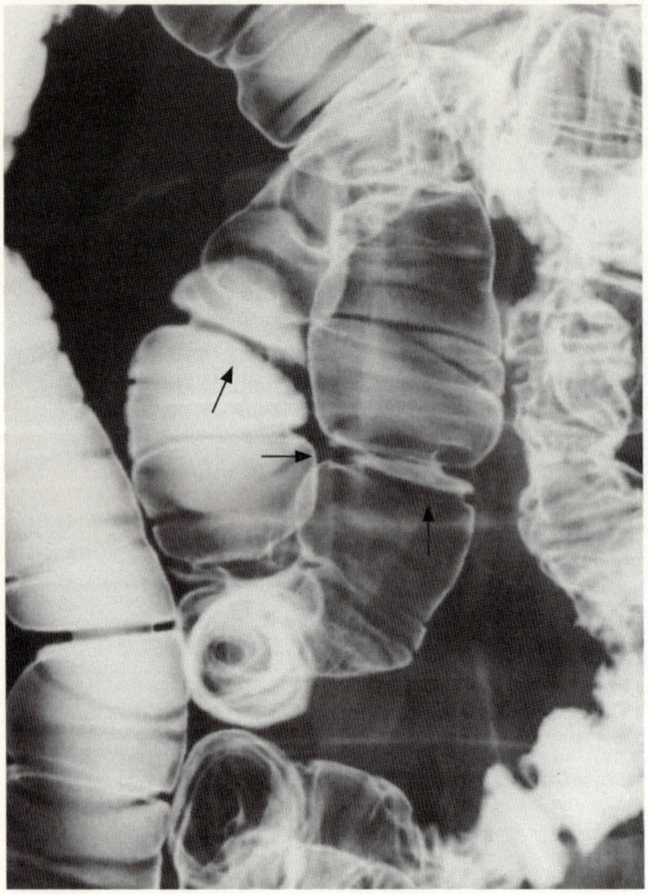

Fig. 19.43 Radiography performed at almost the same time as CE showed bilateral stenosis from the jejunum to the ileum, irregular Kerckring's folds, indentations, and circular ulcers (*arrows*)

19.15.2 Aspirin-Induced Enteropathy (Fig. 19.43)

- This condition can show a variety of symptoms, including epigastric abdominal pain, bloody stool, diarrhea, and abdominal distension. Symptoms are lacking in many cases, however, and the disorder is frequently asymptomatic. In severe cases, hemorrhagic shock, perforation, or similar events may result. It may sometimes be regarded as OGIB.
- Radiography at almost the same time as CE showed multiple bilateral stenoses, with multiple circular ulcers (radiographic image). Stenosis had progressed further by the time DBE was performed (endoscopic image, bottom left), and endoscopic balloon dilation was performed for lesions through which the scope was unable to be passed.
- Similar to ulcers caused by other NSAIDs, those caused by low-dose aspirin range in shape from round or oval through to irregular, punched-out, circular, and other forms.
- Diaphragmatic stenosis may occur.

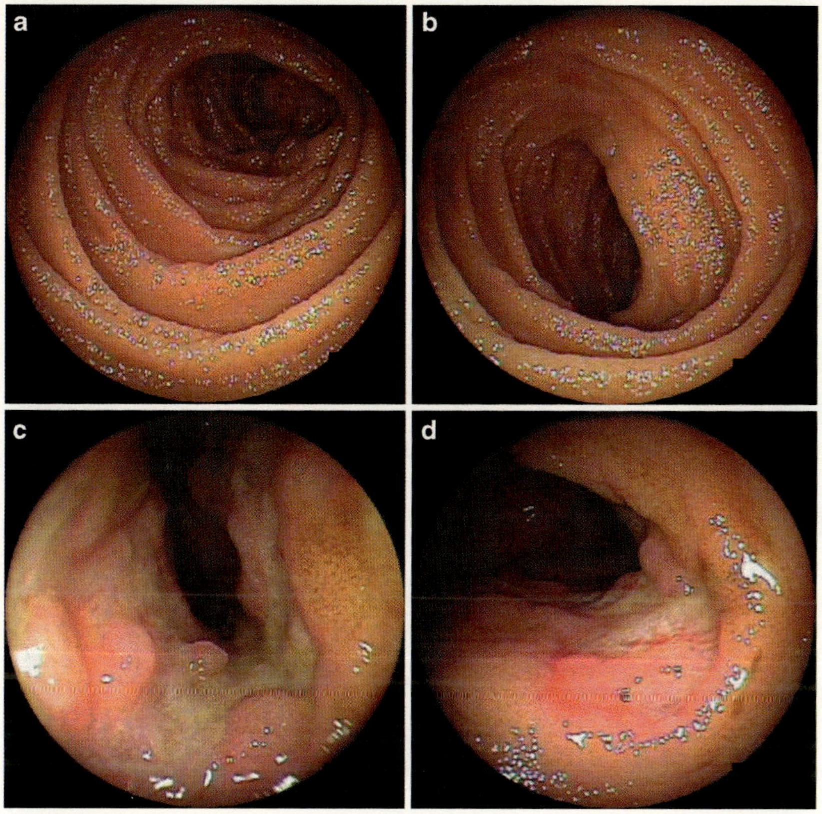

Fig. 19.44

19.16 Case 22 [15]

19.16.1 Male, 20s (Fig. 19.44a–d)

- Onset with fever, abdominal pain, bloody diarrhea, and vomiting. Pronounced anemia, edematous lesion, and petechial purpura on the extremities were evident. The patient had suffered from fever, cold-like symptoms, and elevated anti-streptolysin O antibody two weeks before, and antecedent infection with group A β-streptococcus was suspected.
- Swelling of Kerckring's folds and edematous mucosa were evident in the jejunum (a, b).
- In the ileum, the mucosa was edematous, and geographic ulcers of varying sizes were present. Reddish inflammatory polyps were also visible (c, d).

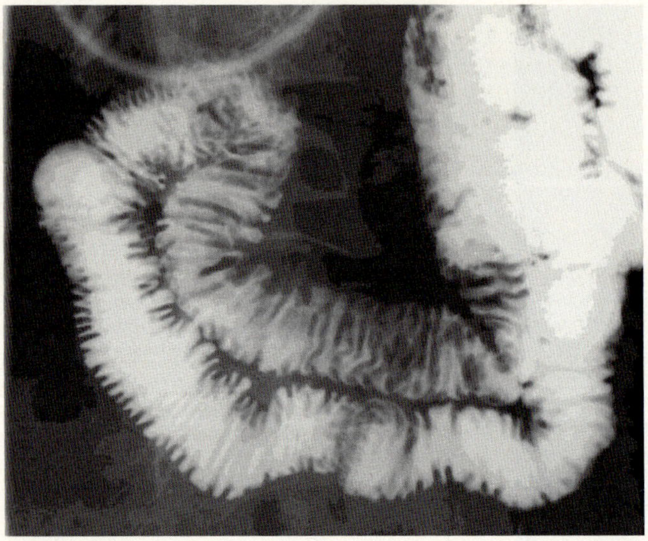

Fig. 19.45 Radiography showed swollen Kerckring's folds due to edema in the ileum

19.16.2 Schönlein-Henoch Purpura (Fig. 19.45)

- Schönlein-Henoch purpura is a disorder in which gastrointestinal symptoms such as abdominal pain and melena occur in addition to purpura in 50 % of patients, with joint pain in 40 %, and nephropathy in 50 %. This pathology is more frequent in children and young people, but occurrence in elderly patients is not uncommon.
- Gastrointestinal lesions may occur in any part of the intestine, from the esophagus to the large intestine, but the duodenum is the most frequently affected site.
- Endoscopic findings include redness, erosion, intramucosal hemorrhage, edema, and ulceration.
- Histopathological findings of gastrointestinal lesions comprise the same angiitis of small vessels such as capillaries and arterioles seen in the pathologic findings of purpura sites, and the fluorescence antibody technique reveals the deposition of immunoglobulin (Ig)A-positive substances in arteriolar endothelium.

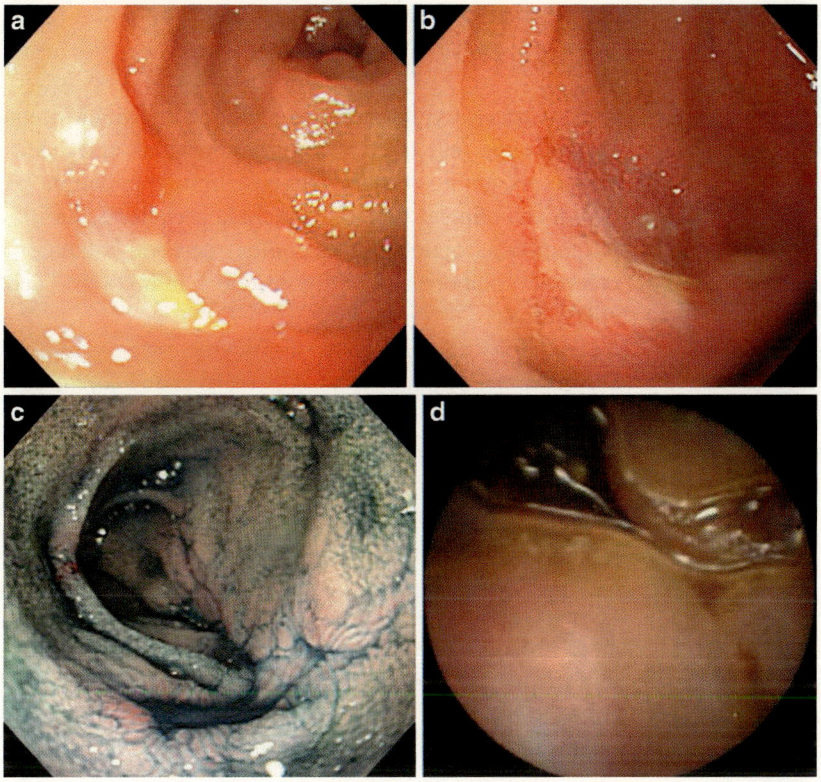

Fig. 19.46

19.17 Case 23 [16]

19.17.1 Male, 40s (Fig. 19.46a–d)

- Numbness in both legs and purpura appeared while the patient was being monitored after eosinophilic pneumonia. Skin biopsy revealed vasculitis with eosinophil infiltration. The patient had been undergoing steroid therapy, but abdominal pain appeared and emergency partial intestinal resection and small intestinal stoma formation were performed to treat multiple small intestinal ulcer perforations. Lesions in the remaining small intestine were observed postoperatively via the stoma.
- Multiple irregularly shaped ulcers were present. There was no deep ulcer, or any obvious longitudinal tendency (a, b).
- An almost completely scarred ulcer. Regenerative epithelium was evident on the mucosa surrounding the ulcer (c).
- During the remission period following surgery for perforation, CE revealed scarring of ulcerative lesions (d).

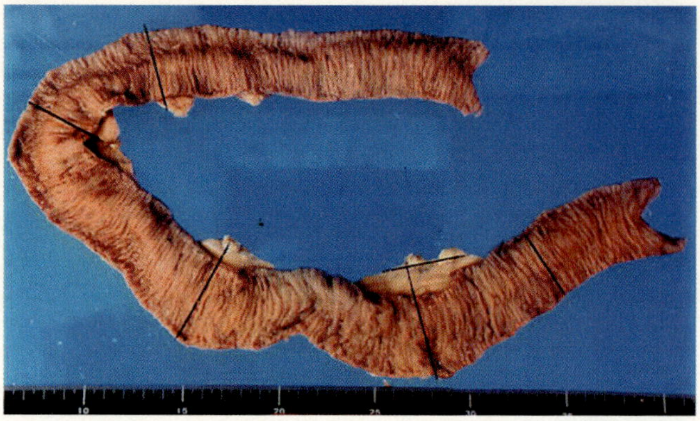

Fig. 19.47 Approximately 80 cm of the small intestine was removed, including the site of perforation. The resected specimen contained a total of five ulcers

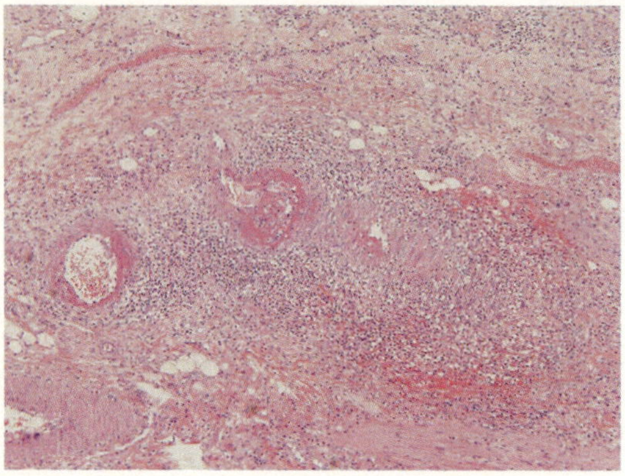

Fig. 19.48 Arteriolitis was present in almost all sections. Arteries with arteritis were around 2 mm in diameter, and fibrinoid necrosis was present within the muscularis propria, submucosa, and subserosa

19.17.2 Churg-Strauss Syndrome (Figs. 19.47 and 19.48)

- Churg-Strauss syndrome is a condition in which bronchial asthma and allergic rhinitis appear as antecedent symptoms, angiitis occurs with eosinophilia in peripheral blood, and clinical symptoms include peripheral neuritis, purpura, gastrointestinal ulceration, cerebral infarction, cerebral hemorrhage, myocardial infarction, and epicarditis.
- Necrotizing angiitis and leukocytoclastic vasculitis accompanied by a pronounced increase in eosinophils are evident in angiitis-affected tissue. At times, extravascular formation of granulomas is observed.
- Elevated erythrocyte sedimentation rate, thrombocytosis, elevated IgE levels, anti-myeloperioxidase antibodies, and elevated eosinophil cationic protein are important as referral findings.
- Gastrointestinal lesions occur in around half of all cases, and are found across a wide area in the stomach, duodenum, small intestine, and large intestine. Irregularly shaped ulcers and small ulcers are evident, with severe redness of the mucosa on the ulcer borders. Ulcers are often deep, and perforation sometimes occurs.

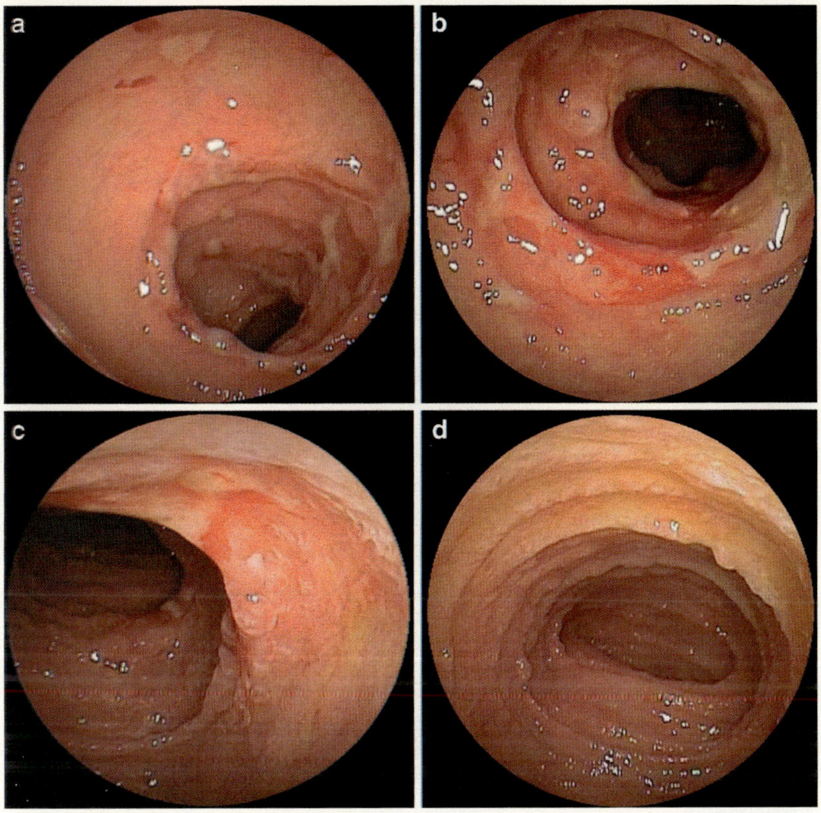

Fig. 19.49

19.18 Case 24 [17]

19.18.1 Male, 50s (Fig. 19.49a–d)

Principal Complaints: Diarrhea, Abdominal Pain, Vomiting

- Protein-losing scintigraphy showed widespread protein loss in the upper small intestine.
- Multiple irregular geographic ulcers, oval or round-shaped ulcers, and erosions were evident, mainly in the jejunum. Ulceration took a variety of forms, with both circular and longitudinal ulcers present (a, b).
- Edema and granular mucosa were apparent in the intervening mucosa (c, d).

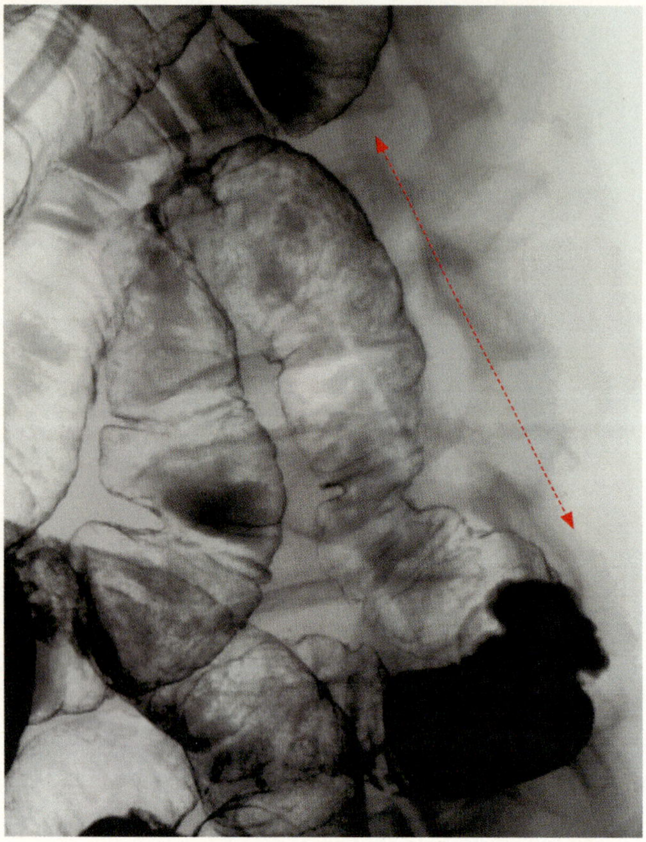

Fig. 19.50 Coarse, granular mucosa and a mild degree of poor distensibility were evident in the jejunum (*arrows*)

19.18.2 Cytomegalovirus Enteritis (Figs. 19.50 and 19.51)

- Latent cytomegalovirus infection may be reactivated in patients who are immunosuppressed due to administration of anticancer drugs or immunosuppressants, or to conditions such as acquired immunodeficiency syndrome, causing damage to organs including the retina, liver, lungs, and intestine.
- A confirmed diagnosis must be based on clinical symptoms, detection of intranuclear inclusion bodies in biopsy tissue, and serological evaluation (such as CMV antigenemia testing).
- Clinical symptoms in the gastrointestinal tract commonly include diarrhea, melena, and abdominal pain.
- Endoscopically, this pathology is characterized by punched-out like ulcers. However, a wide variety of other forms is also possible, including irregular geographic ulcers, edema, aphthae, and redness.

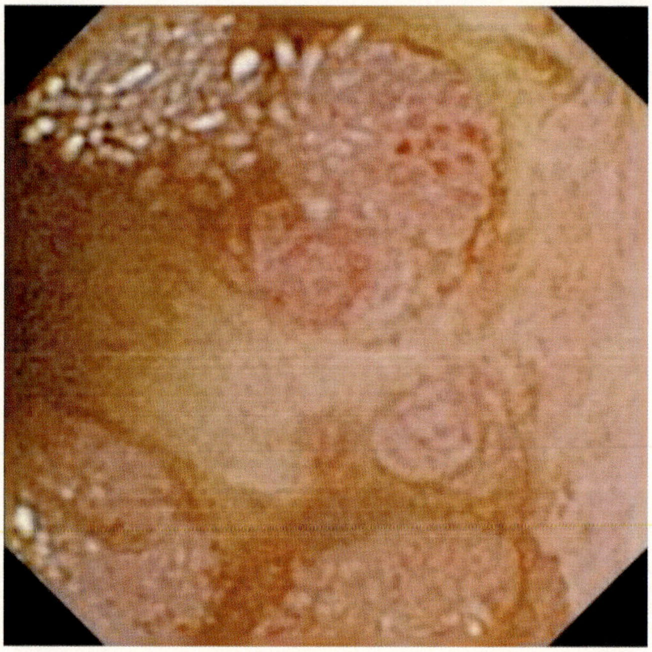

Fig. 19.51 Female, 50s. Multiple organ failure. CE revealed multiple deep geographic ulcers in the jejunum

References

1. Partridge BJ et al. Small bowel cancers diagnosed device-assisted enteroscopy at a U.S. referral center: a five-year experience. Dig Dis Sci. 2011;56:2701–5.
2. Barakat MH. Endoscopic features of primary small bowel lymphoma: a proposed endoscopic classification. Gut. 1982;23:36–41.
3. Matsumoto T et al. Endoscopic diagnosis of malignant enterocolic fistula caused by ileal lymphoma. Gastrointest Endosc. 2000;51:508–9.
4. Matsumoto T et al. Crohn's disease of aphthous type: serial changes in intestinal lesions. Br J Radiol. 2000;73:1046–51.
5. Hizawa K et al. Crohn's disease. Early recognition and progress of aphthous lesions. Radiology. 1994;190:451–4.
6. Hayashi Y et al. Diagnosis and management of mid-gastrointestinal bleeding by double-balloon endoscopy. Ther Adv Gastroenterol. 2009;2:109–17.
7. Sunada K et al. Advances in the diagnosis and treatment of small bowel lesions with Crohn's disease using double-balloon endoscopy. Ther Adv Gastroenterol. 2009;2:357–66.
8. Boltin D et al. Concurrent small bowel adenocarcinoma and carcinoid tumor in Crohn's disease–case report and literature review. J Crohns Colitis. 2011;5:461–4.
9. Lee CR et al. Colonoscopic findings in intestinal Behçet's disease. Inflamm Bowel Dis. 2001;7:243–9.
10. Neves FS et al. Behçet's disease: clinical value of the video capsule endoscopy for small intestine examination. Rheumatol Int. 2009; 29:601–3.
11. Ona FV et al. Diagnosis and management of nonspecific colon ulcer. Arch Surg. 1982;117:888–94.
12. Matsumoto T et al. Chronic non-specific multiple ulcers of the small intestine: a proposal of the entity from Japanese gastroenterologists to Western enteroscopists. Gastrointest Endosc. 2007;66:S99–107.
13. Matsumoto T et al. Endoscopic features of chronic nonspecific multiple ulcers of the small intestine: comparison with nonsteroidal anti-inflammatory drug-induced enteropathy. Dig Dis Sci. 2006;51:1357–63.
14. Mizukami K et al. Aspirin-induced small bowel injuries and the preventive effect of rebamipide. World J Gastroenterol. 2011;17:5117–22.
15. Esaki M et al. GI involvement in Henoch-Schönlein purpura. Gastrointest Endosc. 2002;56:920–3.
16. Venditti D et al. Bowel perforations in a patient affected by Churg-Strauss syndrome under high-dose steroid treatment: will alternative drugs reduce risk of surgery? Rheumatol Int. 2011;31:1239–41.
17. Fujita T et al. A case of cytomegalovirus enterocolitis diagnosed by the double-balloon enteroscopy. Hepatogastroenterology. 2008;55: 2087–90.

20 Case Presentations: Stenosis

Shinji Tsukamoto, Masashi Yamaguchi, Shotaro Nakamura, Takashi Watanabe, Naoya Kubokura, Kensei Ohtsu, Takayuki Matsumoto, and Yoshitaka Tomioka

20.1 Case 1 [1]

20.1.1 Female, 70s (Fig. 20.1a–d)

- Weight loss due to nausea, vomiting, and loss of appetite were present.
- An irregularly shaped ulcer with an ulcer mound was present near the ligament of Treitz, causing severe stenosis. The endoscope was unable to be passed through (a, b).
- The same lesion after dye spraying (c, d).

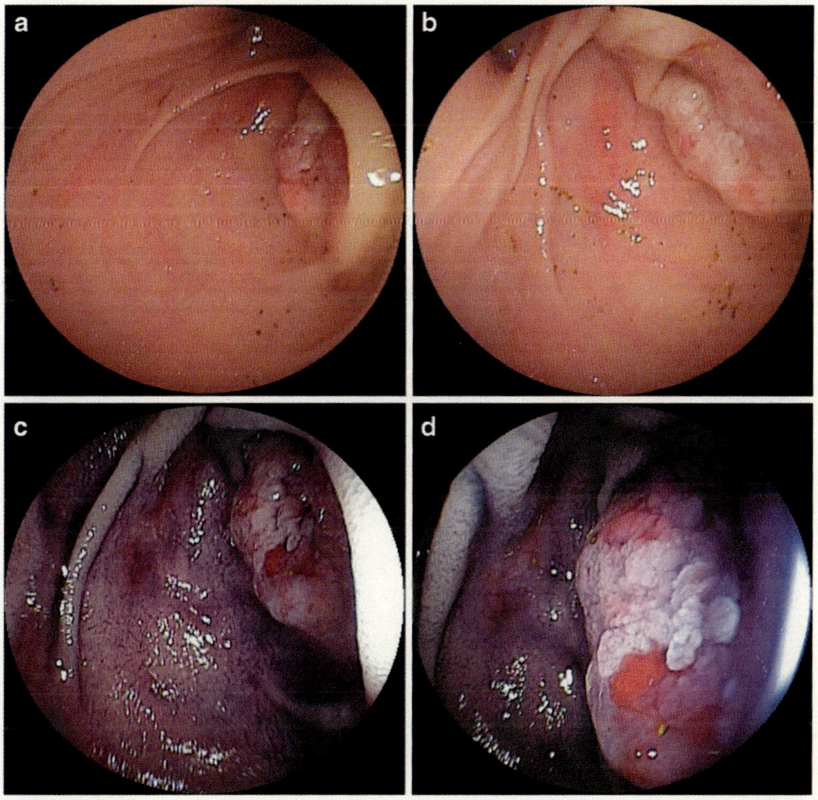

Fig. 20.1

S. Tsukamoto (✉) • M. Yamaguchi • T. Watanabe • Y. Tomioka
Department of Gastroenterology and Medicine, Fukuoka University Faculty of Medicine, 7-45-1 Nanakuma, Jonan-ku, Fukuoka 814 0180, Japan
e-mail: shinshinzi@yahoo.co.jp

S. Nakamura • N. Kubokura • T. Matsumoto
Department of Medicine and Clinical Science, Graduate School of Medicine, Kyushu University, 3-1-1, Maidashi, Higashi-ku, Fukuoka 812-8582, Japan

K. Ohtsu
Department of Gastroenterology, Fukuoka University Chikushi Hospital, 1-1-1 Zokumyoin, Chikushino 818-8502, Japan

T. Matsui et al. (eds.), *Endoscopy in the Diagnosis of Small Intestine Diseases*, DOI 10.1007/978-4-431-54352-7_20, © Springer Japan 2014

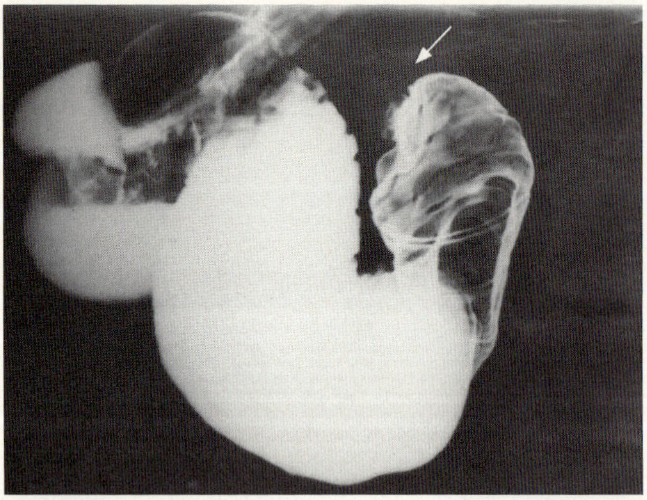

Fig. 20.2 Complete obstruction of the intestine and dilation of the duodenum were evident slightly distal to the ligament of Treitz. In a lateral view of the site of obstruction, an irregular barium fleck was evident in the center, surrounded by nodular filling defects

20.1.2 Small Intestinal Carcinoma (Primary) (Figs. 20.2 and 20.3)

- Clinical symptoms of small intestinal carcinoma include abdominal pain, vomiting, melena, and abdominal distension.
- Endoscopic signs of small intestinal carcinoma comprise irregular tumors and ulcers, with severe stenosis of the lumen frequently evident at the time of discovery.
- Macroscopically, primary small intestinal carcinoma is broadly divided into ulcerative and protrusive types, with the ulcerative type further categorized into concentric stenosis, extraluminal growth, or non-stenotic types. Concentric stenosis is the most common.
- In terms of histological type, well to moderately differentiated adenocarcinoma is common, whereas signet ring cell carcinoma is rare (Fig. 20.4).

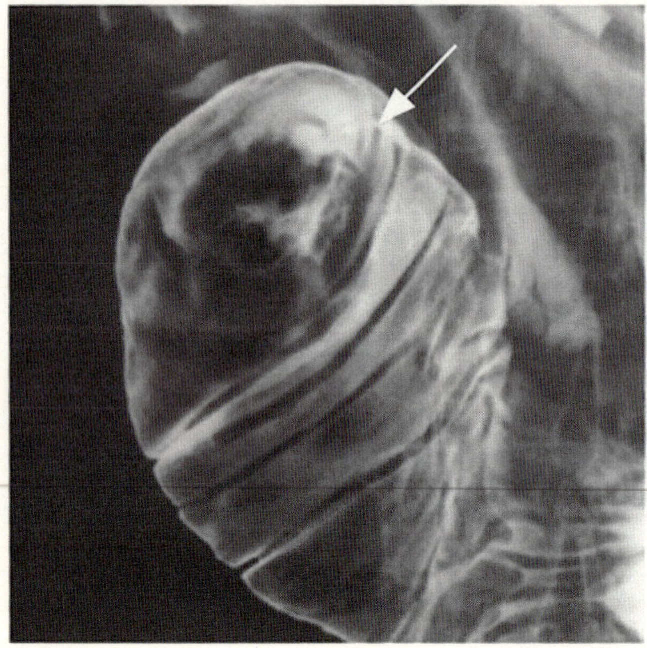

Fig. 20.3 A frontal view of the site of obstruction showed an irregular barium fleck in the center of the filling defect

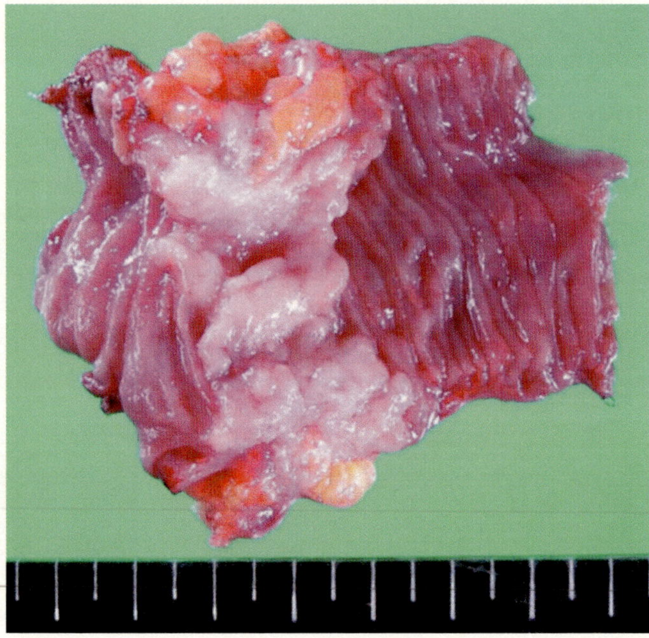

Fig. 20.4 Resected specimen. The tumor measured 5×3 cm, with severe circumferential stenosis, and the morphology exhibited type 2 findings in the form of a central ulcer with an ulcer mound. Histopathological diagnosis was moderately differentiated adenocarcinoma, and the tumor was exposed to the serosa and had invaded as far as the mesenterium

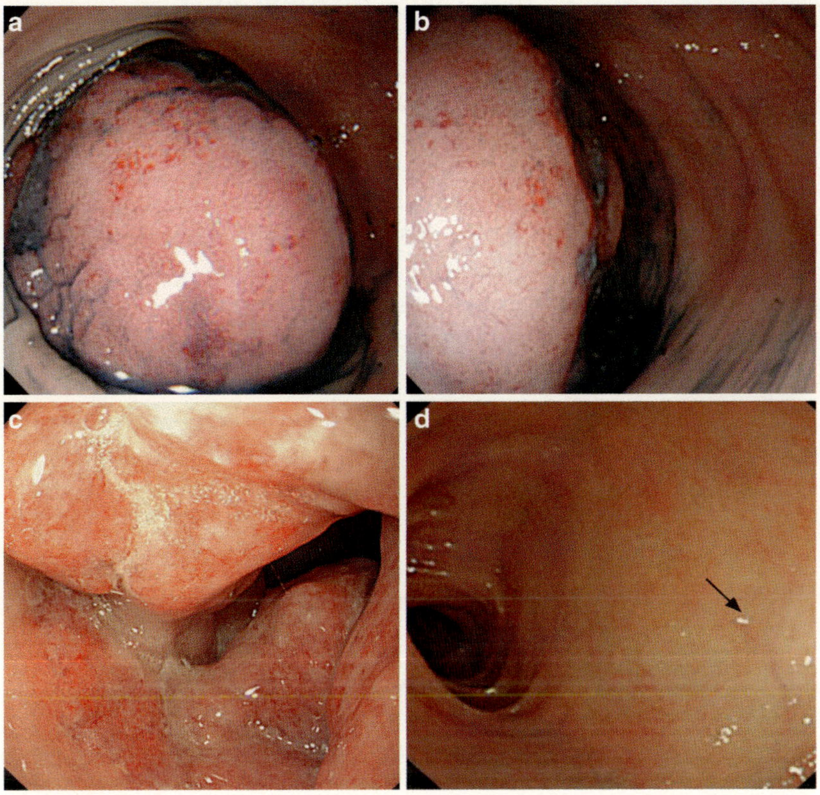

Fig. 20.5

20.2 Case 2 [2]

20.2.1 Male, 80s (Fig. 20.5a–d)

Principal complaints: Abdominal pain, sensation of abdominal distension, soluble IL-2R 3.997 U/mL.

- A large lesion with submucosal elevation in the terminal part of the ileum had escaped to the cecal side (a).
- A shallow ulcer had formed on its peak (b).
- A submucosal tumor-like irregular protrusive lesion was evident in the terminal ileum (c).
- The lesion disappeared following chemotherapy. A scar believed to represent the base of the lesion was present in the terminal ileum (arrow) (d).

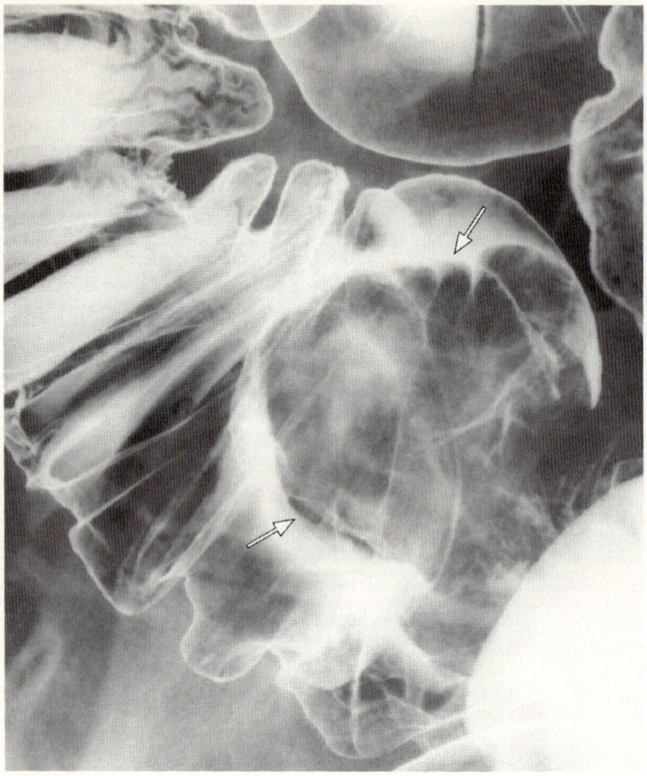

Fig. 20.6 A large submucosal elevation of the terminal ileum had escaped to the cecal side. It was approximately 70 × 50 mm in size

20.2.2 DLBCL (Figs. 20.6 and 20.7)

- This type of tumor is classified as a localized small intestinal malignant lymphoma and is the next most common type after the ulcerated type. It almost always occurs in the ileum.
- Most DLBCLs are sessile with smooth surfaces.
- Most cases are discovered due to abdominal pain, and as tumors enlarge they may become palpable and cause melena and intestinal intussusception.
- Histologically, most are derived from B cells, with DLBCL accounting for the majority of cases.

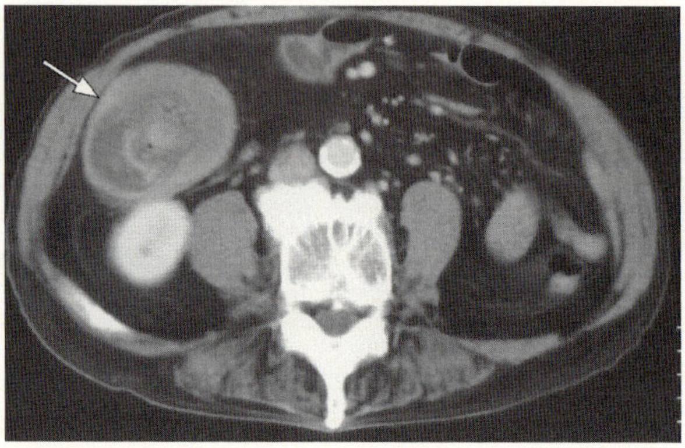

Fig. 20.7 Contrast-enhanced CT. The interior of the lesion exhibited a stratified enhancing effect, and the lesion in the terminal part of the ileum had caused intestinal intussusception

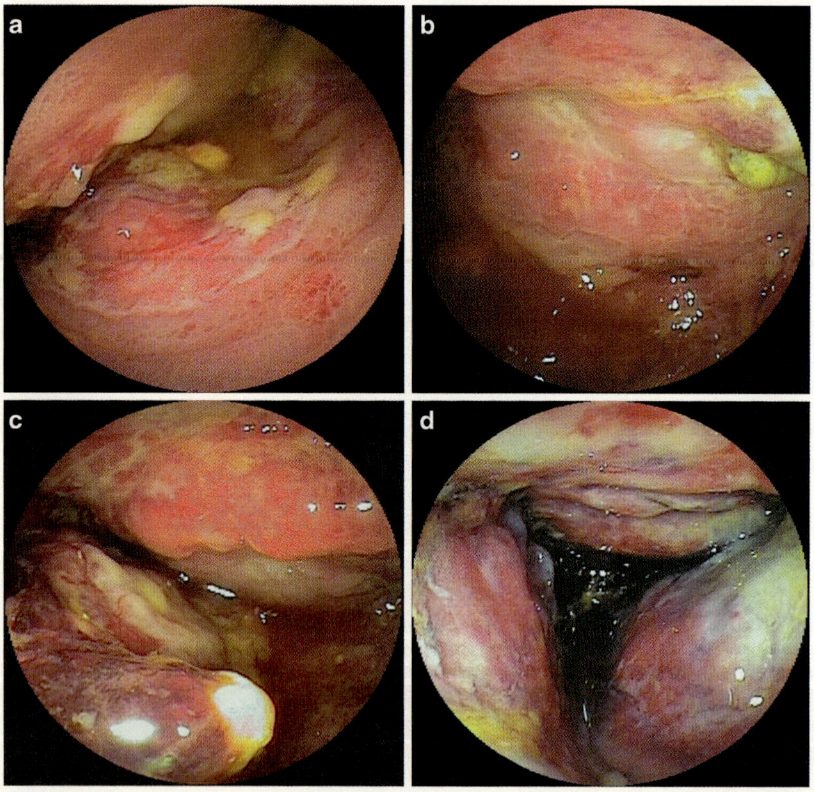

Fig. 20.8

20.3 Case 3 [3]

20.3.1 Male, 60s (Fig. 20.8a–d)

- Admitted to hospital for testing to investigate causes of abdominal pain, vomiting, and weight loss.
- DBE revealed a circumferential ulcerative lesion with clearly demarcated margins in the jejunum (a).
- Although some normal mucosa remained in the center of the lesion (b), stenosis due to a circumferential tumor was present further on the distal side (c, d).

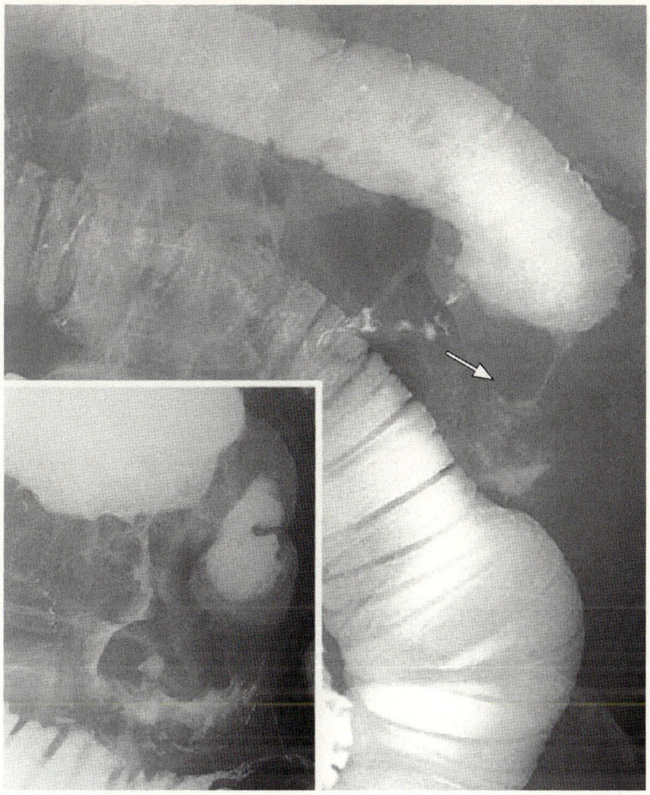

Fig. 20.9 Radiography revealed long luminal narrowing with complex flexion and dilation of the intestine on the proximal side

20.3.2 Malignant Lymphoma: T-Cell Lymphoma (Figs. 20.9 and 20.10)

- In cases of ulcerative-type lymphomas with high proliferative activity such as DLBCL, Burkitt lymphoma, and T-cell lymphoma, the tumor itself may cause intestinal stenosis.
- In the case illustrated here, radiography revealed long luminal narrowing with complex flexion and dilation of the intestine on the proximal side (left). Naso-intestinal tube insertion was required after imaging.
- The resected specimen included remaining normal mucosa between a severely stenotic lesion on the distal side and a lesion on the proximal side (bottom). Histologically, this tumor comprised T-cell lymphoma with no HTLV-1 infection, and there were no clear findings of enteropathy-associated T-cell lymphoma (ETL).

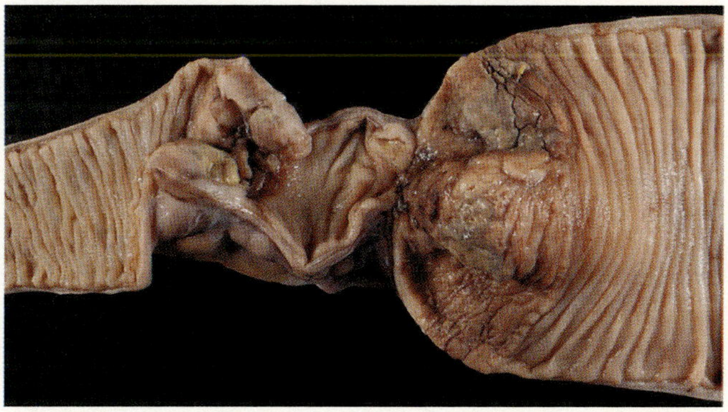

Fig. 20.10 The resected specimen included remaining normal mucosa between a severely stenotic lesion on the distal side and a lesion on the proximal side

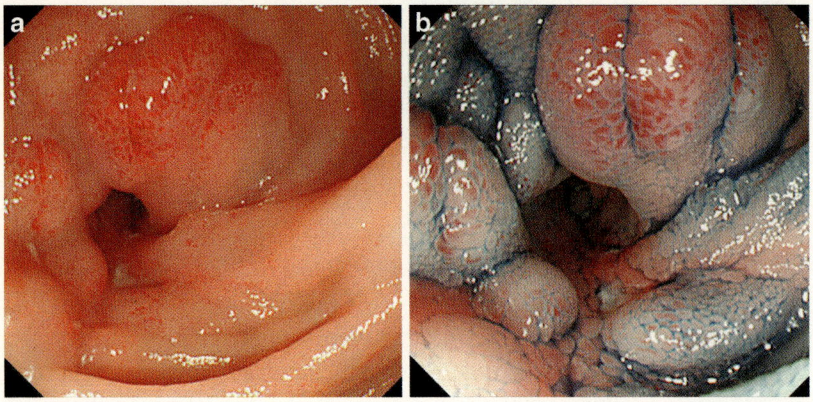

Fig. 20.11

20.4 Case 4, 5 [4]

20.4.1 Male, 30s (Fig. 20.11a, b)

Principal complaint: Abdominal pain

- Stenosis with a unilateral deformity caused by a single longitudinal ulcer was evident in the terminal ileum.
- The endoscope was unable to pass through.

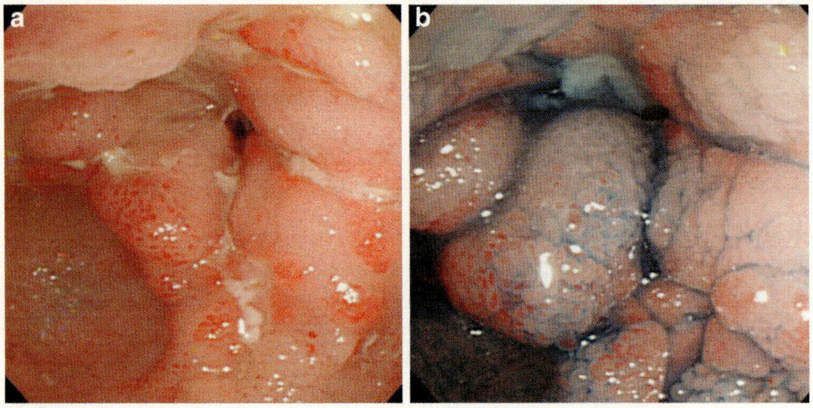

Fig. 20.12

20.4.2 Female, Teens (Fig. 20.12a, b)

Principal complaint: Abdominal pain

- Severe stenosis with several longitudinal ulcers was evident in the terminal ileum.
- The endoscope was unable to pass through.

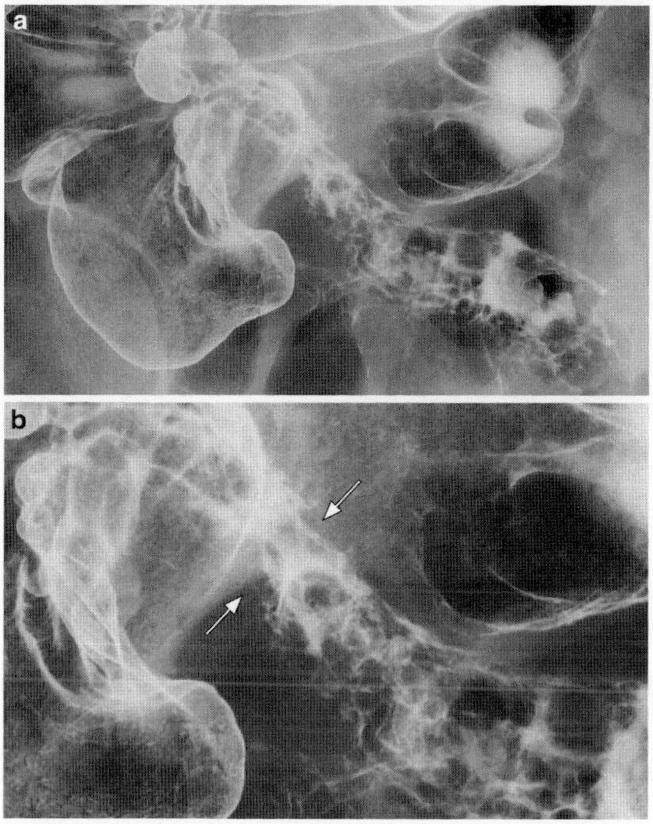

Fig. 20.13 Case 5: Radiographic image (the *bottom image* is a magnification of the *top*). *Arrows* indicate the site of endoscopic observation. Severe stenosis with several longitudinal ulcers was evident (*arrows*). Bilateral deformity due to several longitudinal ulcers was present. On the proximal side, the intestine exhibited a cobblestone appearance

20.4.3 Crohn's Disease (Fig. 20.13a, b)

- Crohn's disease may cause luminal stenosis due to edema or fibrosis as a result of inflammation of the full thickness of the intestine from lesions such as longitudinal ulcers or cobblestone appearance.
- Although stenosis due to edema improves with medical treatment, fibrotic stenosis may respond poorly or even progress, and endoscopic dilation therapy or surgical treatment is indicated.

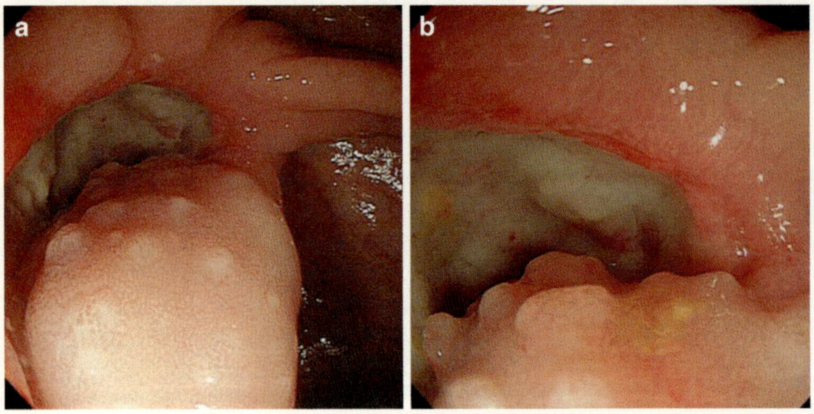

Fig. 20.14

20.5 Case 6, 7 [5]

20.5.1 Male, 40s (Fig. 20.14a, b)

- Abdominal pain had appeared 6 months previously, and colonoscopy was performed because bloody stool was evident.
- An undermining ulcer covered with a thick white coat was present in the terminal part of the ileum.
- This caused dilation of the ileocecal valve and convergence of the folds.
- Luminal narrowing was present, and the endoscope did not pass through.

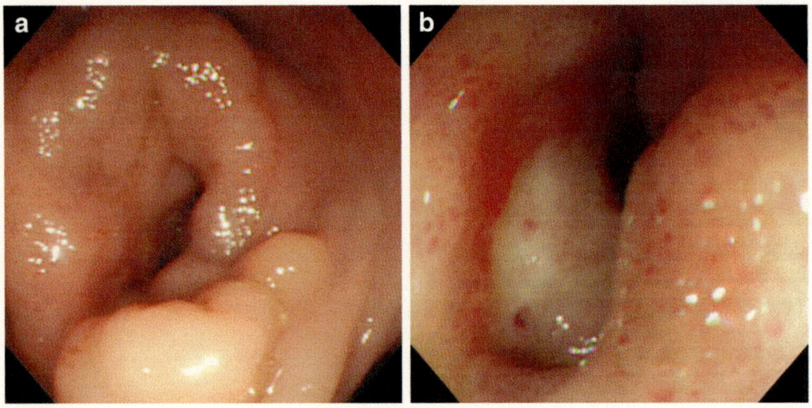

Fig. 20.15

20.5.2 Male, 50s (Fig. 20.15a, b)

Principal complaint: Abdominal pain

- Endoscopy revealed an open ulcer causing severe luminal narrowing at the site of anastomosis.
- Ulcer margins were clearly demarcated, and the surroundings were covered with normal ileal mucosa.

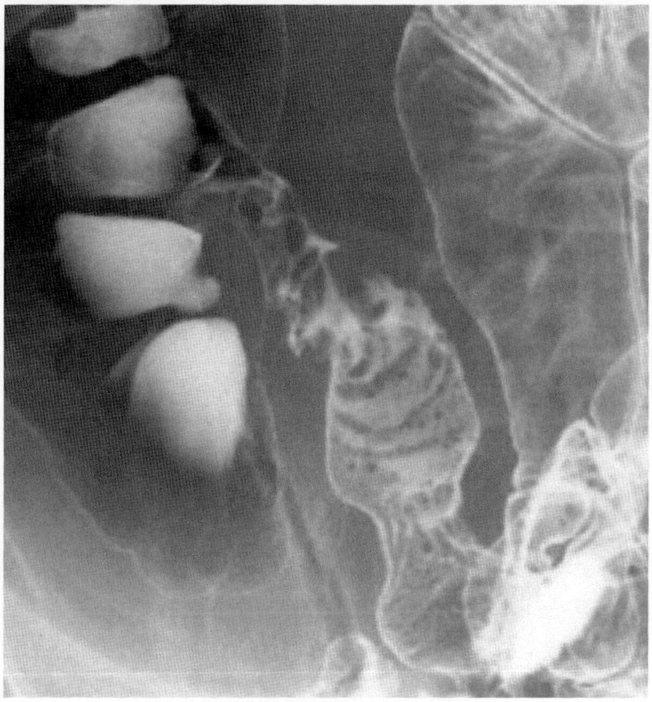

Fig. 20.16 Radiography revealed stenosis of almost the entire circumference of the terminal part of the ileum, with irregular barium flecks

20.5.3 Behçet's Disease (Fig. 20.16)

- Behçet disease is an intractable disorder characterized by recurrent ulceration of the oral mucosa, skin, eyes, and genital area, and intractable iridocyclitis. It may cause refractory ulcers with an undermining tendency, mainly in the ileocecal area. If these are central to the clinical presentation, the condition is known as intestinal Behçet disease.
- Histologically, such ulcers comprise deep Ul-IV ulcers that exhibit non-specific inflammatory findings of chronic activity.
- Bleeding and perforation are common complications, and stenosis may also occur.
- Radiographically, ulcers are visualized as deep, clearly demarcated barium flecks. Dilation of the intestine on the proximal side of the stenosis is rare. Endoscopy reveals ulcers with clear margins at the site of stenosis.

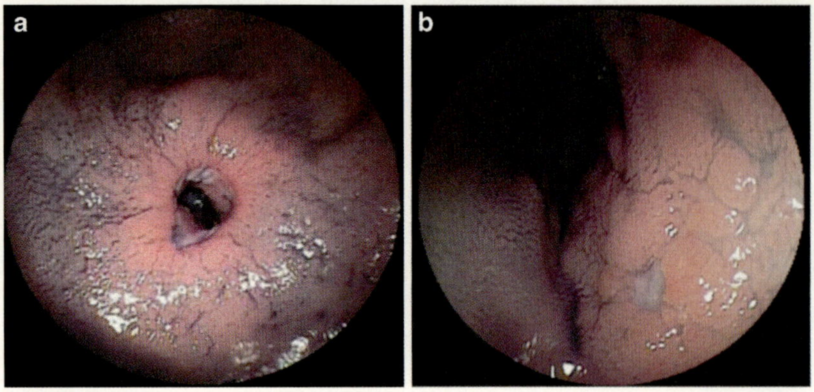

Fig. 20.17

20.6 Case 8, 9 [6]

20.6.1 Confirmed Diagnosis: Male, 60s (Fig. 20.17a, b)

Principal complaints: constipation, sensation of abdominal distension

- Concentric stenosis was evident in the lower small intestine. Active ulceration was present in the center. Biopsy of the ulcer margin did not reveal any specific findings.
- The endoscope was unable to pass through, meaning that the proximal side of the concentric stenosis could not be observed.
- A small ulcer was identified in a Peyer's patch on the distal side, with atrophic scarring area close by.

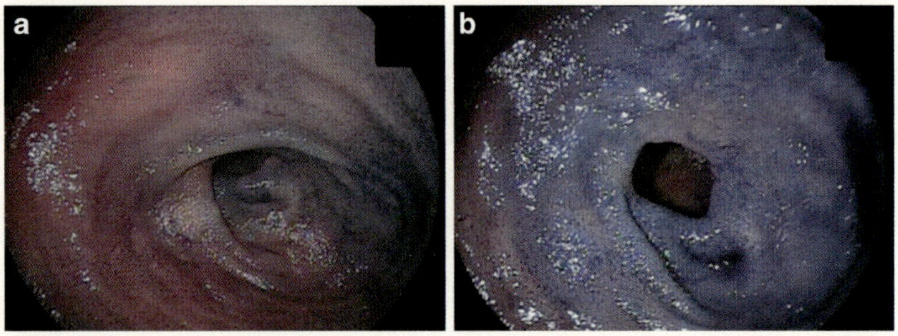

Fig. 20.18

20.6.2 Suspected Diagnosis: Female, 70s (Fig. 20.18a, b)

Principal complaints: stomach pain, vomiting

- Underlying disease: tubercular pleurisy in 1949
- Circular ulcer was evident in the lower small intestine. There was no ulceration in the center, or any clear area of atrophic scarring at any location, including the entire large intestine.
- No abnormality was identified in nearby Peyer's patches.

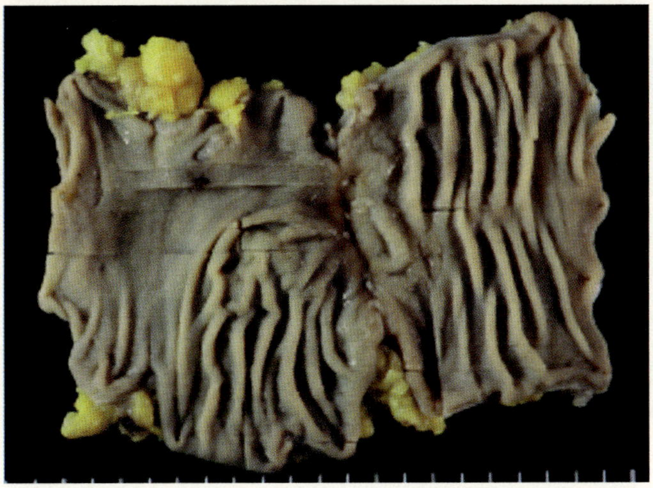

Fig. 20.19 Case 8: Resected specimen. Although this case could not be histologically identified as caseating granuloma, the diagnosis of intestinal tuberculosis was confirmed from the characteristic concentric girdle-like ulcers, areas of atrophic scarring, and multiple stenoses

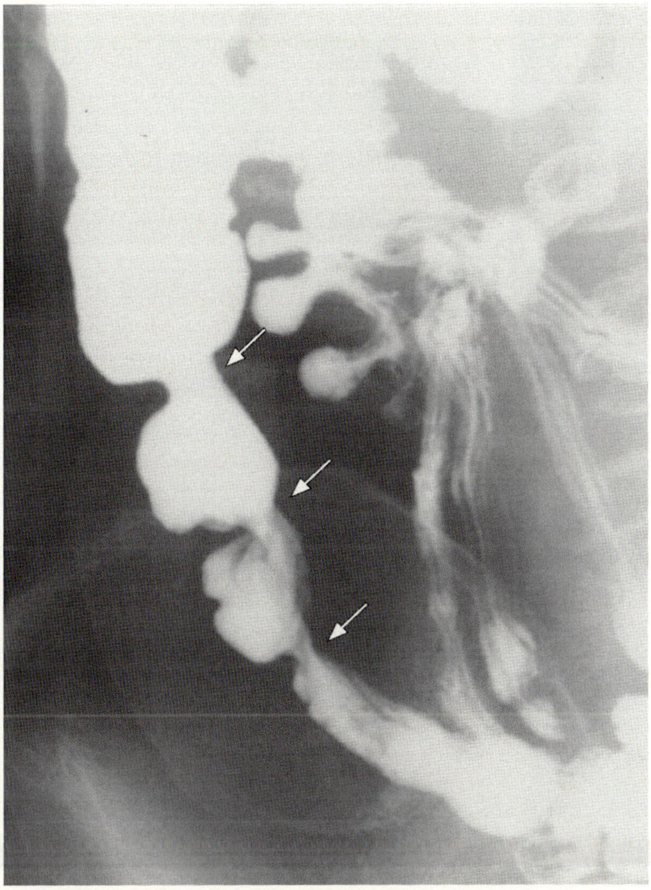

Fig. 20.20 Case 9: Radiography revealed multiple concentric stenoses of the lower small intestine (*arrows*). No other characteristic findings apart from concentric stenosis were present in this case, which was diagnosed as suspected intestinal tuberculosis

20.6.3 Intestinal Tuberculosis (Figs. 20.19 and 20.20)

- Intestinal tuberculosis occurs when Mycobacterium tuberculosis invades intestinal lymphoid follicles, particularly in Peyer's patches, causing the formation of tuberculous nodules and caseating granuloma, which results in mucosal damage and the formation of erosions or ulcers. Concentric stenosis and areas of atrophic scarring form during the mucosal healing process.
- Barium contrast radiography of the small intestine characteristically shows: (1) diverse ulcer morphology; (2) areas of atrophy due to ulcer scarring; and (3) bilateral deformity of the lumen.
- Endoscopically, intestinal tuberculosis is characterized by: (1) areas of atrophic scarring; and (2) concentric stenosis. Stenosis is severe, with the endoscope frequently unable to pass through.

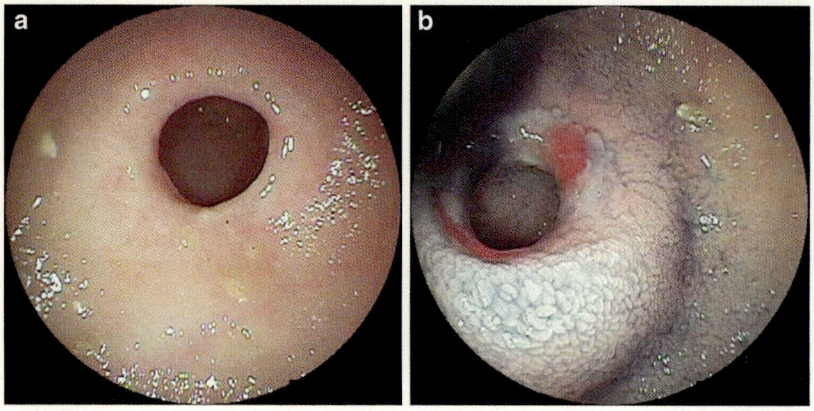

Fig. 20.21

20.7 Case 10, 11 [7]

20.7.1 Female, 50s (Fig. 20.21a, b)

- The patient had suffered from idiopathic iron-deficiency anemia since she was 15 years old, and presented with a principal complaint of abdominal pain.
- A circular ulcer had initially appeared to have scarred with the use of total parenteral nutrition, causing stenosis (a).
- Observations close to the site of stenosis revealed a clearly demarcated shallow open ulcer (b).

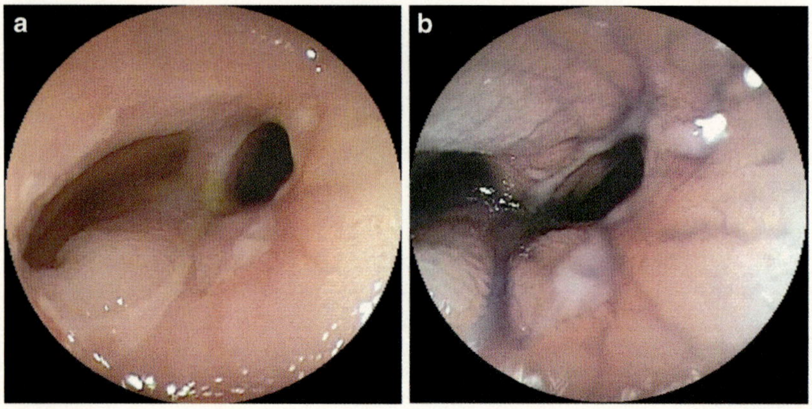

Fig. 20.22

20.7.2 Female, 30s (Fig. 20.22a, b)

- Anemia and hypoproteinemia had been identified at 8 years old, but the cause was unknown.
- The patient was admitted to hospital due to pronounced edema, and technetium scintigraphy revealed protein loss in the lower small intestine.
- DBE revealed severe luminal narrowing and pseudo-diverticulum formation in the pelvic ileum, with shallow, branching ulceration in the same area.

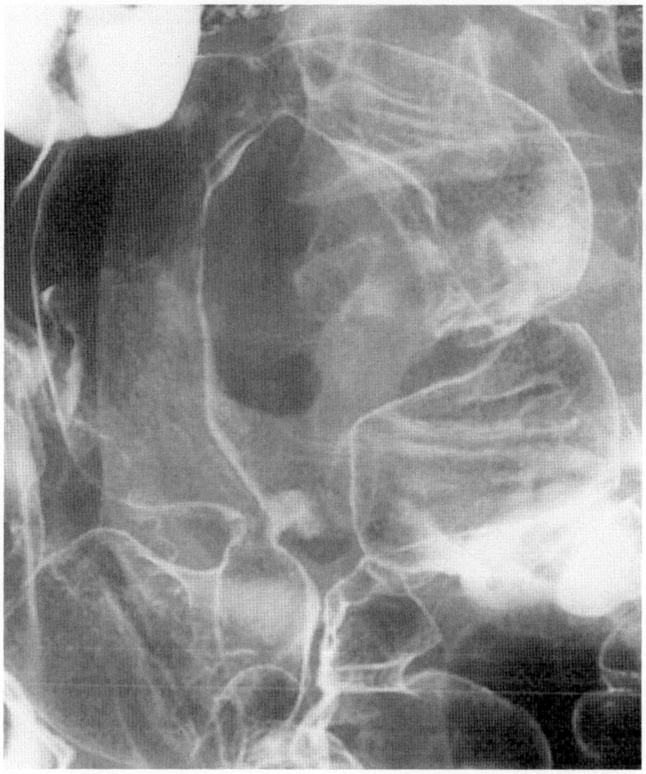

Fig. 20.23 Multiple areas of bi- and unilateral luminal narrowing of the ileum were evident

20.7.3 Chronic Non-specific Multiple Ulcers of the Small Intestine (Fig. 20.23)

- This condition arises in infancy or early childhood and comprises idiopathic ulceration of the small intestine, characterized clinically by persistent positive results for fecal occult blood test and hypoproteinemia.
- Unlike Crohn's disease, inflammatory findings are mild, and ulcers are shallow and clearly demarcated, with a tendency to be circular or oblique. Small intestinal lesions exhibiting a similar clinical profile have also been reported from several other countries, and this is not regarded as a rare condition.
- Ulcers exhibit resistance to medical treatment, and do not scar completely. However, a tendency for healing accompanied by luminal narrowing is evident among patients treated with total parenteral nutrition and in long-term cases. Circular ulcers in particular lead to severe stenosis. In such cases, however, clearly demarcated open ulcers in positions consistent with sites of stenosis are frequently also evident.

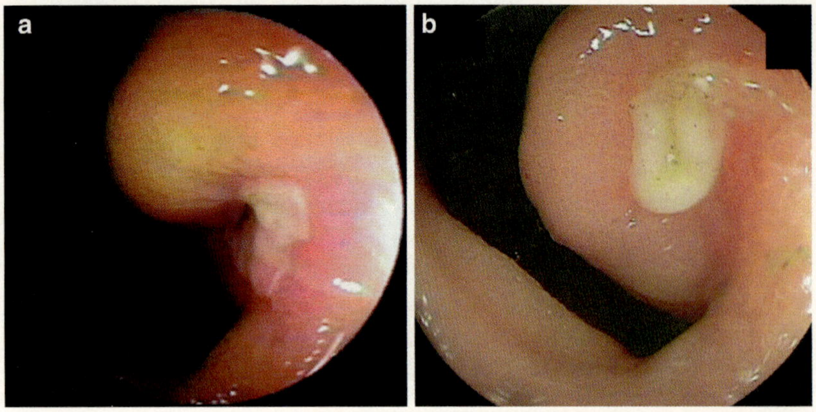

Fig. 20.24

20.8 Case 12 [7]

20.8.1 Female, 50s (Fig. 20.24a, b)

- Anemia and hypoproteinemia were identified at 15 years old.
- DBE performed at 54 years old (a) and 57 years old (b) showed severe stenosis at the flexed site of anastomosis, with a shallow, clearly demarcated open ulcer.

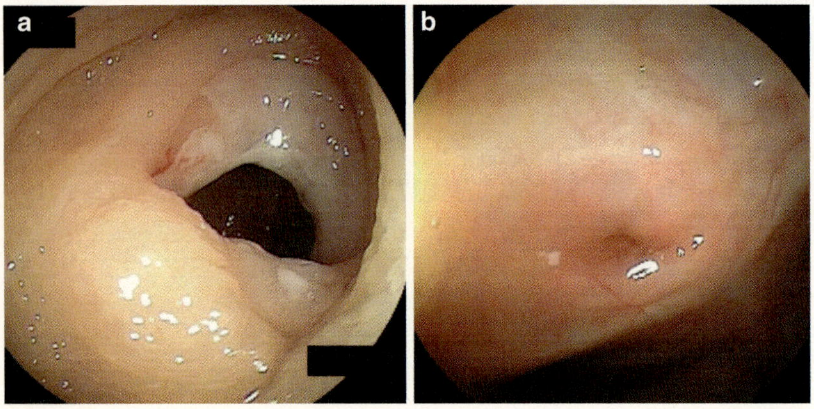

Fig. 20.25

20.8.2 Female, 40s (Fig. 20.25a, b)

- Anemia was identified during junior high school. Ulceration of the small intestine was identified at around 40 years old due to abdominal pain, and the patient twice underwent ileal resection.
- DBE at 2 years after the second surgery identified a circumferential open ulcer at the site of anastomosis (a). When total parenteral nutrition was implemented, the ulcer scarred, leading to severe stenosis (b).

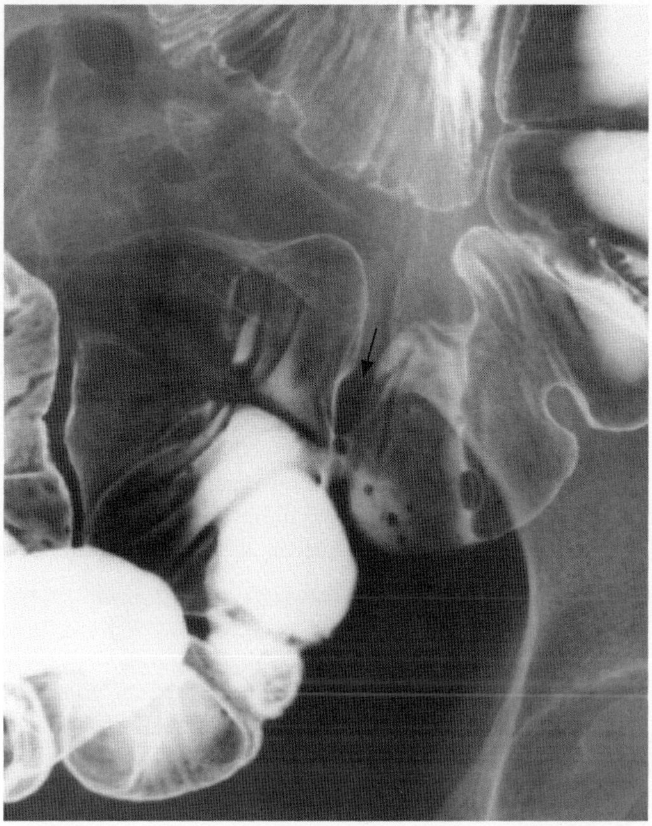

Fig. 20.26 Continuous severe luminal narrowing was evident at the same location as a side-to-side anastomosis in the lower ileum

20.8.3 Chronic non-Specific Multiple Ulcers of the Small Intestine (Fig. 20.26)

- Chronic non-specific multiple ulcers of the small intestine represent an intractable ulcerative condition characterized clinically by persistent anemia and hypoproteinemia, which may require surgical treatment due to stenosis. Even if major lesions are resected, however, ulceration recurs within a short time. There is a particularly high rate of recurrence at the site of anastomosis, and this may be considered to occur in almost all cases.
- Endoscopy reveals circumferential, shallow ulcers with clear borders at the site of anastomosis. Anastomotic ulcers are also resistant to medical treatment, and scar as a result of total parenteral nutrition.
- Scarring of anastomotic ulcers leads to severe stenosis. Such stenosis can be effectively treated with endoscopic balloon dilation.

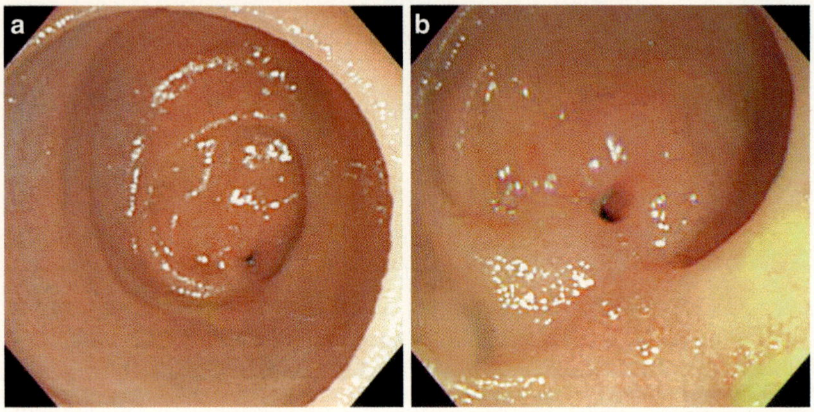

Fig. 20.27

20.9 Case 13 [8]

20.9.1 Male, 70s (Fig. 20.27a, b)

- The patient developed cervical spondylosis following a traffic accident at 40 years old, since which time he had been using indomethacin and diclofenac.
- During this period, intermittent overt bleeding occurred, and recurrent intestinal obstruction had developed a few years previously.
- Endoscopy revealed severe luminal narrowing with convergence of the folds in the middle small intestine (a).
- An open ulcer at the same location was also evident (b).

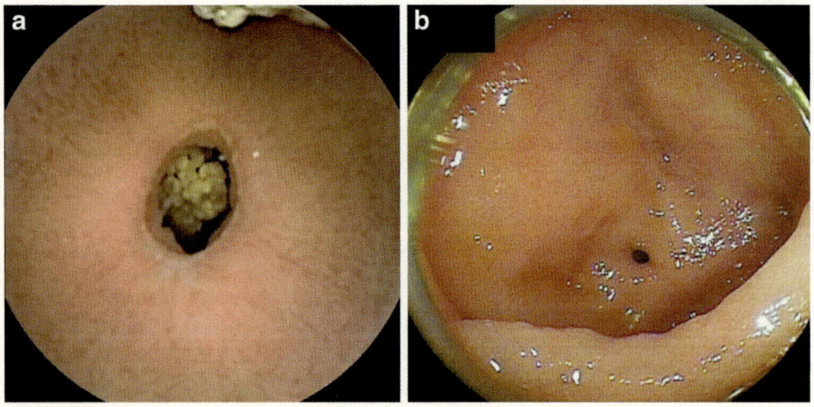

Fig. 20.28

20.9.2 Female, 70s (Fig. 20.28a, b)

- The patient had been undergoing treatment for rheumatoid arthritis since 40 years old. She had also been taking diclofenac for severe pain.
- Constipation and abdominal distension had become pronounced 1 year previously.
- CE showed a circular ulcer and stenosis, with retention (a).
- DBE revealed severe central stenosis, but no open ulcer (b).

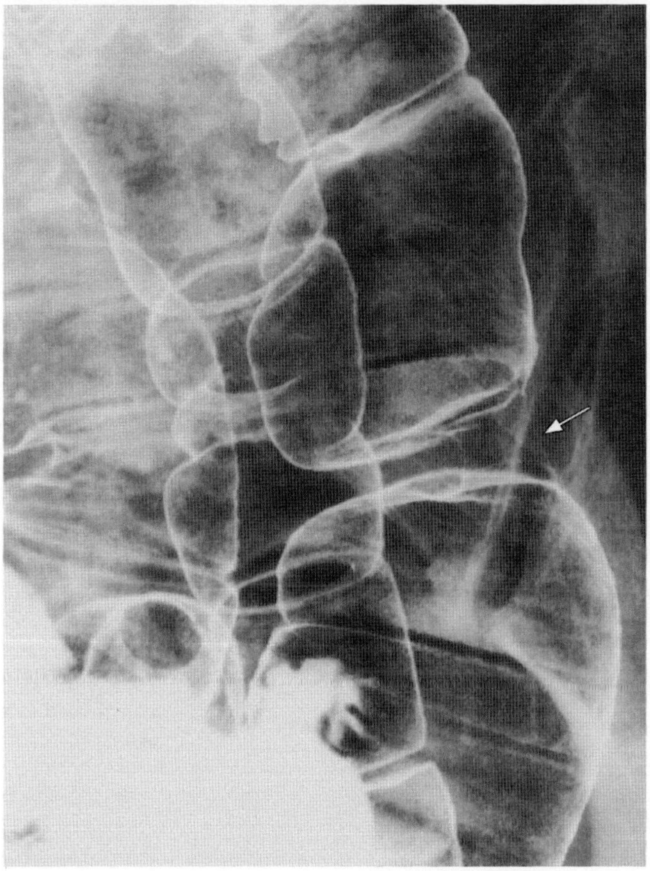

Fig. 20.29 Severe stenosis was evident in the middle small intestine (*arrow*), with prominent folds in neighboring intestinal loops

20.9.3 NSAID-Induced Enteropathy (Fig. 20.29)

- Non-steroidal anti-inflammatory drugs (NSAIDs) are the type of drug that most commonly causes mucosal damage in the small intestine. Patients taking oral NSAIDs exhibit a high rate of small intestinal lesions during small intestinal endoscopy. The most severe type of lesion is diaphragm-like stenosis, which is regarded as the terminal form of small intestinal mucosal damage.
- Endoscopically, diaphragm-like stenosis almost always coincides with healed ulceration.
- This condition occurs more commonly in the middle and lower small intestine, and is visualized radiographically as narrow bilateral luminal narrowing. Multiple healed circular ulcers are also evident at other sites in the small intestine in NSAID-induced diaphragmatic stenosis. Radiographically, at first glance these appear similar to small intestinal folds, and CE should therefore be avoided if the patient has a history of NSAID use.

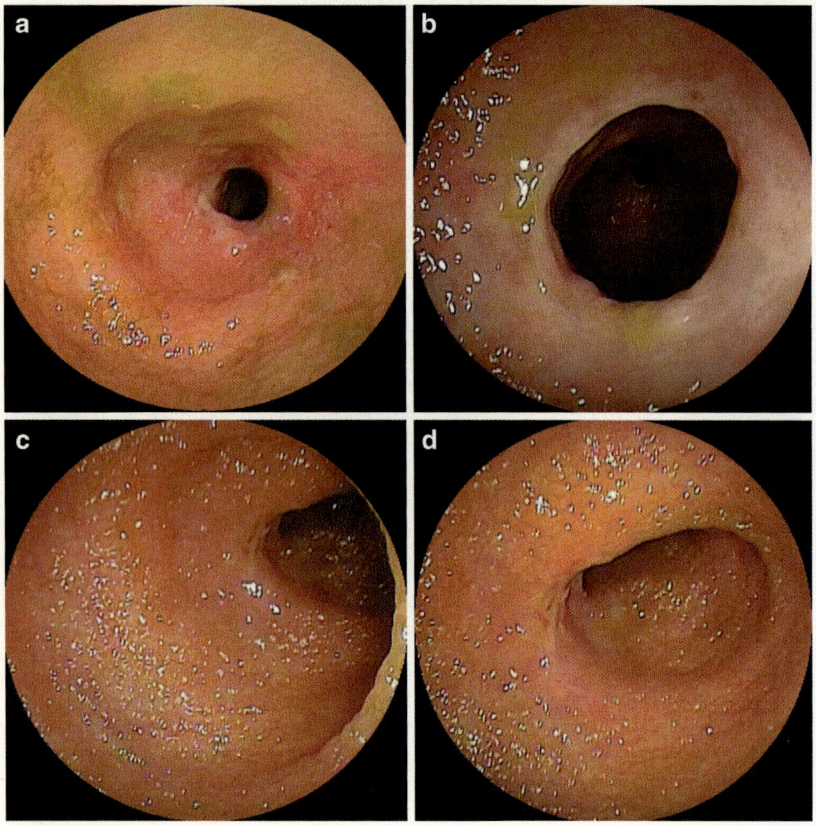

Fig. 20.30

20.10 Case 14 [9]

20.10.1 Male, 50s (Fig. 20.30a–d)

Principal complaints: abdominal pain, vomiting

- The patient had gone into shock due to adrenal failure 2 months previously, with the subsequent appearance of intermittent abdominal pain
- A girdle-like ulcer causing narrowing of the jejunum was evident. Insertion into deeper areas past this site was difficult (a, b).
- The intervening mucosa was edematous and coarse, and Kerckring's folds were indistinct (c, d).

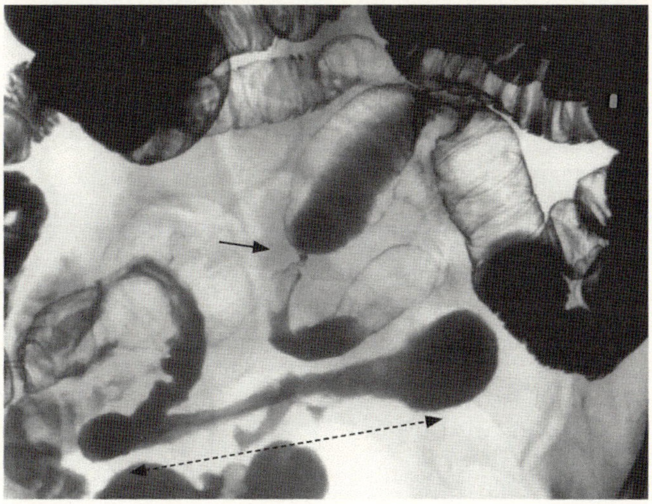

Fig. 20.31 Concentric stenosis (*arrow*), enteric edema, and indistinct Kerckring's folds (*arrow* with *broken line*) were evident

20.10.2 Ischemic Enteritis (Figs. 20.31, 20.32 and 20.33)

- Ischemic enteritis occurs most frequently in men in their 60s.
- Underlying conditions such as hypertension, ischemic heart disease, arrhythmia, and diabetes mellitus are present in around half of cases.
- Principal complaints are abdominal pain, nausea, and melena
- Radiographically, it is characterized by concentric stenosis, edema, and indistinct Kerckring's folds.
- Endoscopic characteristics comprise girdle-like, longitudinal, and circular ulcers, erosions, and granular mucosa.

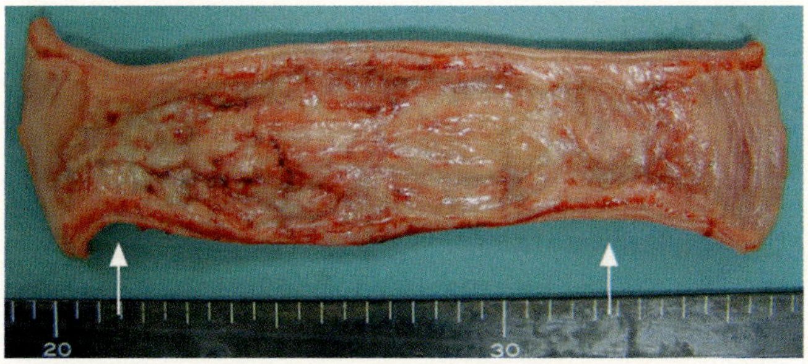

Fig. 20.32 Concentric narrowing, circumferential segmental ulceration, and thickened bowel wall were evident (*arrows*)

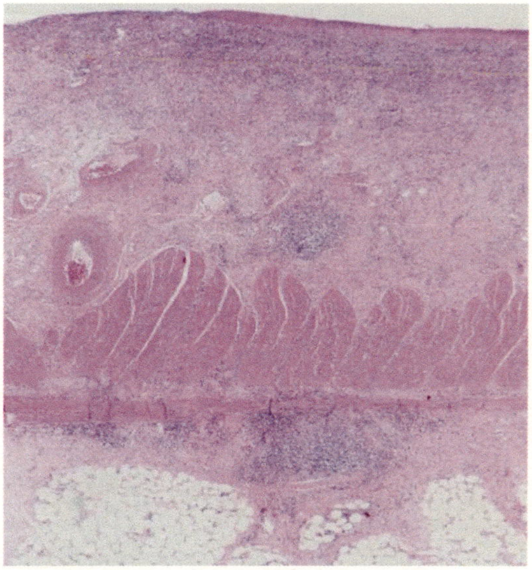

Fig. 20.33 Erosive fibrosis causing thickening of the wall was evident from the submucosa to the subserosa

References

1. Suekane T et al. A case of jejunal choriocarcinoma detected by capsule endoscopy and double-balloon endoscopy. Endoscopy. 2010;42 Suppl 2:E52–3.
2. Coumaros D et al. Diffuse large B-cell lymphoma complicated with jejunal stricture: the palliative role of double-balloon enteroscopy. Am J Gastroenterol. 2008;103:2656–7.
3. Loberant N et al. Enteropathy-associated T-cell lymphoma: a case report with radiographic and computed tomography appearance. J Surg Oncol. 1997;65:50–4.
4. Hirai F et al. Endoscopic balloon dilatation using double-balloon endoscopy is a useful and safe treatment for small intestinal strictures in Crohn's disease. Dig Endosc. 2010;22:200–4.
5. Lee CR et al. Colonoscopic findings in intestinal Behçet's disease. Inflamm Bowel Dis. 2001;7:243–9.
6. Misra SP et al. Ileoscopy in patients with ileocolonic tuberculosis. World J Gastroenterol. 2007;13:1723–7.
7. Matsumoto T et al. Endoscopic features of chronic nonspecific multiple ulcers of the small intestine: comparison with NSAID-enteropathy. Dig Dis Sci. 2006;51:1357–63.
8. Matsumoto T et al. Double-contrast barium enteroclysis as a patency tool for nonsteroidal anti-inflammatory drug-induced enteropathy. Dig Dis Sci. 2011;56:3247–53.
9. Nishimura N et al. Balloon dilation when using double-balloon enteroscopy for small-bowel strictures associated with ischemic enteritis. Gastrointest Endosc. 2011;74:1157–61.

21 Case Presentations: Hemorrhagic Lesions

Tomonori Yano, Mayumi Kodama, Tomohiko Moriyama, and Ken Kinjo

21.1 Case 1 [1]

21.1.1 Male, 50s (Fig. 21.1a–d)

- The patient showed advanced iron-deficiency anemia and persistently positive results from fecal occult blood tests with no overt bleeding.
- Underlying disease: anti-coagulation therapy following valve replacement.
- A small amount of bloody intestinal fluid and a redness 2-mm in size were evident in the distal jejunum (Type 1b) (a, b)
- Oozing started as a result of stimulation by water used for flushing (c)
- Argon plasma coagulation (APC) was performed briefly for diathermy, after physiological saline was injected locally (d).

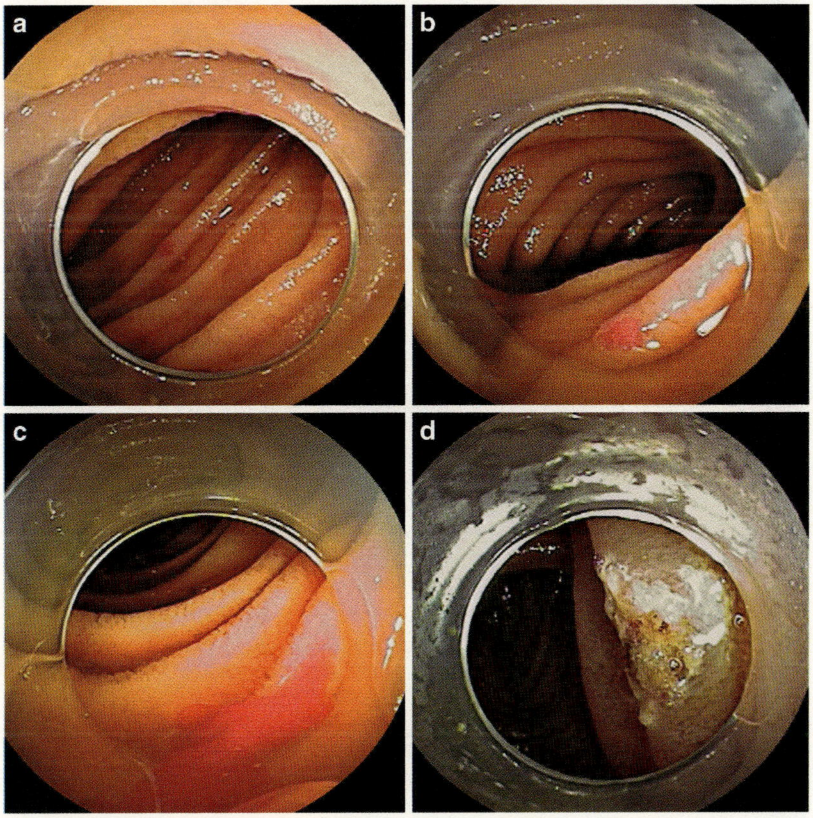

Fig. 21.1

T. Yano (✉)
Department of Internal Medicine, Division of Gastroenterology, Jichi Medical University, 3311-1 Yakushiji, Shimotsuke 329-0498, Japan
e-mail: tomonori@jichi.ac.jp

M. Kodama
Center for Digestive and Liver Diseases, Miyazaki Medical Center Hospital, 2-16 Takamatsu-cho, Miyazaki 880-0003, Japan

T. Moriyama
Department of Medicine and Clinical Science, Graduate School of Medical Sciences, Kyushu University, 3-1-1, Maidashi, Higashi-ku, Fukuoka 812-8582, Japan

K. Kinjo
Department of Gastroenterology, Fukuoka University Chikushi Hospital, 1-1-1 Zokumyoin, Chikushino 818-8502, Japan

T. Matsui et al. (eds.), *Endoscopy in the Diagnosis of Small Intestine Diseases*, DOI 10.1007/978-4-431-54352-7_21, © Springer Japan 2014

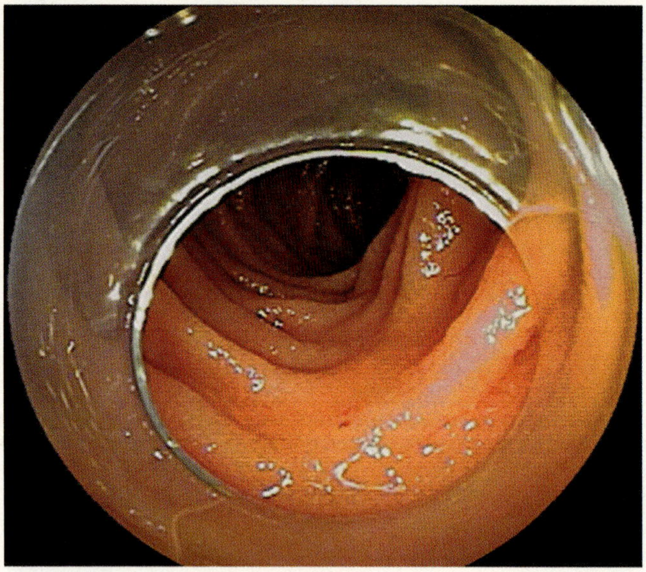

Fig. 21.2

21.1.2 Type 1 Vascular Lesions (Angiodysplasia) of the Small Intestine (Fig. 21.2)

- Among vascular lesions of the gastrointestinal tract, the condition that comprises tortuous abnormal blood vessels with the properties of veins or capillaries composed of a thin vascular wall without an internal elastic lamina is referred to by various different terms, including angiodysplasia, angioectasia, angiectasia, telangiectasia, and vascular ectasia.
- Types 1a and 1b in the endoscopic classification of vascular lesions of the small intestine are regarded as corresponding to this condition, and are considered to represent good candidates for diathermy. Simultaneous and asynchronous multiple occurrence is common, and caution is required.

An examination on the same day revealed endoscopic classification Type 1a petechial redness (vascular lesions of the small intestine) in two places, and diathermy was performed using an argon plasma coagulator (APC).

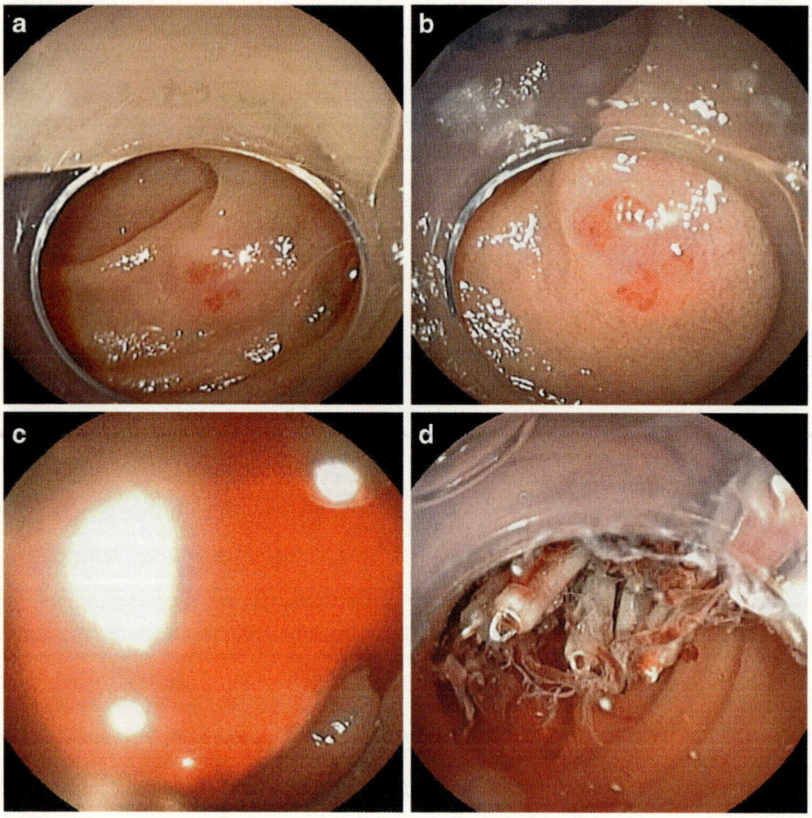

Fig. 21.3

21.2 Case 2 [1]

21.2.1 Female, 80s (Fig. 21.3a–d)

Principal complaints: tarry stool, anemia

- Underlying disease: chronic hepatitis C
- A 3-mm pulsating red protrusion (Type 2b) (a, b) was evident in the proximal jejunum, and was treated with hemostatic clipping.
- Massive bleeding occurred after marking clips had been placed in the area and a hemostatic clip applied, and the field of view deteriorated.
- Clips were added using the relative positions of the marking clips as indicators, and hemostasis was confirmed by underwater observation (c, d).

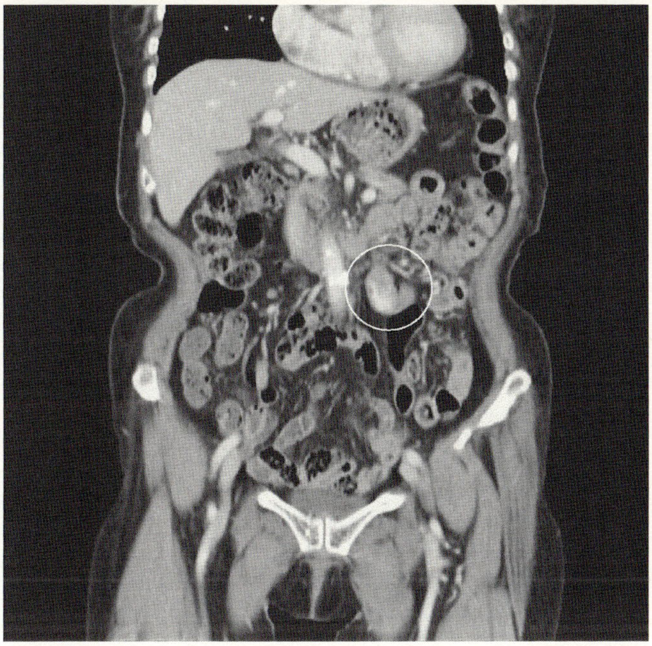

Fig. 21.4

21.2.2 Type 2 Vascular Lesions (Angiodysplasia) of the Small Intestine (Fig. 21.4)

- Among the vascular lesions of the gastrointestinal tract, a condition that comprises the presence of abnormally broad arterial vessels in the submucosa and bleeding from a mucosal defect is known as Dieulafoy's lesion.
- Types 2a and 2b in the endoscopic classification of vascular lesions of the small intestine are regarded as corresponding to this condition, and are considered to represent good candidates for treatment with hemostatic clip.
- Type 2a comprises minute petechial lesions, which are extremely difficult to find once they have stopped bleeding. Timing examinations carefully while lesions are bleeding is therefore important.

Type 2b is considered to involve broader angiodysplasia, and as the field of view may be lost during treatment, it is vital to start treatment after placing marking clips in the neighborhood of the lesion.

Contrast agent leakage (inside circle) was evident in the jejunum in the upper left abdomen.

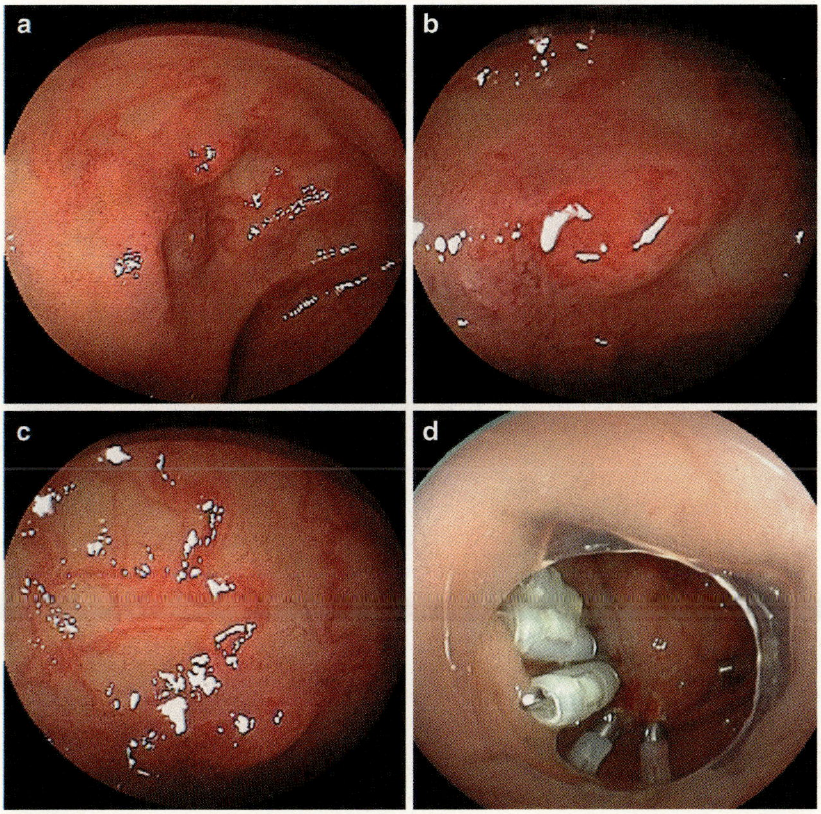

Fig. 21.5

21.3 Case 3 [1]

21.3.1 Female, 70s (Fig. 21.5a–d)

Principal complaint: tarry stool

- Underlying diseases: history of emphysema and cerebral aneurysm
- A pulsatile red protrusion with dilation and tortuosity of the surrounding vessels was present in the distal ileum (a–c).
- Endoscopic ultrasound (EUS) later confirmed feeding vessels, and treatment was carried out by ligation with hemostatic clips (d).

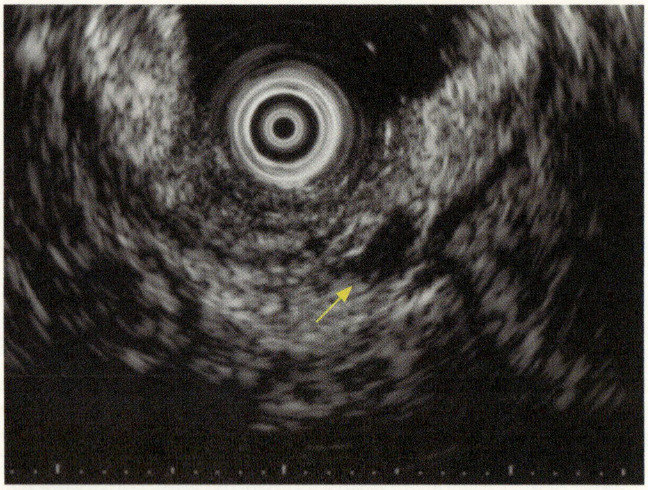

Fig. 21.6

21.3.2 Type 3 Vascular Lesions (Angiodysplasia) of the Small Intestine (Fig. 21.6)

- Among vascular lesions of the gastrointestinal tract, a condition that comprises a reciprocal connection between vessels with arterial properties that possess an internal elastic lamina and vessels with venous properties that do not possess an internal elastic lamina is known as arteriovenous malformation (AVM). Lesions may not be localized to the mucosa or submucosal layers, but extend throughout the entire thickness of the intestinal wall.
- Type 3 in the endoscopic classification of vascular lesions of the small intestine is regarded as corresponding to this condition. Surgical resection or transcatheter arterial embolization should be considered for large lesions, but treating comparatively small lesions endoscopically by ligating feeding vessels with clips may be possible.

A structure believed to constitute a feeding vessel from outside the intestinal wall and a drainage vessel was evident (*arrow*).

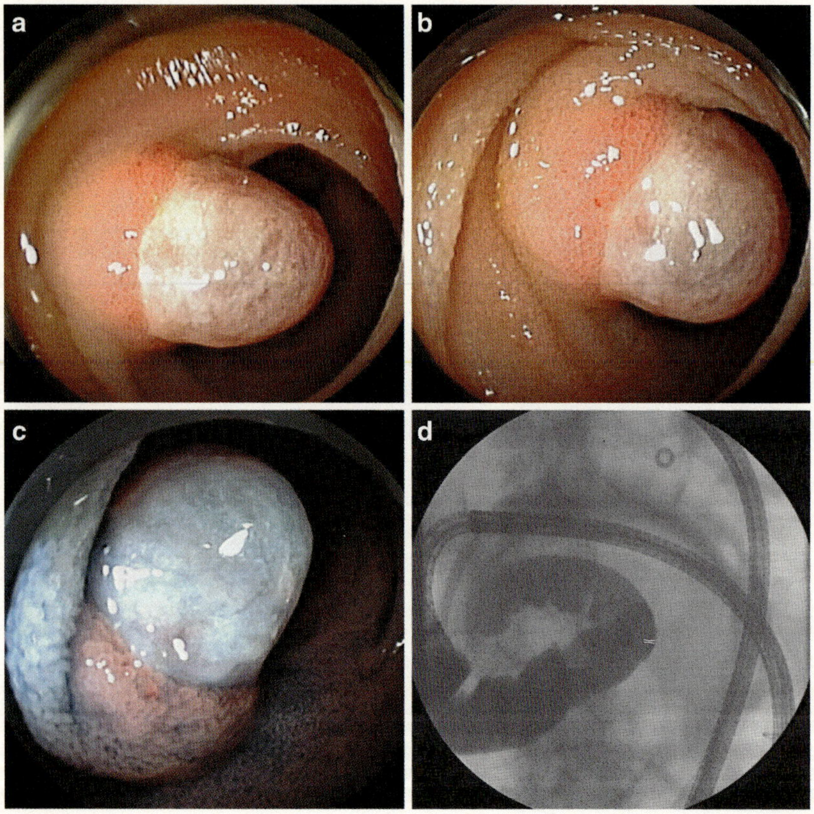

Fig. 21.7

21.4 Case 4 [2]

21.4.1 Male, 60s (Fig. 21.7a–d)

Principal complaint: tarry stool

- Underlying disease: none
- A bluish-white protruding lesion 10 mm in size protruding from the submucosa was evident in the proximal ileum (a, b).
- Examination after spraying with indigo carmine. The mucosa had detached and appeared translucent (c).
- Selective contrast with the balloon at the tip of the DBE inflated showed a 10-mm protruding lesion (d).
- After tattooing and marking clip placement, laparoscopy-assisted partial ileal resection was performed.

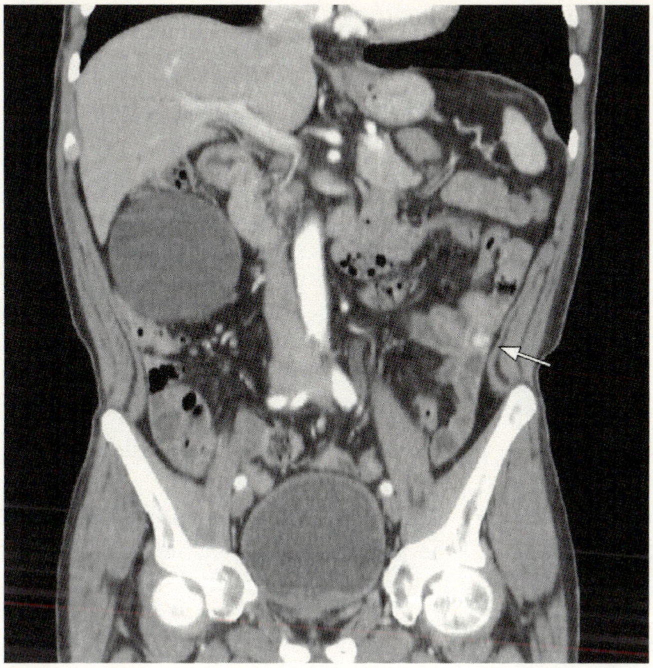

Fig. 21.8 A small, contrasted tumor was evident in the intestine of the left lower abdomen (*arrow*)

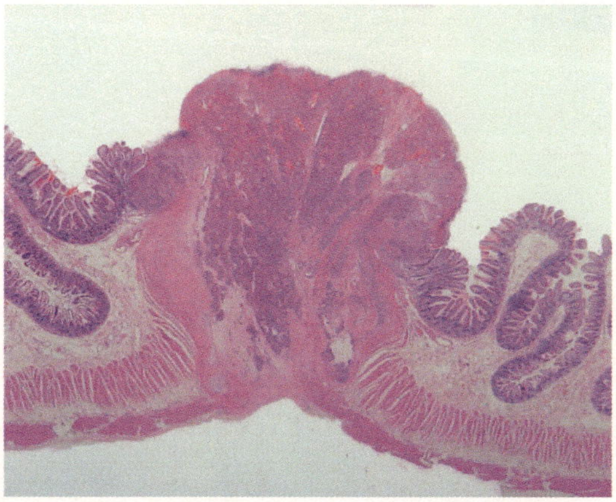

Fig. 21.9 The mucosa was detached, and there was prominent internal inflammatory cell infiltration

21.4.2 Pyogenic Granuloma (Figs. 21.8 and 21.9)

- Hemangiomas are benign lesions formed by the proliferation of blood vessels, and are broadly divided into capillary hemangioma, cavernous hemangioma, mixed type, and pyogenic granuloma. Pyogenic granuloma characteristically arises more commonly on the skin of the hands and feet or in the oral mucosa, appearing as a pronounced protrusion from the surface of the skin or mucosa that exhibits a lobular structure, with ulceration frequently forming in the surface layer. Lesions are believed to grow rapidly until they reach a certain size. Pyogenic granuloma in the intestine has been reported, albeit rarely, and in such cases the lesions adopt a polypoid morphology, frequently with surface ulceration.
- Histologically, capillary proliferation and formation of granulation tissue with infiltration by inflammatory cells, including neutrophils, is evident (Fig. 21.9).

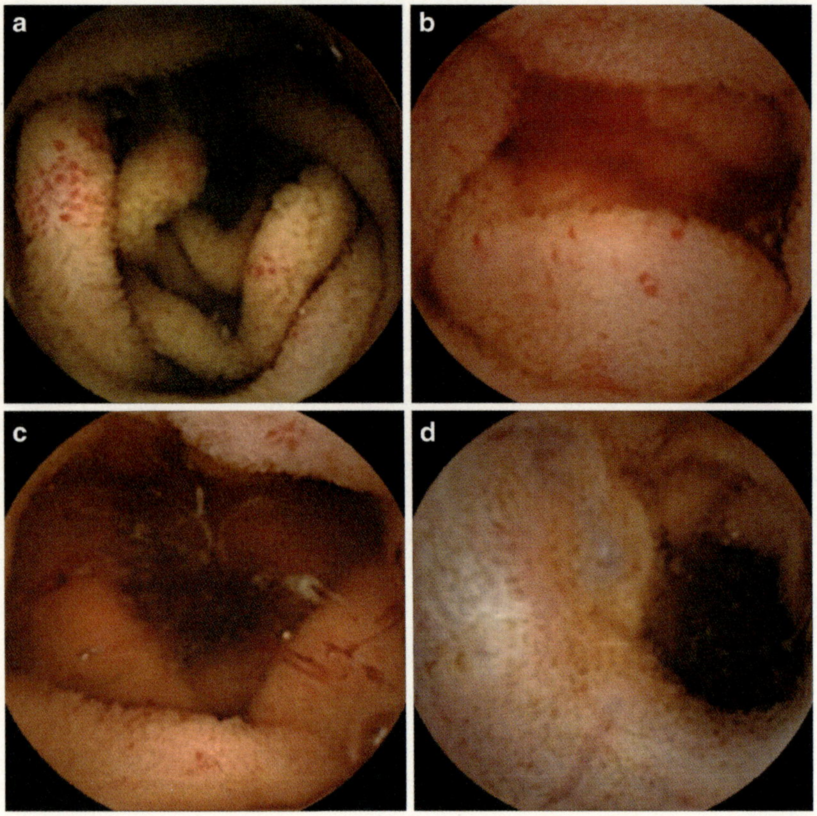

Fig. 21.10

21.5 Case 5 [3]

21.5.1 Female, 80s (Fig. 21.10a–d)

- Principal complaints were anemia and positive results for fecal occult blood testing. Upper gastrointestinal endoscopy and colonoscopy were unable to identify the source of bleeding in this case
- Underlying disease: liver cirrhosis (type C virus)
- CE revealed erosive edema of the small intestinal villi, with multiple reddened villi and bleeding (a–c).
- There were multiple points of bleeding in the jejunum and ileum, and varices were evident in the ileum (d).

21.5.2 Portal Hypertensive Enteropathy (Fig. 21.11a–c)

- Liver cirrhosis, extrahepatic portal vein obstruction, and other underlying diseases causing portal hypertension may cause small intestinal lesions. Principal complaints are melena or anemia. This condition may be suspected in patients exhibiting obscure gastrointestinal bleeding in whom the source of bleeding has not been identified by upper and lower gastrointestinal examinations.
- Characteristic endoscopic findings comprise: (1) diffuse abnormality of small intestinal villi (villous edema, villous redness, villous atrophy); and (2) diffuse vascular lesions (angiodysplasia-like findings, dilation/proliferation of arterioles, varices) (Figs.21.11 and 21.12)

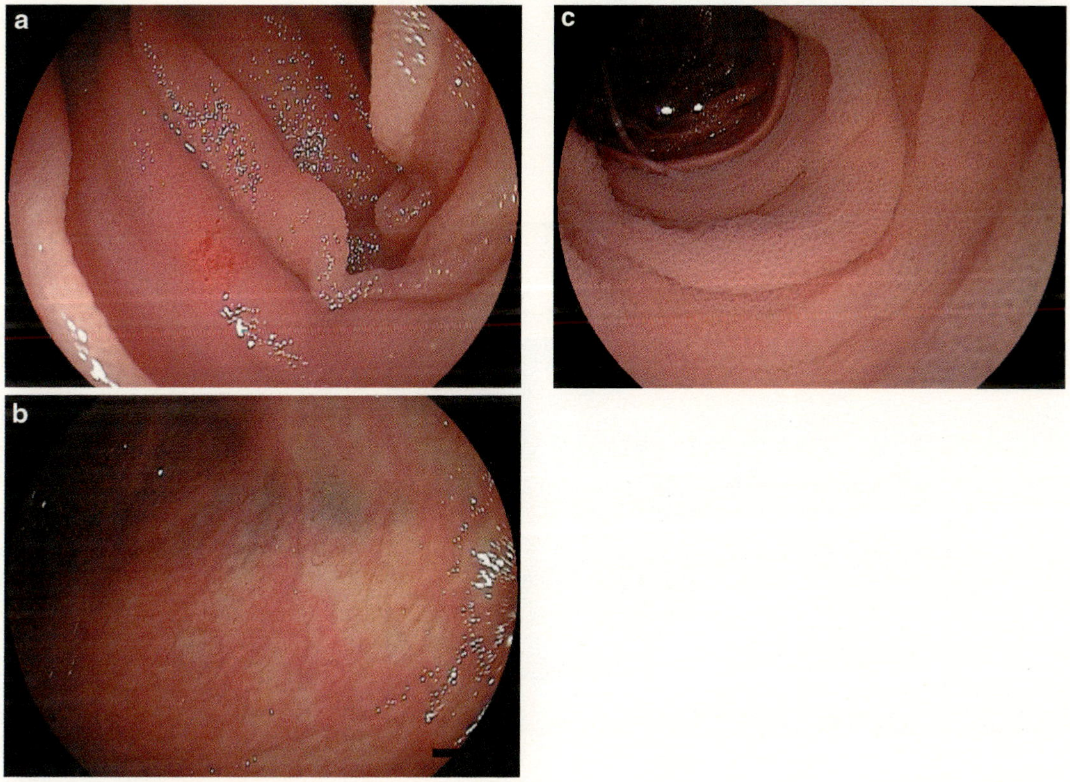

Fig. 21.11 (**a**) Villi were edematous, with bleeding from angiodysplasia-like findings. (**b**) Findings of dilation/proliferation of arterioles. (**c**) Observation of villous edema by the submersion method

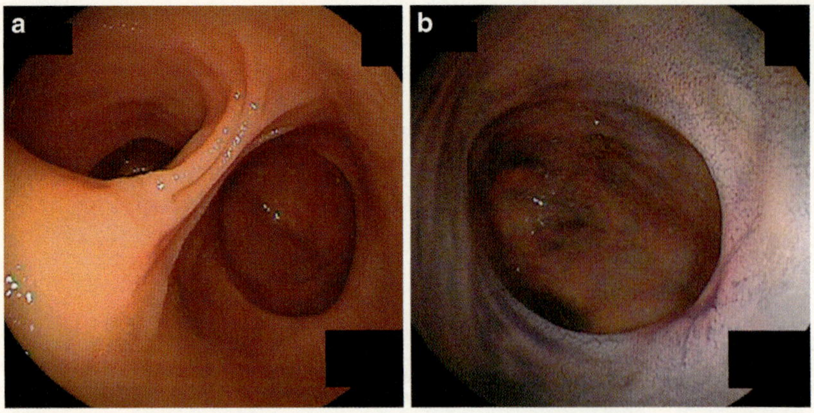

Fig. 21.12

21.6 Case 6, 7 [4]

21.6.1 Male, 40s (Fig. 20.12a, b)

Principal complaints: fresh melena, anemia

- A luminal structure protruding from the small intestinal lumen was evident in the lower ileum. The protruding lumen formed a blind loop.
- The blind loop contained an almost healed ulcer causing mild deformation.
- Only villous epithelium was present within the blind loop, and there were no findings suggesting ectopic gastric mucosa.

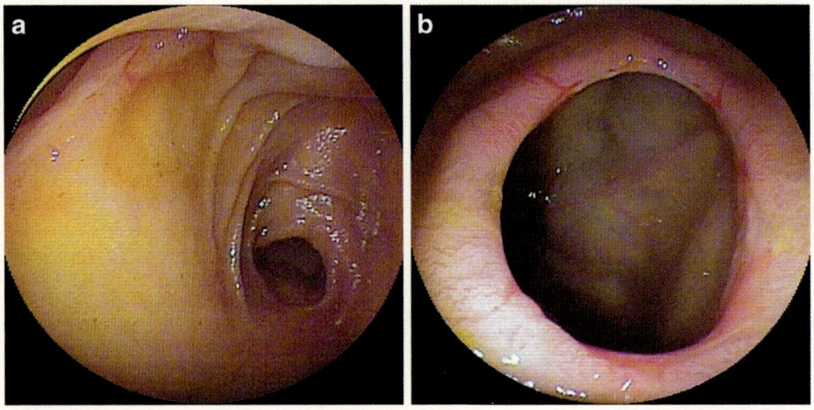

Fig. 21.13

21.6.2 Female, 40s (Fig. 21.13a, b)

Principal complaint: Fresh melena. The patient was taking NSAIDs for abdominal pain.

- A dilated cystic lumen branched off from the ileum, forming a blind loop.
- The cystic lumen contained a narrow, clearly demarcated circular ulcer, causing narrowing.
- The villi surrounding the circular ulcer had a flattened appearance. The lumen did not contain any ectopic gastric mucosa.

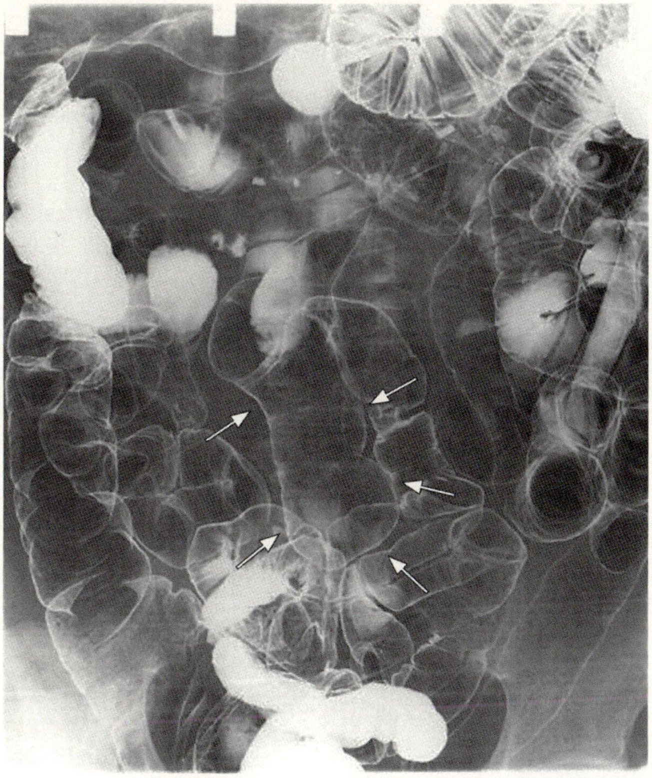

Fig. 21.14 A clavate diverticulum branching off the ileum was evident (*arrows*). The interior of the diverticulum was deformed by bow-shaped injury scarring

21.6.3 Meckel's Diverticulum (Figs. 21.14 and 21.15)

- This is a congenital true diverticulum caused by persistence of the yolk duct, which is present on the antimesenteric side.
- It occurs in 1–2 % of the total population, with a male–female ratio of 1:1 in autopsy cases.
- Aberrant heterotopic tissue is present in over 50 % of cases, and frequently comprises gastric tissue
- The majority of cases are asymptomatic, but melena may occur in patients with erosions or ulceration within the diverticulum or the neighboring ileum.
- It can be recognized both radiographically and endoscopically as a blind pocket branching off the ileum.
- Inversion may also occur, albeit rarely, in which case the structure is visualized as a soft, clavate tumor.

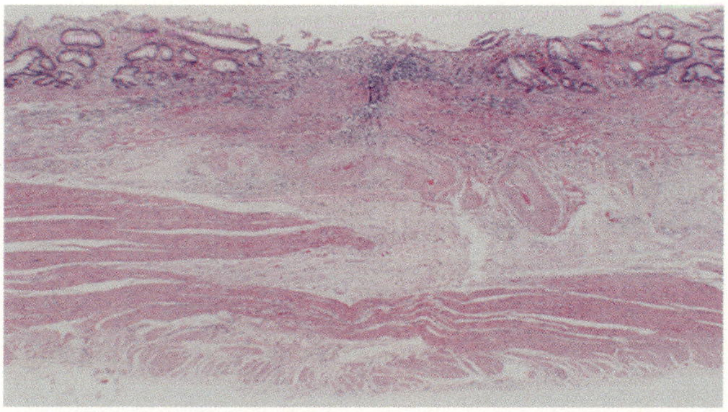

Fig. 21.15 This diverticulum was a true diverticulum with a muscle layer, thickening of part of the muscularis mucosa and disruption of the laminar structure, as well as shallow ulceration and fibrosis

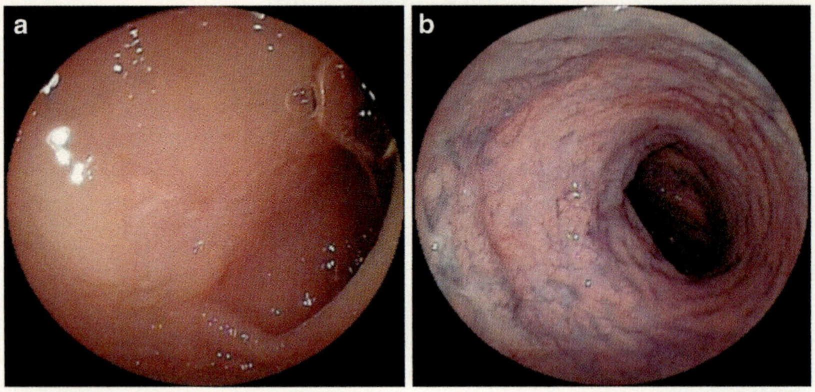

Fig. 21.16

21.7 Case 8, 9

21.7.1 Female, 70s (Fig. 21.16a, b)

- Abdominal pain, diarrhea. Positive results were obtained from fecal occult blood testing, and anemia was evident (Hb 8.6 g/dL).
- A 4-mm round erosion covered in a white coat was evident in the terminal ileum, with coarse surrounding mucosa.
- The coarse mucosa was clearly visualized by dye spraying, and was mildly granular.
- Biopsy showed only non-specific inflammatory findings.

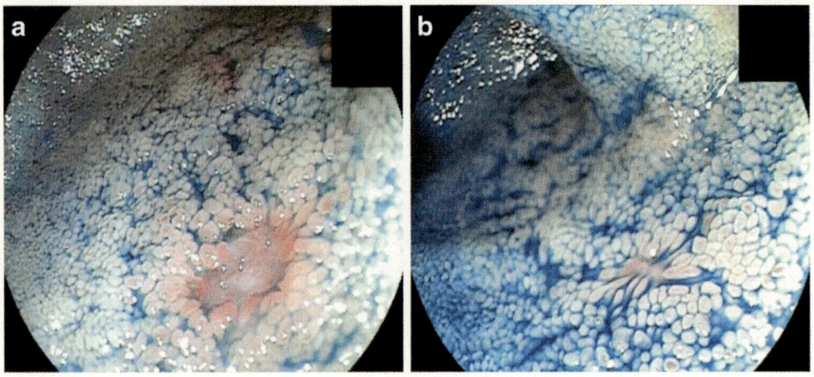

Fig. 21.17

21.7.2 Male, 30s (Fig. 21.17a, b)

- The principal complaint was diarrhea that had continued for 2 years
- The ileal mucosa was coarse.
- The left-hand image shows a 3- to 4-mm erosion in the terminus of the ileum, with a thin white coat within the depression.
- The right-hand image shows a small erosion around 1 mm in diameter in the ileum, with loss of villous structure in the center.

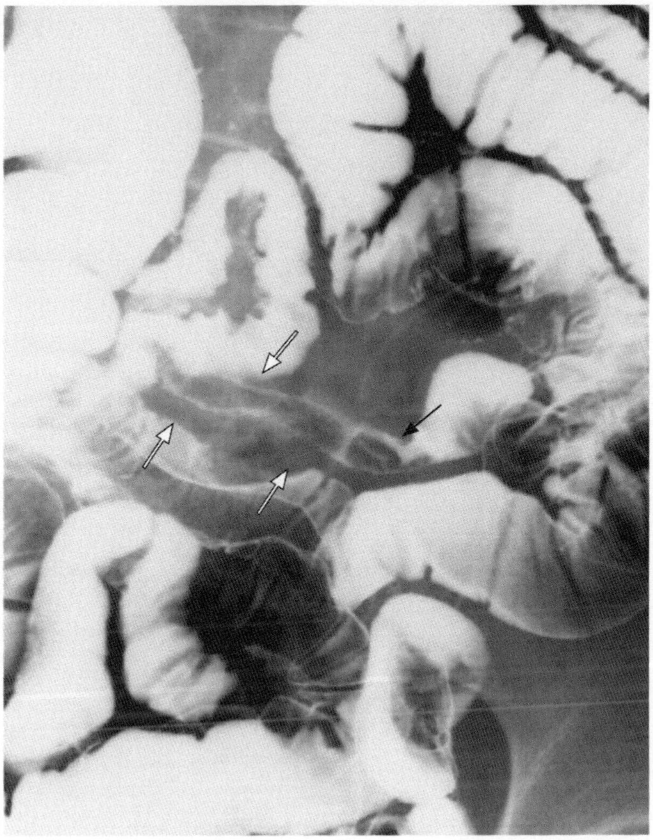

Fig. 21.18 Case 8: An erosion (*black arrow*) containing a barium fleck and filling defect was evident in the terminal ileum in a location consistent with the endoscopic findings on the *left-hand page*. The small intestinal wall also showed a fluffy appearance (*white arrows*), and the mucosa displayed a coarse appearance

21.7.3 Lesions of Unknown Etiology (Fig. 21.18)

- Small lesions (aphthae, redness, and small erosions) are of low radiographic detectability. The spread of small intestinal endoscopy, however, has enabled the acquisition of good-quality images. This has led to an increase in the detection of small intestinal lesions of unknown etiology without the presence of major lesions.
- Non-specific small lesions constitute a mild inflammatory condition, and most are transient.
- In cases of lesions of unknown etiology, lesions frequently comprise only aphthae/erosions with no tendency to regular arrangement. Single ulcers or erosions may also be of unknown etiology, and differentiation from specific diseases (such as Crohn's disease and ulcerative colitis) must be made.

References

1. Yano T et al. Endoscopic classification of vascular lesions of the small intestine (with videos). Gastrointest Endosc. 2008;67:169–72.
2. Shinozaki S et al. Long-term outcome of patients with obscure gastrointestinal bleeding investigated by double-balloon endoscopy. Clin Gastroenterol Hepatol. 2010;8:151–8.
3. Kodama M et al. Endoscopic characterization of the small bowel in patients with portal hypertension evaluated by double balloon endoscopy. J Gastroenterol. 2008;43:589–96.
4. Turgeon DK, Barnett JL. Meckel's diverticulum. Am J Gastrotenterol. 1990;85:777–81.

22 Case Presentations: Reddened Lesions

Ken Kinjo, Satoshi Ishikawa, Takahiro Beppu, Mitsue Sogawa, and Kenji Watanabe

22.1 Case 1 [1]

22.1.1 Male, 20s (Fig. 22.1a–d)

- The patient had pain in the right knee, with the appearance of purpura on both legs. Abdominal pain was subsequently evident.
- Upper gastrointestinal endoscopy revealed no esophageal or gastric abnormalities.
- Severe mucosal redness was evident in the duodenal bulb (a, b).
- Pronounced friability, redness, edema, and ulceration were present from the second part of the duodenum.
- CE was performed the day before upper gastrointestinal endoscopy to investigate small intestinal lesions in detail.
- Petechial redness and aphthae were visible from the upper jejunum to the ileum (c, d).

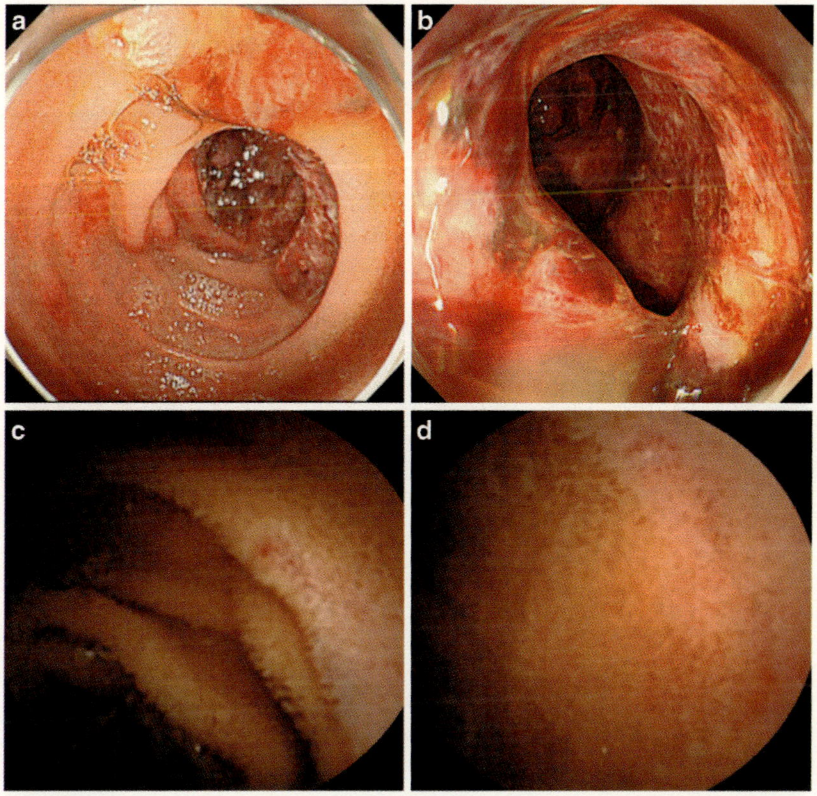

Fig. 22.1

K. Kinjo (✉) • S. Ishikawa • T. Beppu
Department of Gastroenterology, Fukuoka University Chikushi Hospital, 1-1-1 Zokumyoin, Chikushino 818-8502, Japan
e-mail: kentamabukuro@yahoo.co.jp

M. Sogawa • K. Watanabe
Department of Gastroenterology, Osaka City University Graduate School of Medicine, 1-4-3 Asahi-machi, Abeno-ku, Osaka 545-8585, Japan

T. Matsui et al. (eds.), *Endoscopy in the Diagnosis of Small Intestine Diseases*,
DOI 10.1007/978-4-431-54352-7_22, © Springer Japan 2014

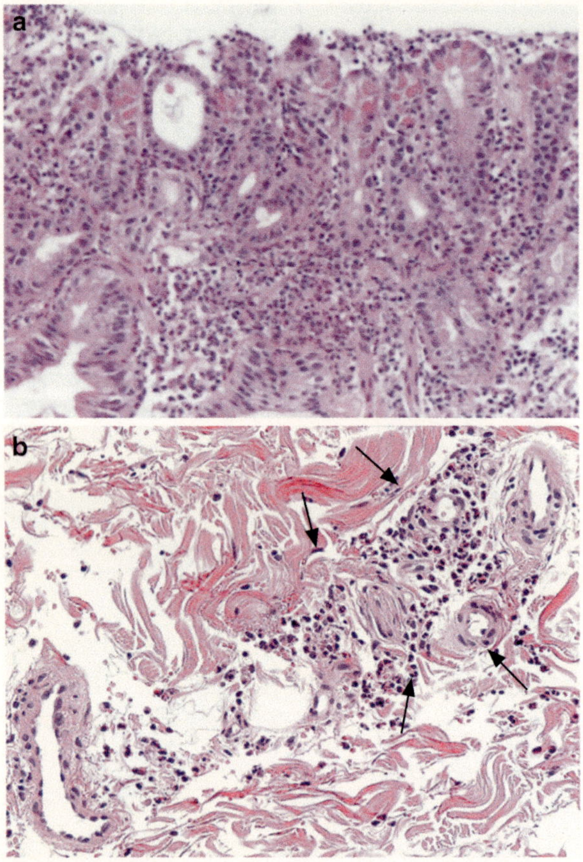

Fig. 22.2 (**a**) Histopathological findings from duodenal biopsy revealed inflammatory cells (neutrophils) in the epithelium. (**b**) Skin biopsy revealed findings of leukocytoclastic vasculitis (neutrophils surrounding blood vessels, destuctecd neutrophils, and fibrin deposits)

22.1.2 Schönlein-Henoch Purpura (Figs. 22.2 and 22.3)

- This condition is caused by an allergic reaction to group A streptococcus infection, drugs, or metal, resulting in Ig A-induced vasculitis.
- This condition frequently occurs in children, and is rare in adults (children, 1 in 10,000 people; adults, 1 in 1–10 million people).
- It often causes purpura on the legs, joint pain, and abdominal pain, but may also cause gastrointestinal symptoms such as vomiting, bloody stool, and constipation, as well as renal symptoms such as hematuria and proteinuria.
- Endoscopically, it is characterized by changes similar to those seen in ischemic colitis, with mucosal edema, redness, erosions, bleeding, and irregular ulceration.

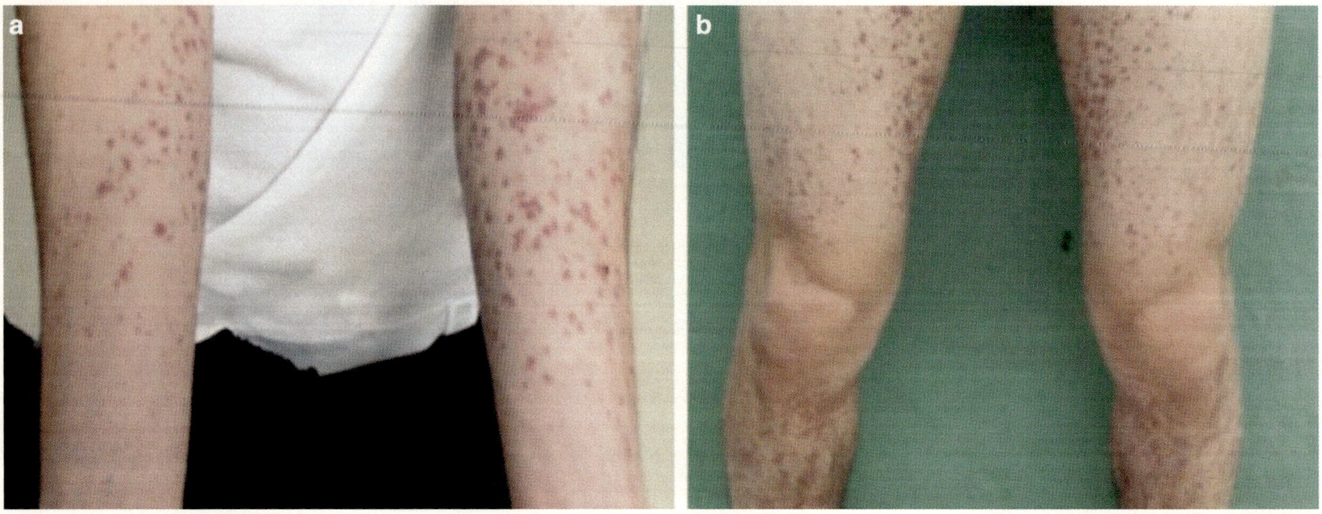

Fig. 22.3 Purpura was present on both legs

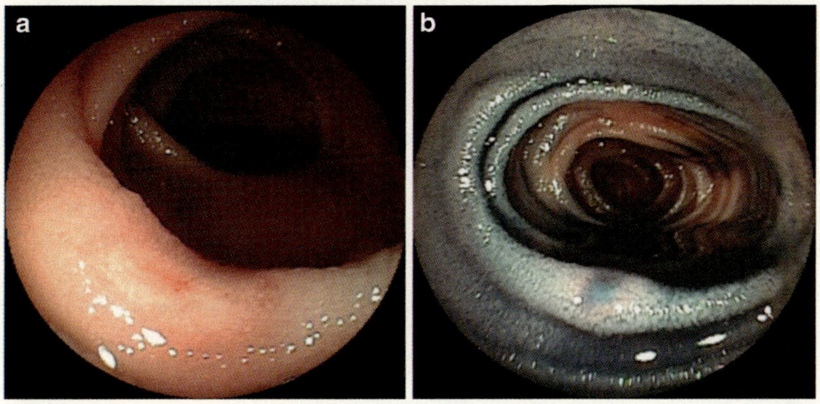

Fig. 22.4

22.2 Case 2, 3 [2]

22.2.1 Female, 70s (Fig. 22.4a, b)

Principal complaints: abdominal pain, bloody stool

- The patient was taking low-dose aspirin for an old cerebral infarction and angina pectoris.
- DBE revealed scattered oval or round small ulcers and erosions in the ileum, some of which were friable.

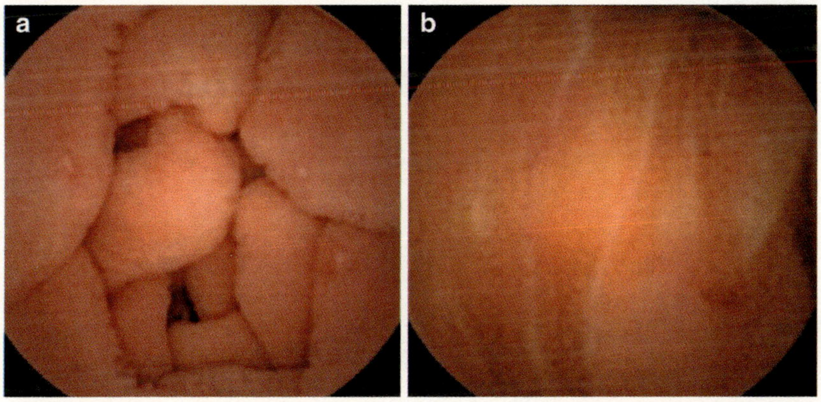

Fig. 22.5

22.2.2 Female, 50s (Fig. 22.5a, b)

Principal complaint: positive fecal occult blood test

- The patient suffered from conditions including hypertension and hyperlipidemia, and had been taking low-dose aspirin long-term to prevent thrombosis.
- Colonoscopic observation of the small intestine revealed redness and aphthae in the large intestine, and CE was performed.
- Redness, aphthae, and small erosions were scattered throughout the small intestine (b), and ulceration was also evident (a).

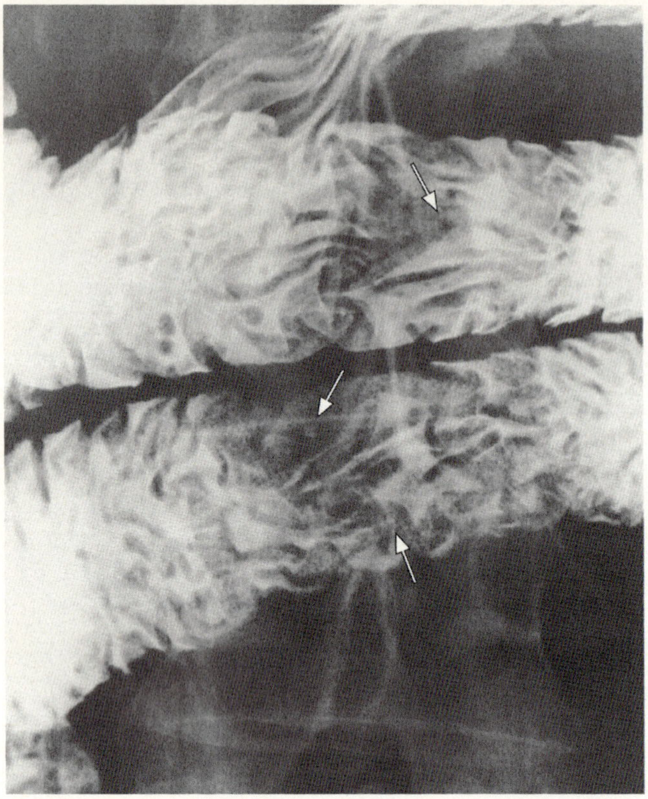

Fig. 22.6 Case 3: radiographic image prior to endoscopy. Aphthae were scattered from the jejunum to the ileum (*arrows*)

22.2.3 Aspirin-Induced Enteropathy (Fig. 22.6)

- This condition may be lacking in symptoms.
- Lower gastrointestinal endoscopy was performed due to positive results of fecal occult blood testing, and the small intestine was examined as redness and aphthae were scattered in the large intestine. Radiography showed aphthae in the small intestine, and the same lesions were also evident on CE.
- There was a tendency for multiple redness, erosions, and ulceration, and lesions were found in both the jejunum and ileum. There was no consistent positional relationship with the mesentery.
- Treatment basically consists of discontinuation of medication.
- Histopathologically, apoptotic bodies, congestion, edema, lymphangiectasia, and epithelial juvenilization are seen comparatively frequently.

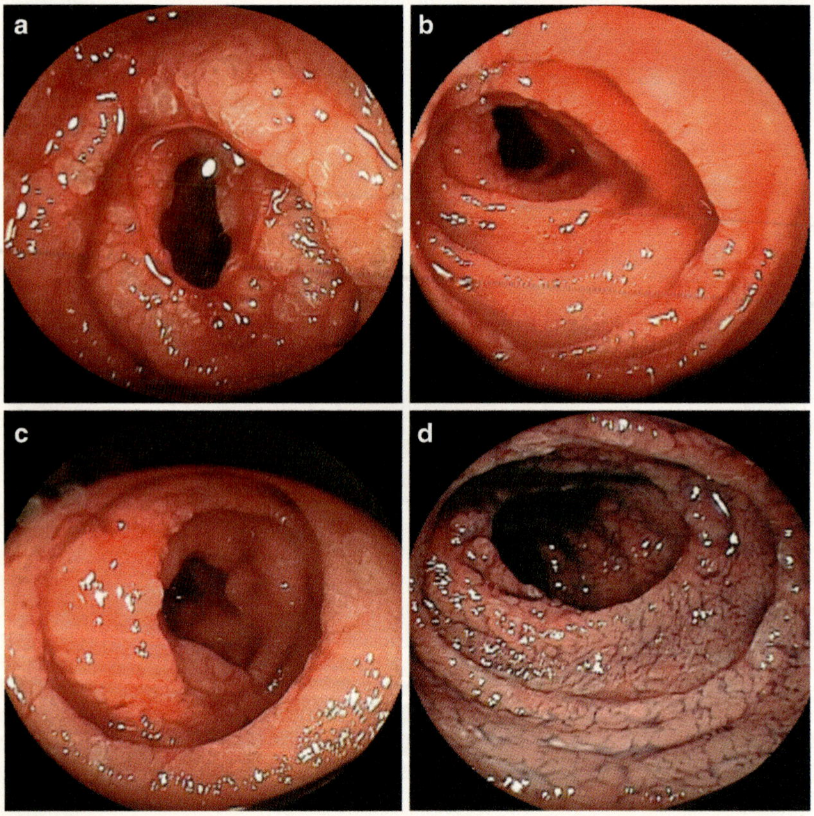

Fig. 22.7

22.3 Case 4 [3]

22.3.1 Male, 60s (Fig. 22.7a–d)

- Onset occurred with acute abdominal pain.
- Coarse, granular mucosa that displayed continuous redness and was friable was evident in the jejunum (a, b).
- Mild luminal narrowing was present, but there was no severe stenosis and DBE passage was easy.
- Reddened mucosa and erosions covered with a thin layer of white mucus were evident (c).
- Dye spraying revealed granular/edematous mucosa (d).

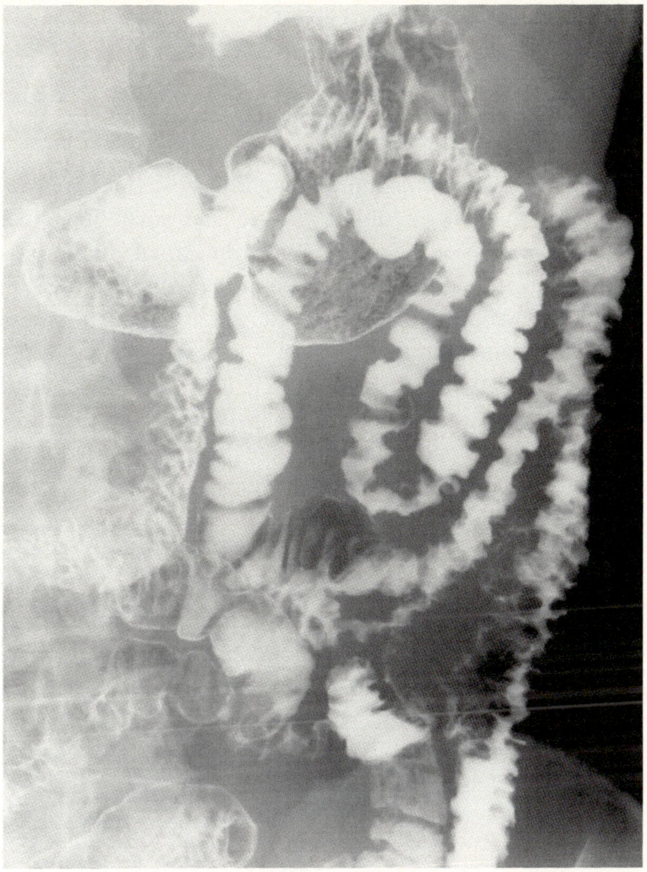

Fig. 22.8 The thumbprinting sign, mild tubular stenosis, thickening of Kerckring's folds, and granular filling defects were evident across a wide area from the jejunum to the middle small intestine

22.3.2 Ischemic Enteritis (Fig. 22.8)

- Ischemic enteritis commonly occurs in men in their 60s. Principal complaints include sudden abdominal pain, nausea, and melena. In its transient form, symptoms disappear and patients improve within a few days to 3 weeks.
- Radiographic imaging of the small intestine shows the thumbprinting sign, mild tubular stenosis, enteric edema, thickening of Kerckring's folds, and granular filling defects across a wide area of the jejunum. Lesions were continuous from the jejunum to the middle small intestine.
- Macroscopically, characteristics of this pathology include concentric stenosis, circumferential segmental ulceration, comparatively pronounced thickening of the intestinal wall at the site of stenosis, and granular changes to the surface.

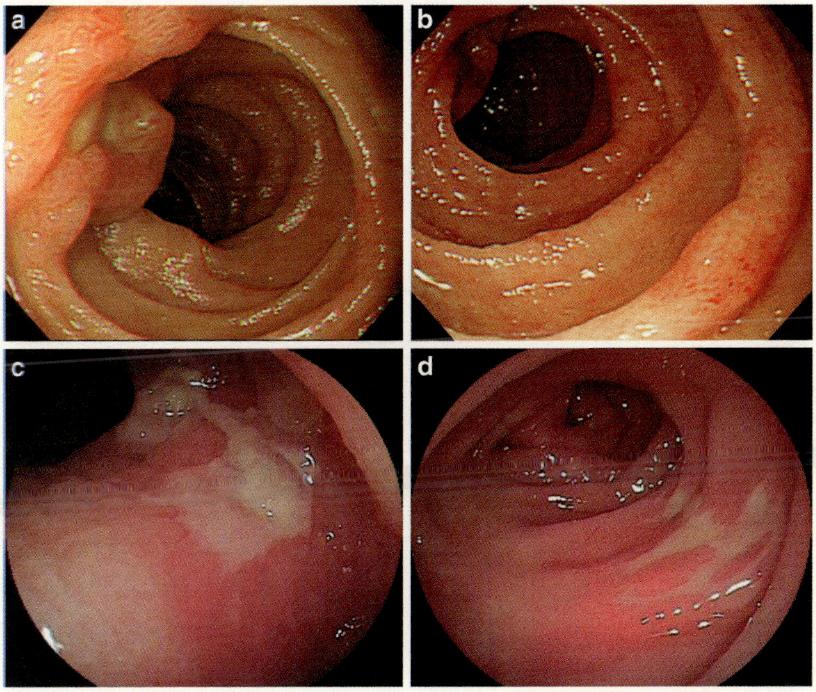

Fig. 22.9

22.4 Case 5 [4]

22.4.1 Male, 70s (Fig. 22.9a–d)

- Onset occurred with drug-induced generalized erythema, watery diarrhea, and abdominal pain. Peripheral blood eosinophilia (27 %, 3,348/μL) was present.
- Ulceration and a reddened protrusion were present in the second part of the duodenum. The mucosa of the entire second part was edematous, with scattered redness (a, b).
- DBE revealed multiple geographic ulcers with a white coat and mucosal redness in the lower ileum (c, d).

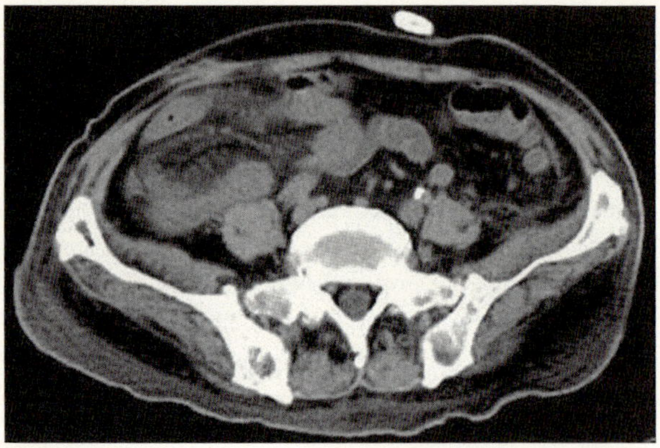

Fig. 22.10 Biopsy histopathology revealed infiltration by a large number of eosinophils

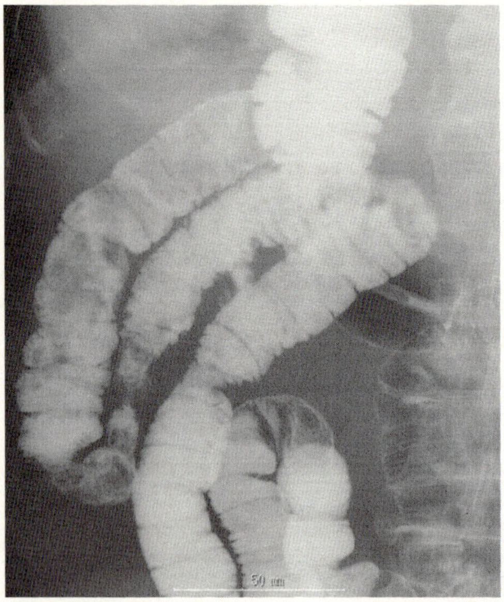

Fig. 22.11 Looping shadows of the mesentery were evident, together with fluid accumulation and edematous thickening of the intestinal tract

22.4.2 Eosinophilic Enteritis (Figs. 22.10, 22.11 and 22.12)

- Eosinophilic enteritis occurs more commonly in men aged from their 20s to their 50s.
- Together with peripheral eosinophilia, eosinophil infiltration is evident mainly in gastric and small intestinal mucosal tissue, causing gastrointestinal symptoms including abdominal pain, vomiting, and diarrhea as well as abnormal test results such as anemia and hypoproteinemia.
- In a few patients, the condition is localized to the small intestine, exhibiting no findings on upper or lower gastrointestinal endoscopy, and there are therefore hopes for the contribution of small intestinal endoscopy (Endo H, et al.: Digestion 83:134–58, 1990).
- Diagnostic criteria (Talley et al.: Gut 31:54–58, 1990): (1) presence of gastrointestinal symptoms; (2) either eosinophil infiltration evident from gastrointestinal biopsy, or peripheral blood eosinophilia and characteristic radiographic findings; and (3) exclusion of diseases revealing eosinophilia caused by parasites and other factors.

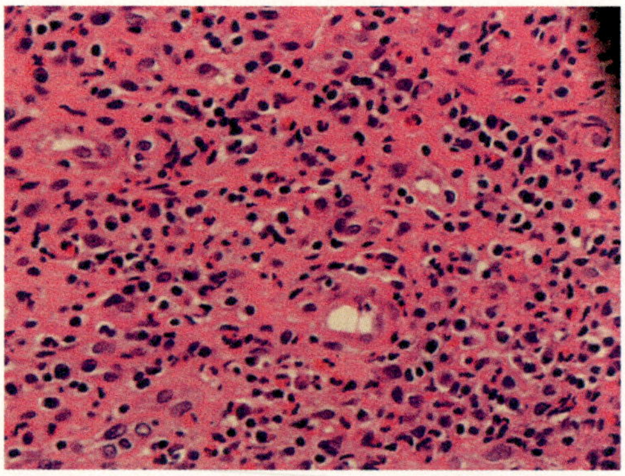

Fig. 22.12 The lower ileum exhibited mucosal irregularity and poor distensibility

References

1. Weiss PF et al. Effect of corticosteroid on Henoch- Schönlein purpura: a systemic review. Pediatrics. 2007;120:1079–87.
2. Watanabe T et al. Small bowel injury by low-dose enteric-coated aspirin and treatment with misoprostol: a pilot study. Clin Gastroenterol Hepatol. 2008;6:1279–82.
3. Nishimura N et al. Balloon dilation when using double-balloon enteroscopy for small-bowel strictures associated with ischemic enteritis. Gastrointest Endosc. 2011;74:1157–61.
4. Endo H et al. Capsule endoscopic evaluation of eosinophilic enteritis before and after treatment. Digestion. 2011;83:134–5.

Case Presentations: Edematous Lesions

23

Takayuki Matsumoto, Kensei Ohtsu, Naoki Ohmiya, Kouichi Asano, Yasuhiro Takaki, Kunihiko Aoyagi, Fukunori Kaneshiro, Kazuto Kishimoto, Takashi Hisabe, Yasuhito Takaki, Motohiro Esaki, Koichi Eguchi, and Takahiro Beppu

23.1 Case 1 [1]

23.1.1 Female, 50s (Fig. 23.1a–d)

- The patient had eaten raw squid as part of her meal the previous evening. She then went to sleep as usual, but acute abdominal pain and vomiting appeared the following morning. As these persisted, she visited the hospital.
- She complained of intermittent pain around the navel, and very slight muscle guarding was evident. CT and abdominal ultrasonography revealed pronounced thickening of the wall of the middle small intestine and a small volume of ascites.
- Symptoms disappeared without treatment after 3 days. Anti-anisakis antibody levels measured 2 weeks later were elevated to 320-fold.
- DBE performed on day 2 revealed segmental edema and swelling of the folds of the pelvic small intestine. The proximal border of the lesion was comparatively clearly demarcated (a), and the endoscope passed through easily.
- No obvious ulcer formation or parasite bodies could be identified on the mucosal surface (b–d).

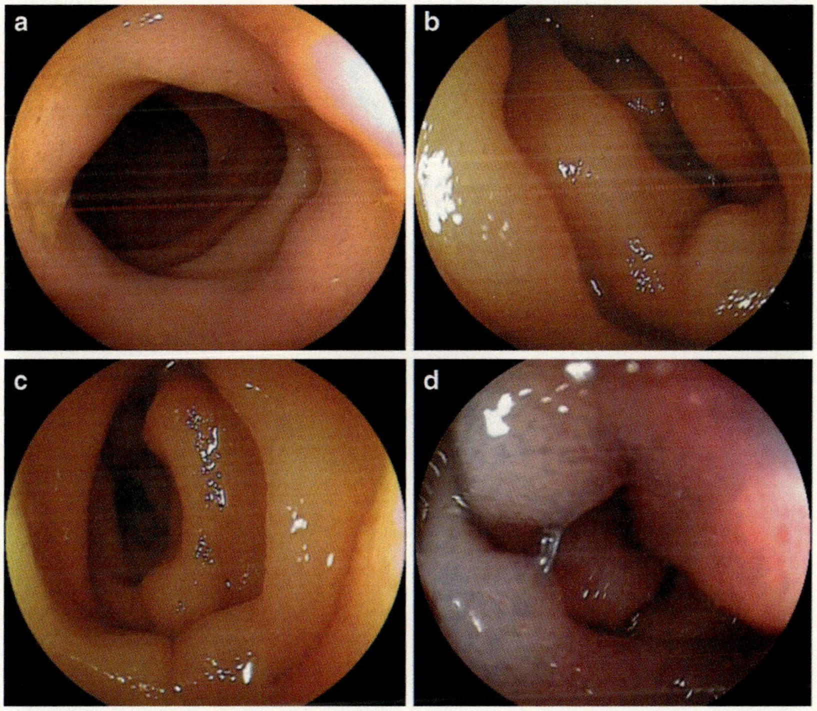

Fig. 23.1

T. Matsumoto (✉) • K. Asano • M. Esaki
Department of Medicine and Clinical Science, Graduate School of Medicine, Kyushu University, 3-1-1 Maidashi, Higashi-ku, Fukuoka 812-8582, Japan
e-mail: matane@intmed2.med.kyushu-u.ac.jp

K. Ohtsu • Y. Takaki • T. Hisabe • Y. Takaki • T. Beppu
Department of Gastroenterology, Fukuoka University Chikushi Hospital, 1-1-1 Zokumyoin, Chikushino 818-8502, Japan

N. Ohmiya
Department of Gastroenterology, Nagoya University Graduate School of Medicine, 65 Tsurumai-cho, Showa-ku, Nagoya 466-8550, Japan

K. Aoyagi • K. Eguchi
Department of Gastroenterology and Medicine, Fukuoka University Faculty of Medicine, 7-45-1 Nanakuma, Jonan-ku, Fukuoka 814-0180, Japan

F. Kaneshiro • K. Kishimoto
Department of Endoscopy, Faculty of Medicine, University of the Ryukyus, 207 Uehara, Nishihara, Okinawa 903-0215, Japan

T. Matsui et al. (eds.), *Endoscopy in the Diagnosis of Small Intestine Diseases*, DOI 10.1007/978-4-431-54352-7_23, © Springer Japan 2014

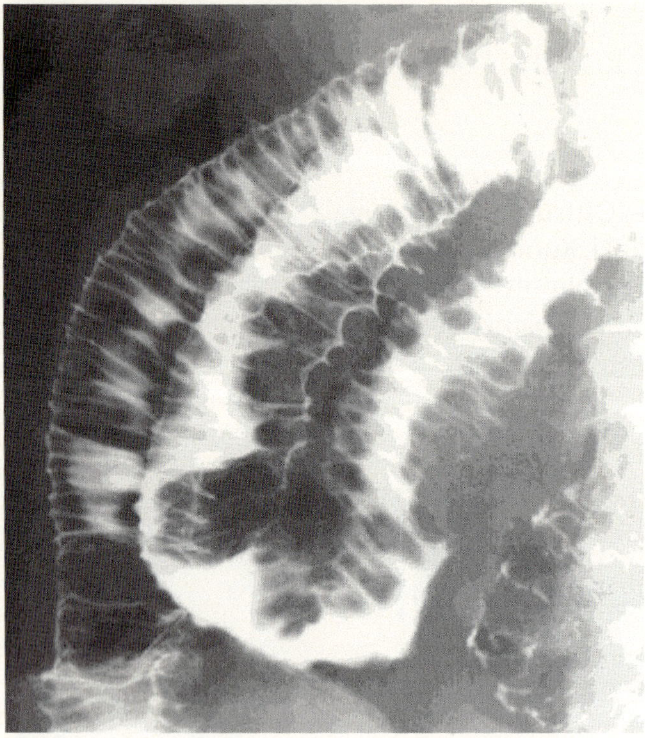

Fig. 23.2 The thumbprinting sign was evident segmentally in the middle small intestine

23.1.2 Anisakiasis (Fig. 23.2)

- Anisakiasis is caused by oral ingestion of nematodes belonging to the genera Anisakis or Terranova, which are parasitic in fish and shellfish. As humans are not the final host for nematodes, long-term parasitosis does not result.
- The upper gastrointestinal tract is normally affected, but in rare cases a parasite may penetrate the small intestinal wall, causing an acute edematous lesion. Typically, acute abdomen occurs within a few hours after eating raw seafood.
- Edema of the submucosal layer, rather than mucosal damage, comprises the main lesion. Radiographically and endoscopically, it appears as edematous stenosis causing regional poor distensibility. Mucosal lesions such as erosions and ulceration are not evident on endoscopy.
- Although there is pronounced edema at the site of parasite penetration, the parasite itself is not easy to detect.

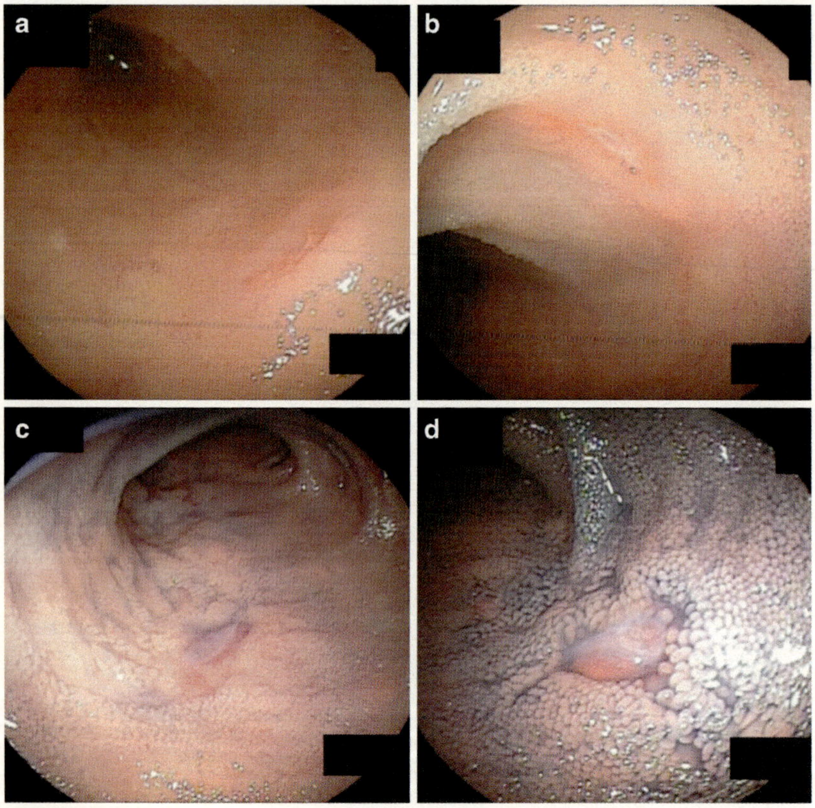

Fig. 23.3

23.2 Case 2

23.2.1 Male, 70s (Fig. 23.3a–d)

Principal complaints: tarry stool, anemia

- The patient was regularly using the NSAID sodium loxoprofen for a broken rib.
- Upper and lower gastrointestinal endoscopy revealed no obvious abnormalities.
- Retrograde DBE with the objective of investigating small intestinal lesions showed multiple small ulcerations on Kerckring's folds in the terminal ileum and middle and lower small intestine. Ulcer margins were slightly edematous (a, b).
- Multiple small ulcers were evident in the middle and lower small intestine.
- Ulcers were located on Kerckring's folds, were comparatively shallow and oval or round-shaped, and had clearly demarcated margins, constituting discrete ulcers against almost normal background mucosa (c, d).

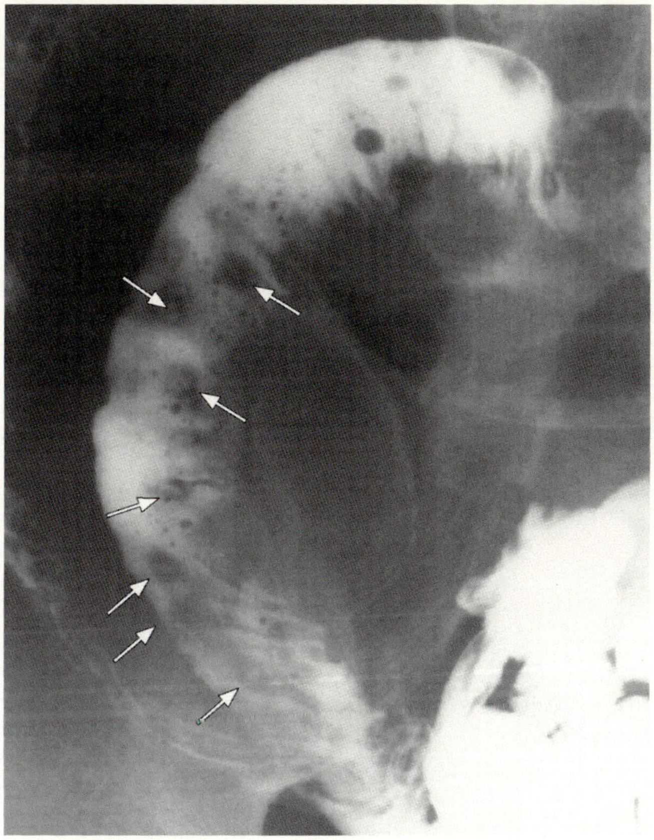

Fig. 23.4 In this radiographic image, small barium flecks and surrounding filling defects were visualized in the middle to lower small intestine (*arrows*)

23.2.2 NSAID-Induced Enteropathy (Fig. 23.4 and 23.5)

- A form of drug-induced enteritis that occurs in patients taking NSAIDs. NSAID-induced enteropathy causes small ulcers of varying sizes that do not exhibit a regular arrangement.
- Radiographically, this pathology is characterized by the visualization of clearly demarcated small, round barium flecks. The intervening mucosa of the small intestine is normal, with no areas of atrophic scarring or cobblestone appearance.

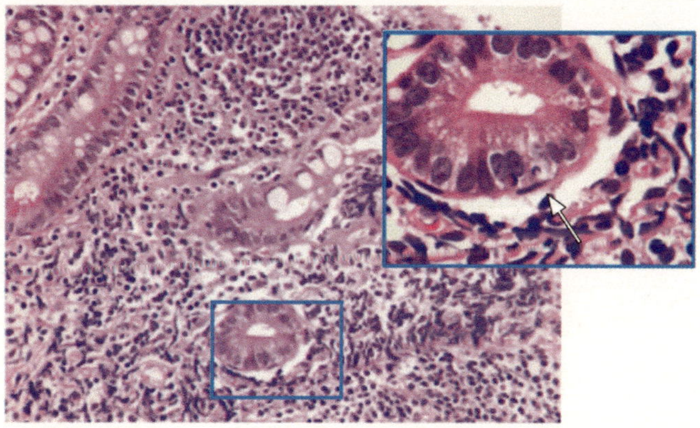

Fig. 23.5 There are no specific histopathological findings of NSAID-induced enteropathy, with only non-specific inflammatory cell infiltration being evident. Apoptotic bodies (*arrow*) are reportedly frequently present in deeper parts of the crypts of ulcerative lesions

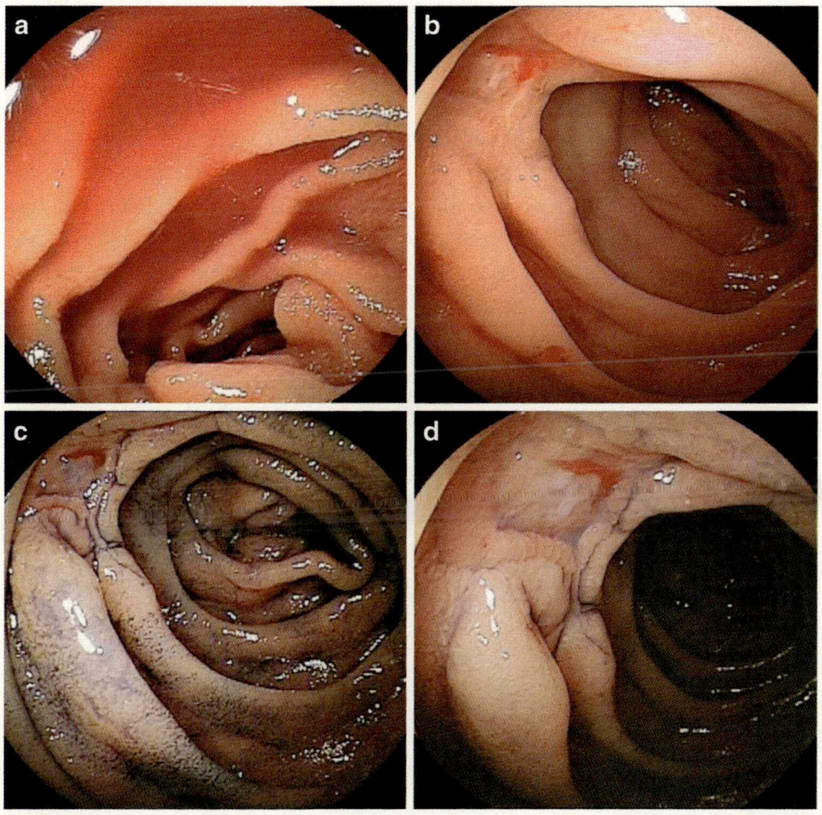

Fig. 23.6

23.3 Case 3 [2]

23.3.1 Male, 50s (Fig. 23.6a–d)

- Onset was marked by black stool and dizziness on standing. The patient had been taking Bufferin OTC medication every time he had a headache since the previous year.
- Underlying disease: none
- An accumulation of blood was evident in the upper jejunum, with a single ulcer in the same area (a, b). Convergence of folds and regenerative epithelium were already apparent in the ulcers, but oozing was seen from the ulcer beds (c, d).

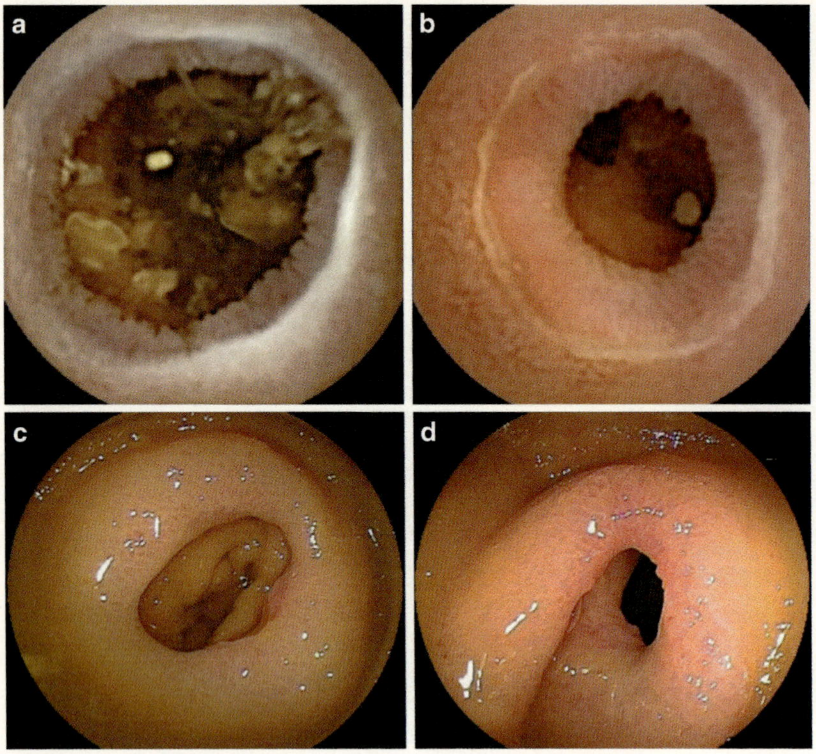

Fig. 23.7

23.3.2 Aspirin-Induced Enteropathy

- NSAIDs are used long-term not only as analgesics and pain relievers to deal with chronic pain, but also as anti-thrombotics to prevent the recurrence or onset of heart disease and cerebral infarction.
- One side effect of NSAIDs is damage to the gastrointestinal mucosa, causing bleeding from erosions and ulcers, perforation, and obstruction. Numerous reports have described upper gastrointestinal lesions due to NSAIDs, and the spread of capsule endoscopy of the small intestine has revealed a high incidence of such lesions (a, b).
- NSAID-induced enteropathy frequently occurs on the ileal side, whereas aspirin-induced enteropathy may also cause lesions in the upper small intestine (c, d).

23.4 Case 4 [3]

23.4.1 Active Stage

Patient: Male, 60s (Fig. 23.7a–d)

Principal complaints: abdominal tenderness, general malaise

- Medication history: regular use of diclofenac sodium, a NSAID, for lumbar spinal canal stenosis
- Capsule endoscopy revealed multiple circumferential, narrow circular ulcers on Kerckring's folds. Some wide circular ulcers were also present.

23.4.2 Healing Stage

- A second examination by retrograde small intestinal endoscopy was performed on day 15 after discontinuation of diclofenac sodium.
- The sites of the shallow multiple circular ulcers had scarred. No inflammatory polyps were identified.
- Concentric diaphragmatic stenosis had appeared at the site of a wide ulcer on Kerckring's folds. Ulceration was apparent at the peak of the stenosis. The endoscope was unable to pass through, and endoscopic dilation therapy was performed.

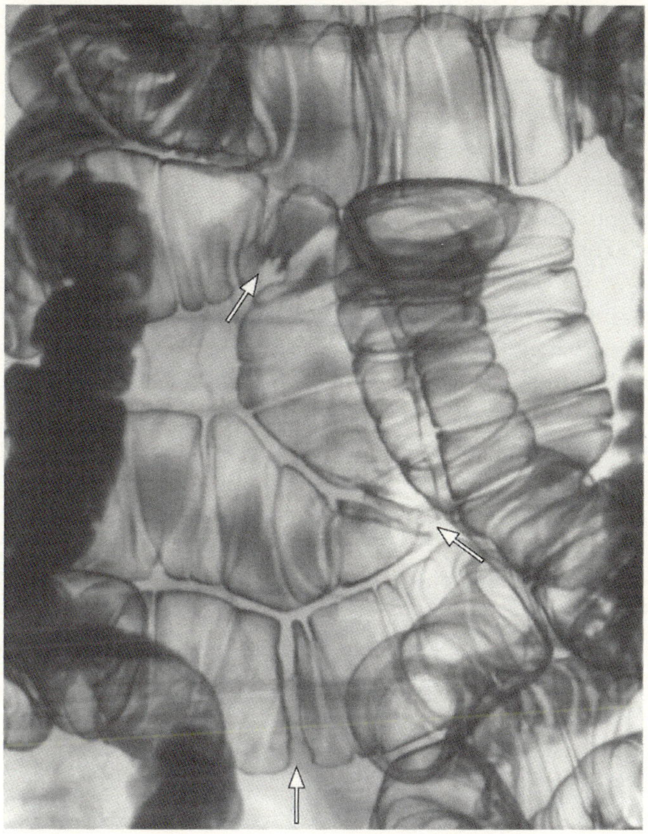

Fig. 23.8

23.4.3 NSAID-Induced Enteropathy (Fig. 23.8)

- NSAID-induced enteropathy characteristically causes lesions comprising circular ulcers on Kerckring's folds or concentric diaphragm-like stenoses.
- In the case illustrated here, it was possible to observe the process leading to stenosis.
- In many cases, the endoscope is unable to pass through, making observation of the small intestinal lesions difficult, and radiography is important for evaluating the location and distribution of lesions, luminal changes, and the degree of luminal narrowing.
- Severely stenotic lesions that prevent passage of the endoscope require treatment with surgery or endoscopic dilation therapy.

Multiple stenotic lesions were evident in the middle small intestine.

Unilateral stenosis (arrows) and luminal stenosis (arrows) were present.

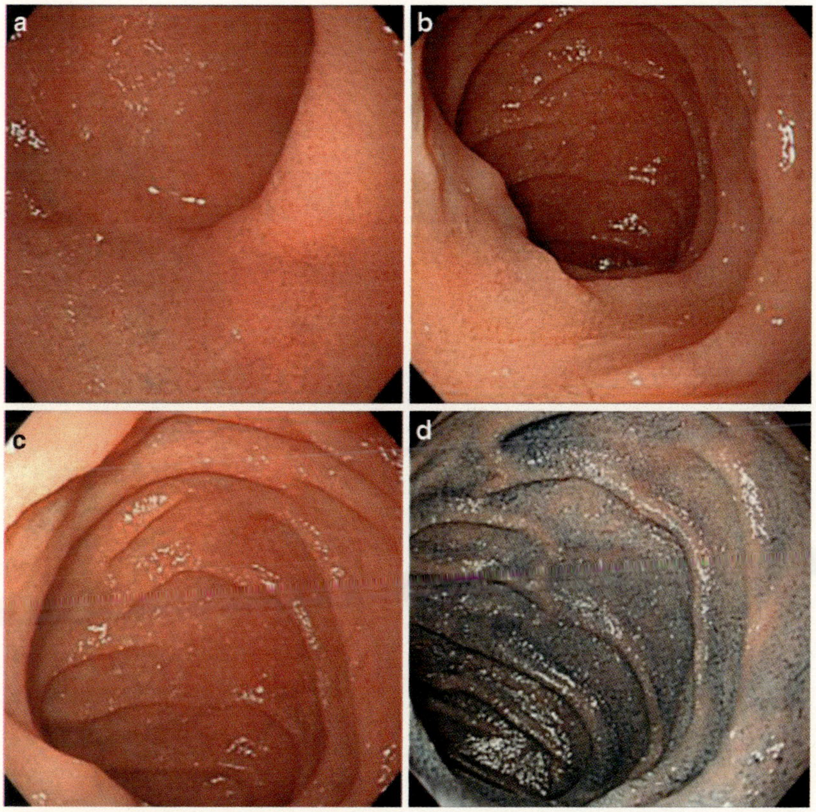

Fig. 23.9

23.5 Case 5 [4]

23.5.1 Female, 50s (Fig. 23.9a–d)

- The patient was being treated for systemic lupus erythematosus (SLE) as an outpatient, and was admitted to hospital with the principal complaints of sudden abdominal pain, vomiting, and diarrhea.
- Duodenal endoscopic findings comprised slight enlargement of Kerckring's folds (a, b).
- Slightly edematous mucosa was apparent in the horizontal duodenum. There was no mucosal damage such as erosions or ulceration (c, d).

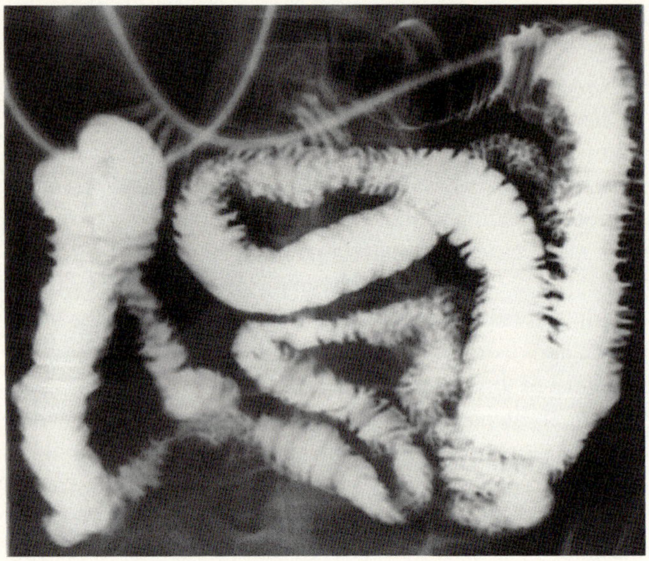

Fig. 23.10 Radiography. Enlargement of Kerckring's folds and a dentate appearance were evident across a wide area of the small intestine

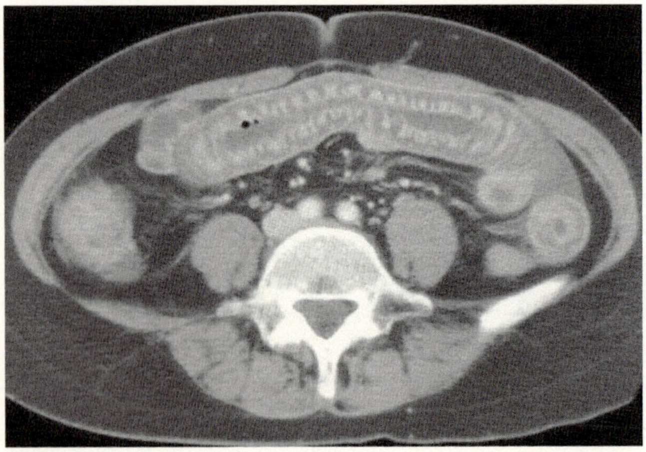

Fig. 23.11 Abdominal contrast-enhanced CT. Edematous thickening of the intestinal wall was apparent

23.5.2 Lupus Enteritis (Figs. 23.10 and 23.11)

- This term is used to describe the intestinal damage that occurs as a complication in 0.2 % of cases of systemic lupus erythematosus (SLE), and is broadly categorized into three types: ulcerative enteritis, ischemic colitis, and protein-losing enteropathy.
- The ischemic colitis type causes small vasculitis and serositis, with widespread edematous lesions in the small intestine. This may be complicated by damage to the urinary tract (lupus cystitis).
- Mucosal damage is mild in this type, which does not cause ulceration.
- Radiography and abdominal CT are more useful for diagnosis than endoscopy. Severe enlargement of Kerckring's folds and a dentate appearance are visualized radiographically.
- Diagnosis must distinguish this condition from others causing acute edematous lesions such as idiopathic ischemic enteritis, Schönlein-Henoch purpura, eosinophilic gastroenteritis, and anisakiasis.
- Systemic steroid administration is effective, but recurrence is common.

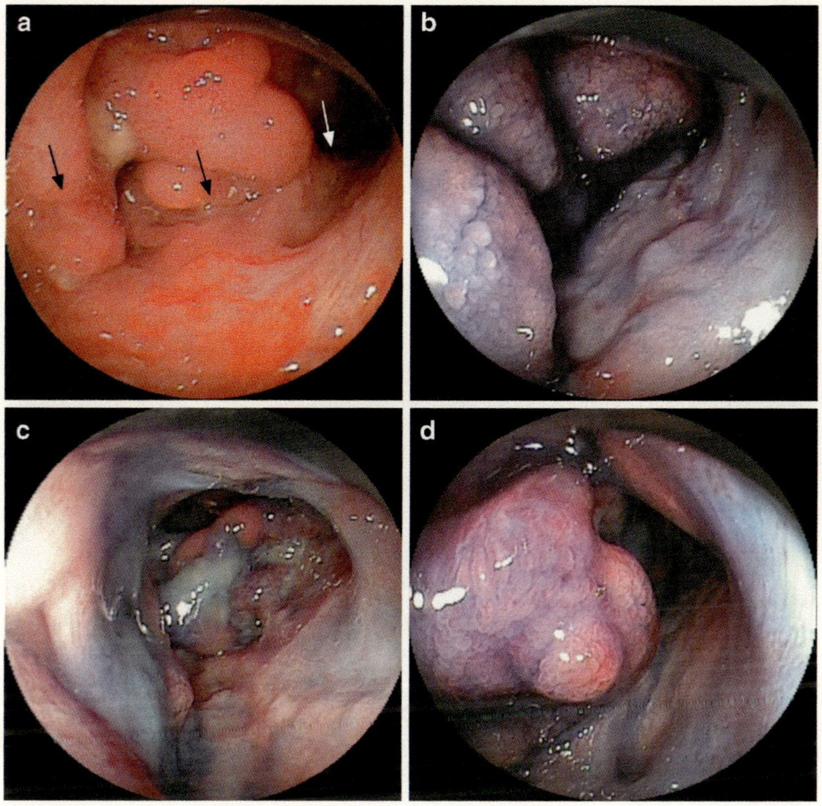

Fig. 23.12

23.6 Case 6 [5]

23.6.1 Male, 40s (Fig. 23.12a–d)

Principal complaints: abdominal pain, fever, no oral aphthae

- There was a massive ulcer on the proximal side of the site of anastomosis following resection of the ileocecal area. It was clearly demarcated (arrow) (a).
- Image after indigo carmine spraying (b).
- Image of the entire ulcer (c).
- The ulcer was massive, occupying the entire lumen of the ileum.
- A fistula was evident in the ulcer bed. A tight adhesion to the neighboring ileum was also present in the resected specimen (d).

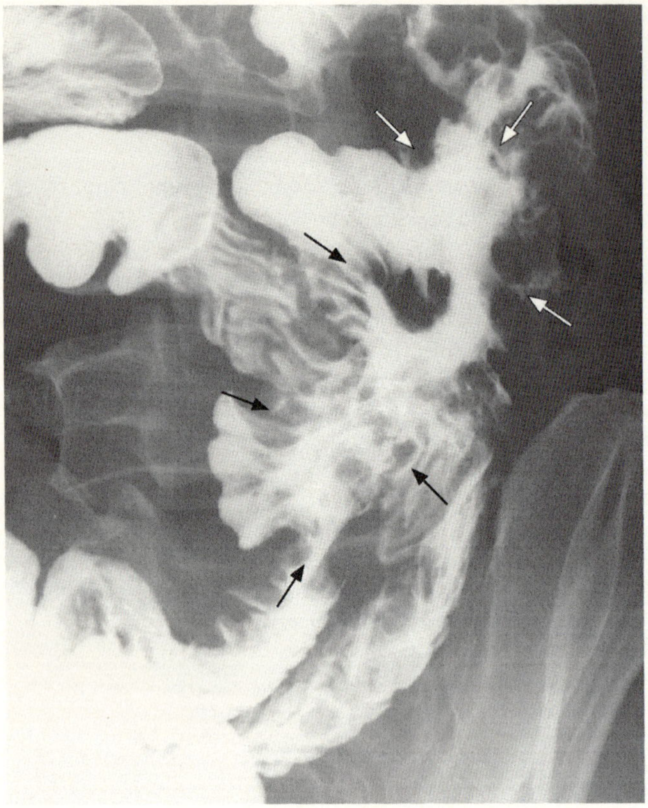

Fig. 23.13 A large undermining ulcer causing intestinal deformity and convergence of the folds was evident on the proximal side of the site of anastomosis following resection of the ileocecal area at another hospital (*arrows*). Tight adhesion between the ulcer site and neighboring loop of ileum was also present

23.6.2 Simple Ulcer (Fig. 23.13)

- Among the non-specific ulcers frequently seen in the large and small intestines, simple ulcers (SUs) tend to occur in the ileocecal area, and those that comprise characteristic punched-out ulcers are regarded as a separate disease concept.
- Pathological macroscopic findings comprise round to egg-shaped punched-out ulcers with an undermining tendency, which histologically mainly exhibit UI-IV non-specific chronic active inflammation.
- They therefore closely resemble typical intestinal Behçet disease (BD) lesions, and it is difficult to distinguish these two conditions on the basis of common sites of occurrence, macroscopic appearance, and histopathology.
- Although SUs tend to be localized to the ileocecal area compared with intestinal BD, there is no consensus view on the difference between these conditions, and in terms of diagnosis, opinion is divided on whether to classify only ulcers that do not exhibit any symptoms of intestinal BD, including oral aphthae, as SUs, or to include suspected cases of BD that do not meet the BD diagnostic criteria. Similarly to typical intestinal BD lesions, SU is also resistant to treatment, constituting an intractable condition that easily recurs.

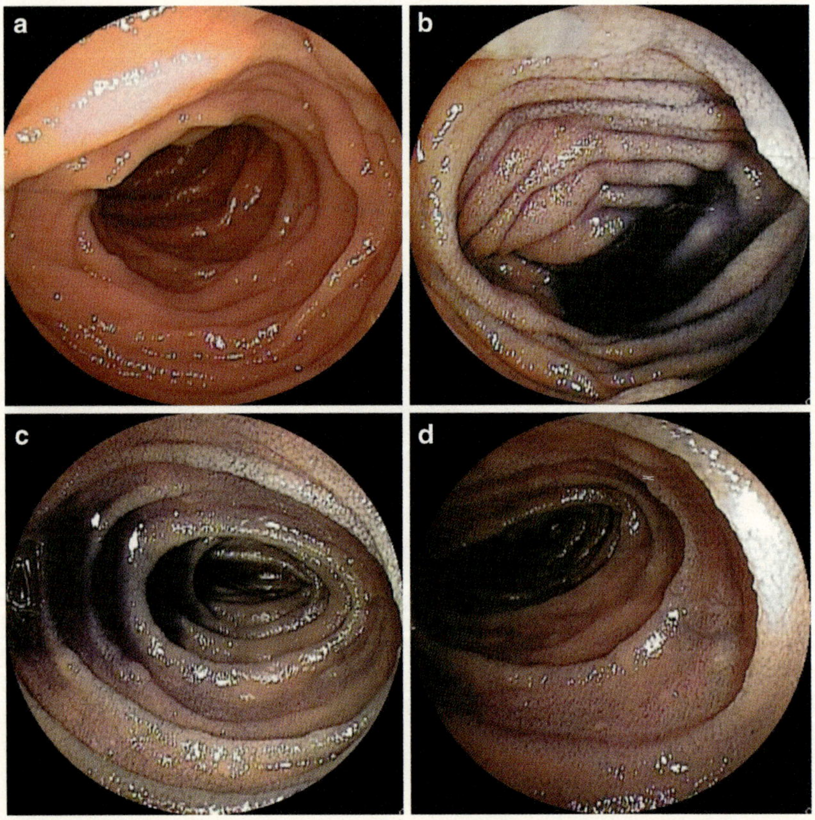

Fig. 23.14

23.7 Case 7 [6]

23.7.1 Male, 30s (Fig. 23.14a–d)

Principal complaint: abdominal pain

- Somewhat uneven enlargement of the folds was evident in the jejunum (a, b).
- A fine granular appearance was evident in part of the jejunum. Small white patches were also present (c, d).

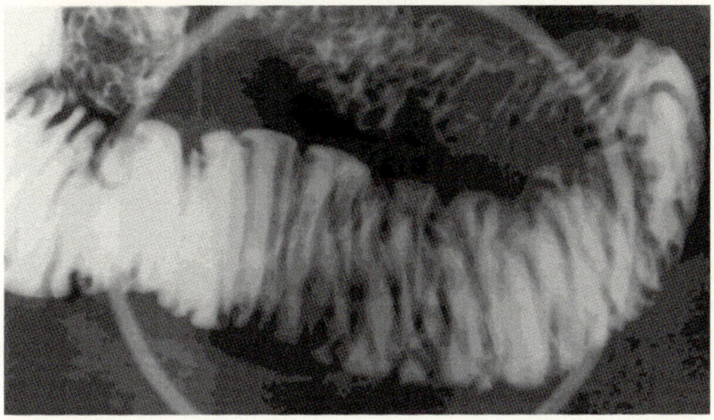

Fig. 23.15 Radiography. Under compression, Kerckring's folds in the jejunum exhibited comparatively even, mild enlargement

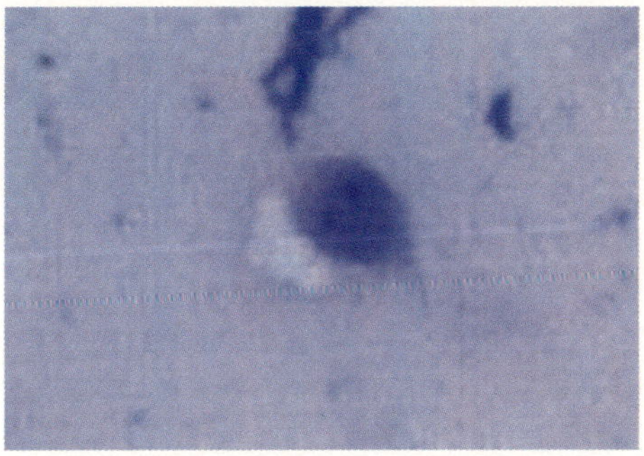

Fig. 23.16 Microscopic examination of stool revealed pear-shaped Giardia. This was the trophozoite, with a nucleus with a shape that resembled spectacles

23.7.2 Giardiasis (Figs. 23.15 and 23.16)

- Giardiasis is caused by Giardia lamblia, a protozoan that parasitizes the upper small intestine and biliary tract. It infects humans via oral ingestion of cysts, excysts into its trophozoite form and proliferates in the small intestine, and encysts from the trophozoite form into the cyst form from the lower small intestine to the large intestine. The trophozoite form is detected in duodenal intestinal fluid or diarrheal stool, and the cyst form is found in formed stool.
- Principal complaints include diarrhea, nausea, upper abdominal discomfort, sensation of abdominal distension, and abdominal pain. It may cause malabsorption syndrome, with the appearance of steatorrhea.
- Radiographically, giardiasis is characterized by coarse granular mucosa from the duodenum to the small intestine, mild edema, and indistinct Kerckring's folds, but as these findings are mild, they are frequently not recognized as abnormal.
- Endoscopically, this condition is characterized by coarse granular mucosa from the duodenum to the upper small intestine, redness, erosion, and white patches.

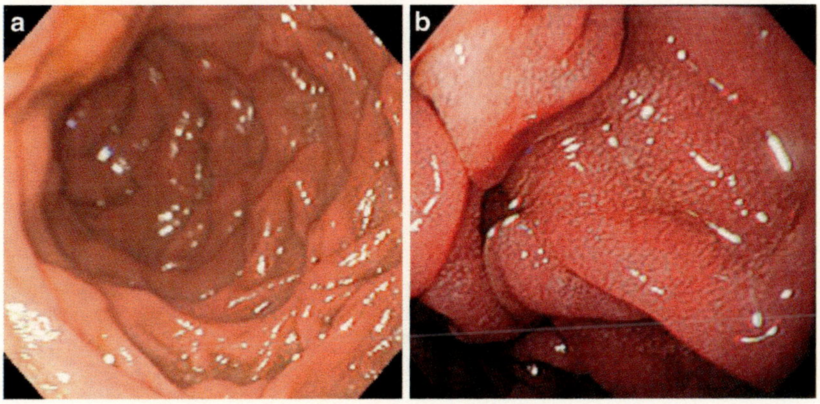

Fig. 23.17

23.8 Case 8, 9, 10, 11 [7]

23.8.1 Male, 50s (Fig. 23.17a, b)

Principal complaints: loss of appetite/weight loss

Underlying disease; diabetes mellitus, HTLV-1(+)

- The patient had been receiving treatment for diabetes mellitus for 17 years, and had a history of treatment for strongyloidiasis diagnosed by fecal testing 4 years and 2 years previously.
- Duodenal endoscopy revealed enlargement of the mucosal folds due to edema, with the presence of white villi.

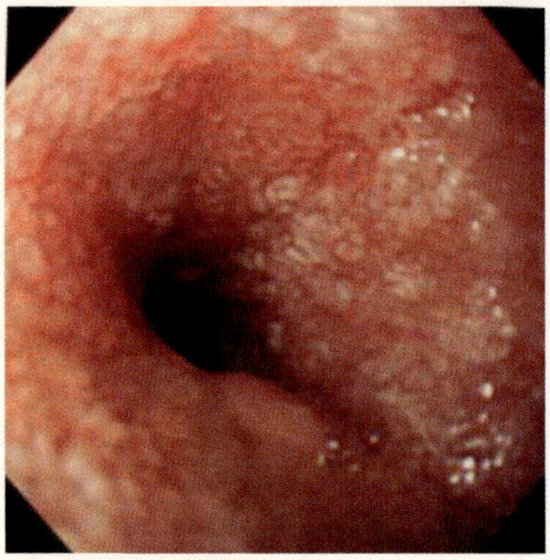

Fig. 23.18

23.8.2 Female, 50s (Fig. 23.18)

- The patient suffered from abdominal pain and vomiting. She also had gallstones and showed positive results for HTLV-1.
- Loss of the duodenal mucosal folds, prominent white villi, and narrowing of the lumen were evident.

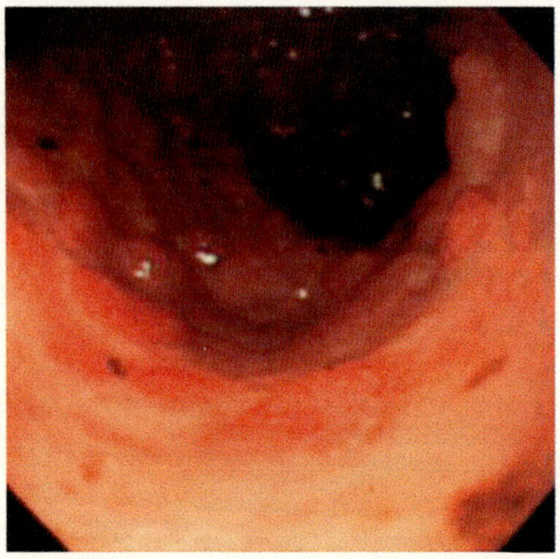

Fig. 23.19

23.8.3 Male, 40s (Fig. 23.19)

- The patient was undergoing treatment for malignant lymphoma, with obstructive symptoms and gastrointestinal bleeding. He waspositive for HTLV-1.
- Loss of the duodenal mucosal folds and inflammatory polyps with diffuse erosive ulceration and redness were present.

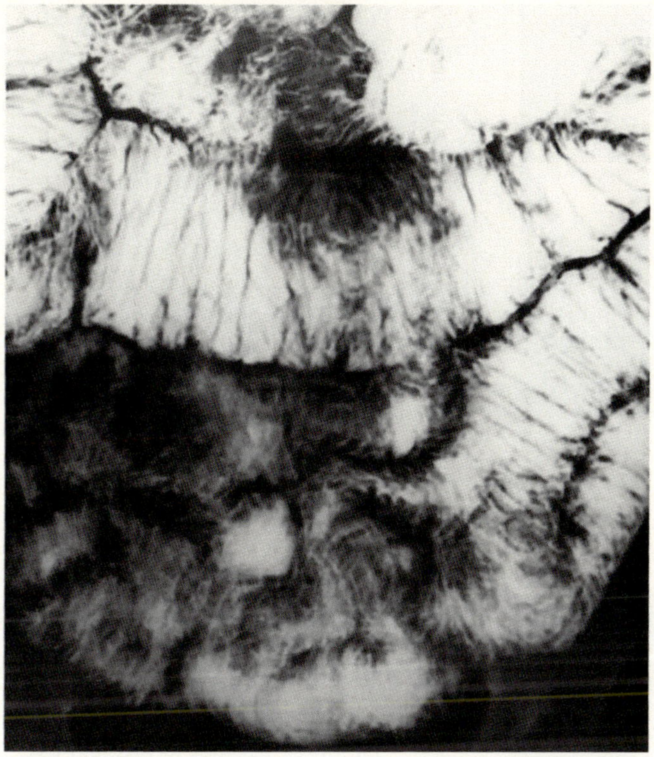

Fig. 23.20 Case 8: The upper small intestine was dilated, and the mucosal folds were enlarged. In more severe cases, ulceration and luminal narrowing become apparent

23.8.4 Strongyloidiasis (Figs. 23.20 and 23.21)

- Infection is common among members of the baby boom generation and older age groups born in Okinawa and the Amami Islands of Kagoshima Prefecture.
- Strongyloidiasis is an opportunistic infection that should be kept in mind in patients with an underlying condition or pathology that renders them immunocompromised.
- Radiographic characteristics of severe strongyloidiasis include thickening of the mucosal folds of the duodenum and upper jejunum and luminal dilation, and loss of the mucosal folds and lead pipe narrowing are evident in more severe cases.
- Endoscopic findings include white villi, edema, redness, erosion, ulceration, enlargement or disappearance of folds, and inflammatory polyps. Luminal dilation, narrowing, or stenosis may also occur.

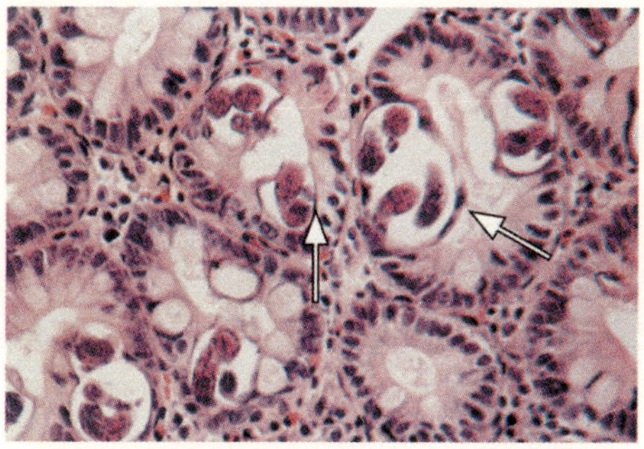

Fig. 23.21 Case 11: Biopsy of the duodenal mucosa may reveal Strongyloides in crypts, but even in severe cases this is only seen in approximately 65 % of patients

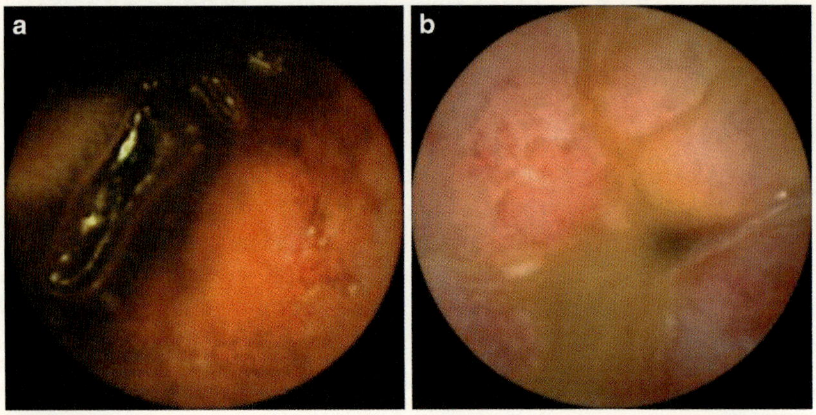

Fig. 23.22

23.9 Case 12, 13

23.9.1 Male, 40s (Fig. 23.22a, b)

- The patient had developed inflammatory ulcerative colitis of the entire colon in 1999. This was resistant to medical treatment, and the entire large intestine was removed in October 2007.
- CE revealed a single erosion in the middle small intestine, and edematous mucosa and diffuse erosions in the lower small intestine.

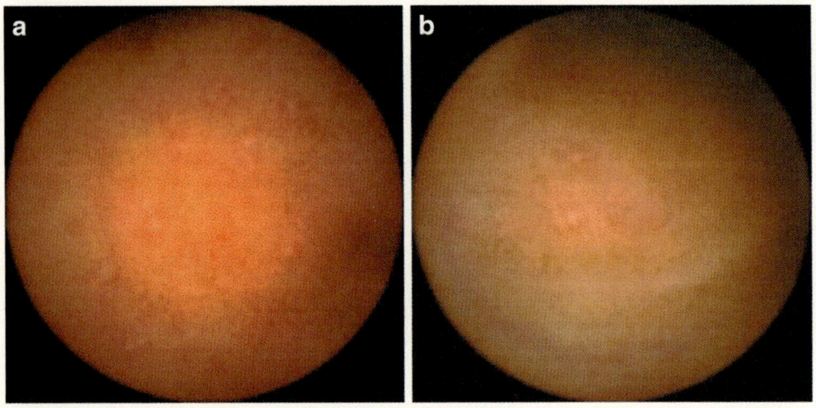

Fig. 23.23

23.9.2 Male, 20s (Fig. 23.23a, b)

- The patient had developed inflammatory ulcerative colitis of the entire colon in 2001. This was resistant to medical treatment, and the entire large intestine was removed in October 2004.
- CE revealed diffuse aphthae from the middle to the lower small intestine.

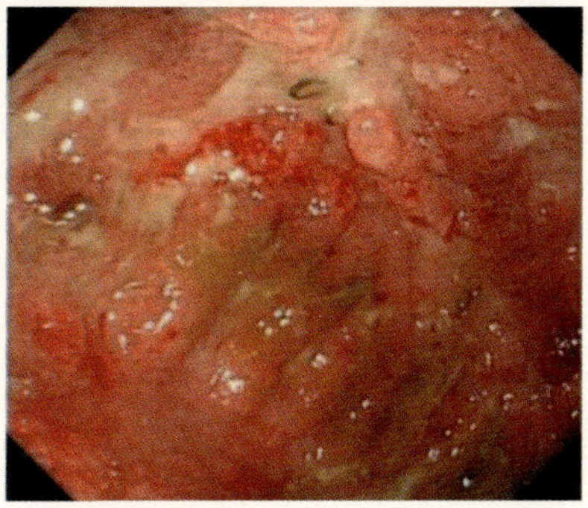

Fig. 23.24 Sigmoidoscopy of Case 12. Diffuse edema and redness were evident in mucosa with severe pouchitis, with multiple friable irregularly shaped ulcers

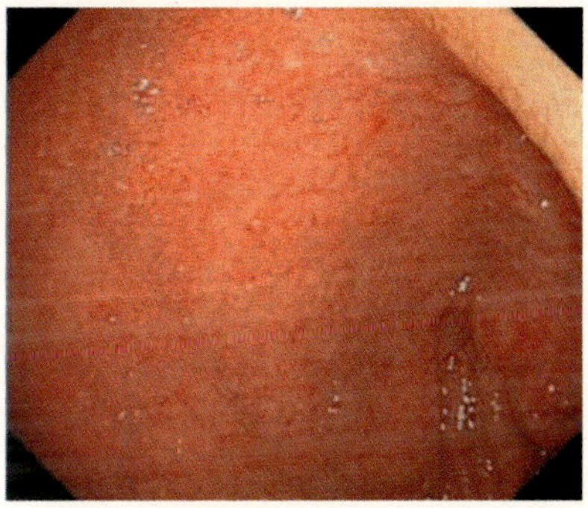

Fig. 23.25 Sigmoidoscopy of Case 13. Vascular transparency was lost in mucosa with moderate pouchitis, which was reddened and edematous, and diffuse aphthae were also present

23.9.3 Ulcerative Colitis-Associated Intestinal Lesion (Figs. 23.24 and 23.25)

- Pouchitis (inflammation of the ileal pouch) is a nonspecific inflammation of the ileal pouch that occurs in patients who have undergone (partial) total removal of the large intestine with a conserved natural anus. The etiology is unknown.
- Endoscopically, mild cases are characterized by edema, granular mucosa, loss of vascular transparency, and mild redness; moderate cases by aphthae, erosion, ulceration, and friable purulent mucosa; and severe cases by widespread ulceration, multiple ulcers, diffuse redness, and natural bleeding. Staple line ulcers must be distinguished from pouchitis.
- Pre-pouch ileitis, in which inflammation extends into the small intestine on the proximal side of the pouch, may be present.
- Small intestinal lesions may occur even if pouchitis is not present. This frequently occurs in patients with colitis of the entire colon.

23.10 Case 14 [5]

23.10.1 Male, 60s (Fig. 23.26a–d)

- A clearly demarcated punched-out ulcer extended from the ileocecal valve to the cecum. Enlargement and convergence of the folds was present at the ulcer margins (a).
- Image after indigo carmine spraying (b).
- DBE image of pelvic small intestinal lesions performed during a recurrence 8 months after the images above. A clearly demarcated, egg-shaped punched-out ulcer with pronounced convergence of the folds was present (c).
- Image after indigo carmine spraying (d).

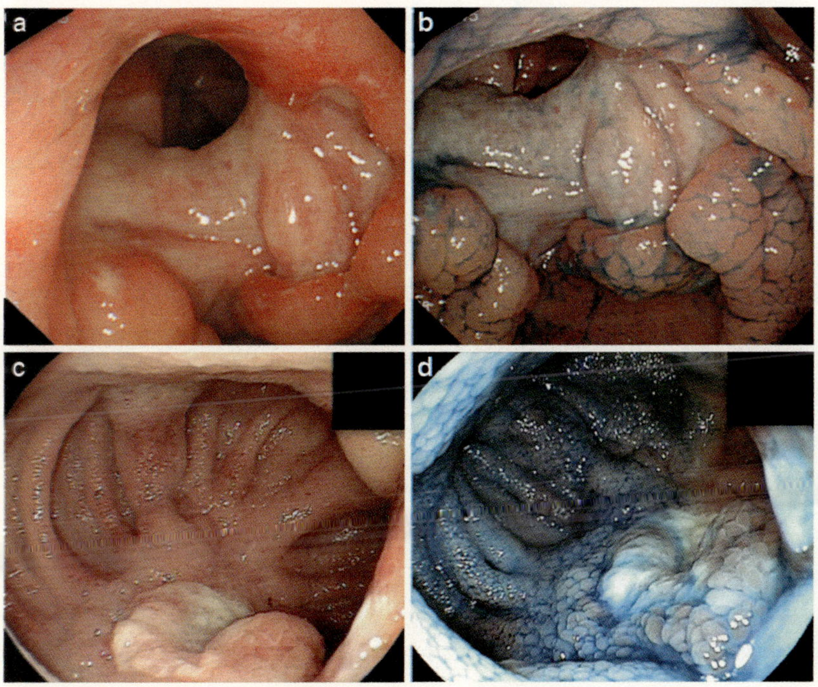

Fig. 23.26

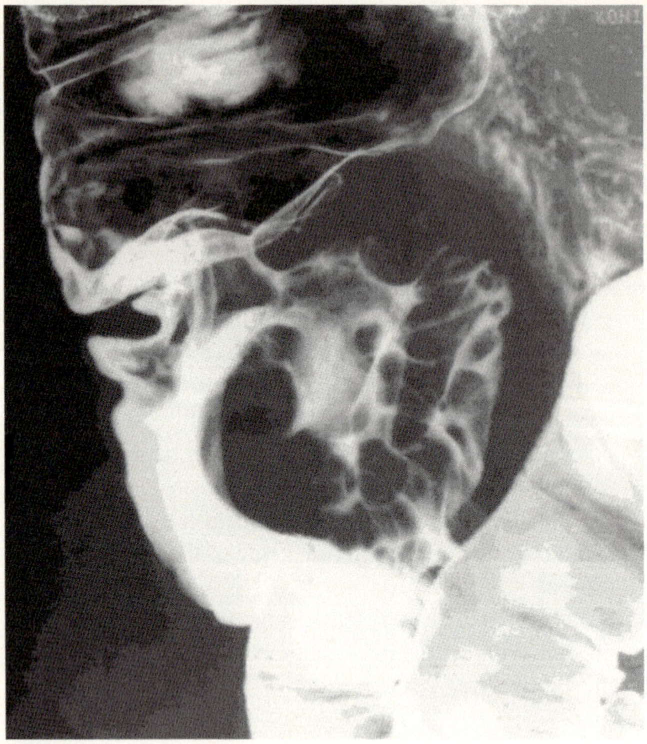

Fig. 23.27 This represents a suspected case of BD with recurrent oral aphthae and cutaneous symptoms. Typical lesions were present in the terminal part of the ileum, as were clear barium flecks with sharp borders. At the margin, convergence of the edematously enlarged folds was evident at the tip

23.10.2 Behçet Disease (Fig. 23.27)

- Behçet disease (BD) is a systemic, intractable disease of unknown etiology with four main symptoms: recurrent aphthous ulcers of the oral mucosa; cutaneous symptoms; ophthalmologic symptoms; and genital ulcers. Ulceration of the intestine may occur during its course, and intestinal BD is regarded as a specific type of BD alongside other types such as neurological and vascular BD.
- In terms of the diagnostic criteria set out by the Japanese Ministry of Health, Labour and Welfare, gastrointestinal lesions are more common in incomplete or suspected cases.
- Principal symptoms are abdominal pain, fever, and bloody stool, and the characteristic lesions are punched-out ulcers in the ileocecal area that tend to be deeply undermining, with ulcer mounds and convergence of the folds. Perforation may sometimes occur, and refractory and recurrent cases are common.

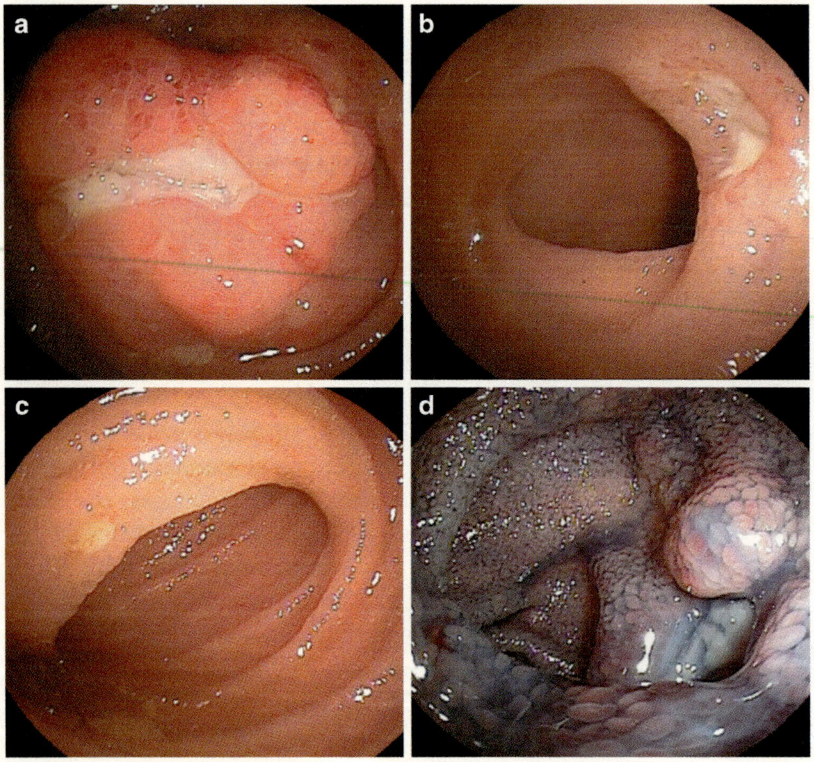

Fig. 23.28

23.11 Case 15 [8]

23.11.1 Male, 20s (Fig. 23.28a–d)

Principal complaints: recurrent oral aphthae, ophthalmologic symptoms, genital ulcers

- Findings from DBE performed at the time of recurrence, 3 years and 4 months after surgery.
- A clearly demarcated, deep ulcer with an ulcer mound was present at the site of anastomosis. There were also multiple small to medium-sized ulcers up to 50 cm distant from the anastomosis on the proximal side (a).
- Medium-sized, clearly demarcated oval or round shaped ulcer (b).
- Small, round-shaped ulcer. Characteristically, such ulcers are clearly demarcated and similar to punched out-like ulcers even when small. There was no inflammation of the intervening mucosa (c).
- Clearly demarcated, deep egg-shaped ulcer (d).

23.11.2 Behçet Disease (Figs. 23.29 and 23.30)

- In addition to typical lesions in the ileocecal area, Behçet disease (BD) may also rarely cause atypical lesions in any part of the gastrointestinal tract, from the esophagus to the rectum. Relatively common among these are esophageal ulceration, ulceration in the ileum distant from the ileocecal valve, and small multiple ulcers in the large intestine. Although these are all atypical lesions, they frequently comprise clearly demarcated, deep punched-out ulcers that resemble typical lesions, albeit small, with normal intervening mucosa.
- In the diagnosis of atypical lesions, caution is required when distinguishing them from other conditions including infections such as cytomegalovirus and herpes, as well as ulceration of the large intestine due to systemic conditions such as Crohn's disease, drug-associated enteritis, rheumatism, and SLE.

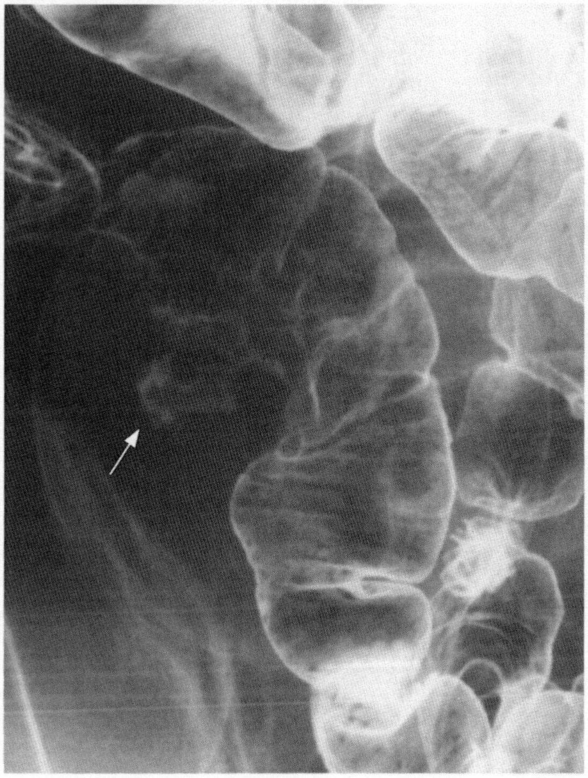

Fig. 23.29 A case of incomplete BD. A prominent undermining ulcer was present in the terminal ileum (*arrow*)

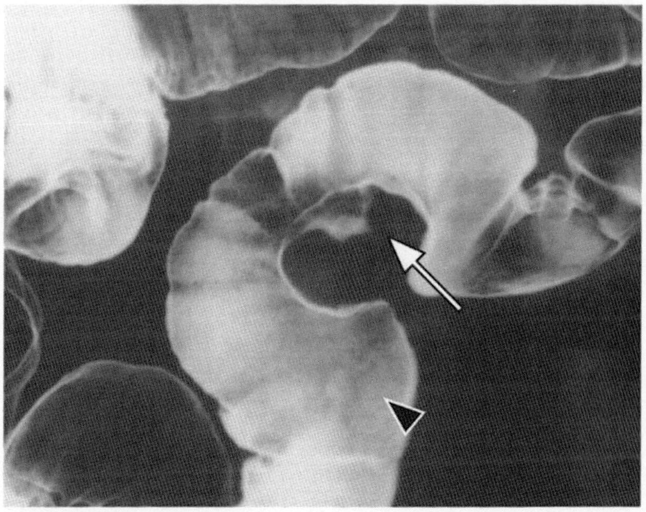

Fig. 23.30 A typical punched-out ulcer was also evident distant from the ileocecal area in the proximal side of the pelvic small intestine (*arrow*). Another clearly demarcated, small punched-out ulcer was also evident adjacent to this on the distal side (*arrowhead*)

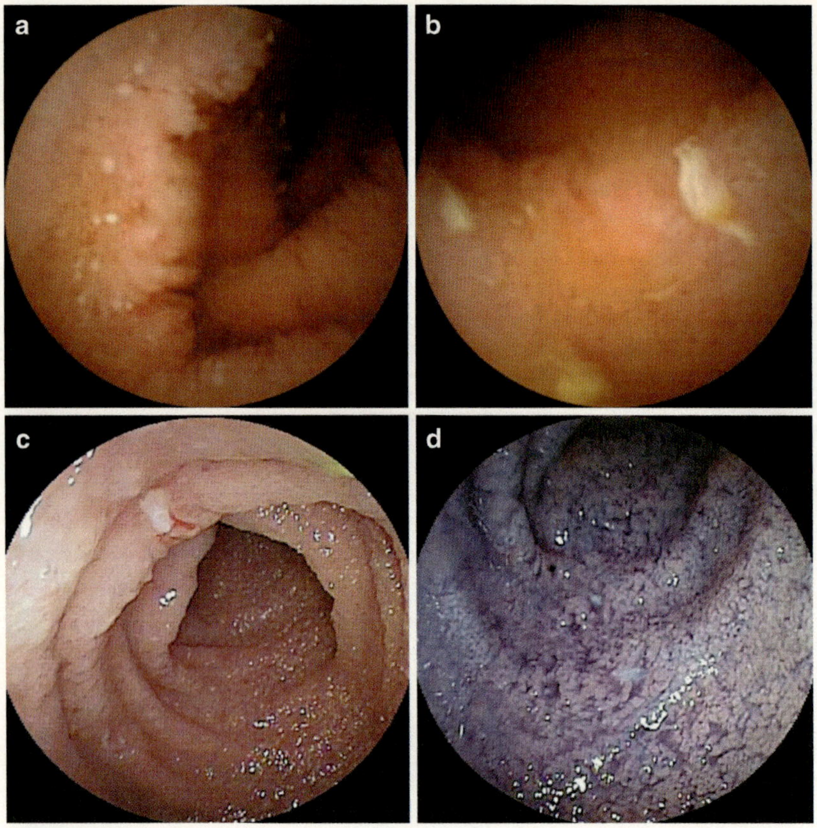

Fig. 23.31

23.12 Case 16 [9]

23.12.1 Female, 50s (Fig. 23.31a–d)

- The patient was admitted for detailed testing with symptoms of general malaise, edema of the legs, and weight loss. She was diagnosed on the basis of oral aphthous ulcers, pleural effusion, positive antinuclear antibodies, positive anti-double-stranded DNA antibodies, and hypocomplementemia.
- Blood biochemical tests showed pronounced hypoproteinemia, with serum protein 4.4 g/dL and serum albumin 12 g/dL.
- CE revealed villous enlargement and multiple white spots from the middle to lower small intestine, with aphthous lesions in the lower small intestine (a, b).
- Retrograde DBE showed multiple aphthae and erosions in the ileum, with coarse mucosa (c, d).

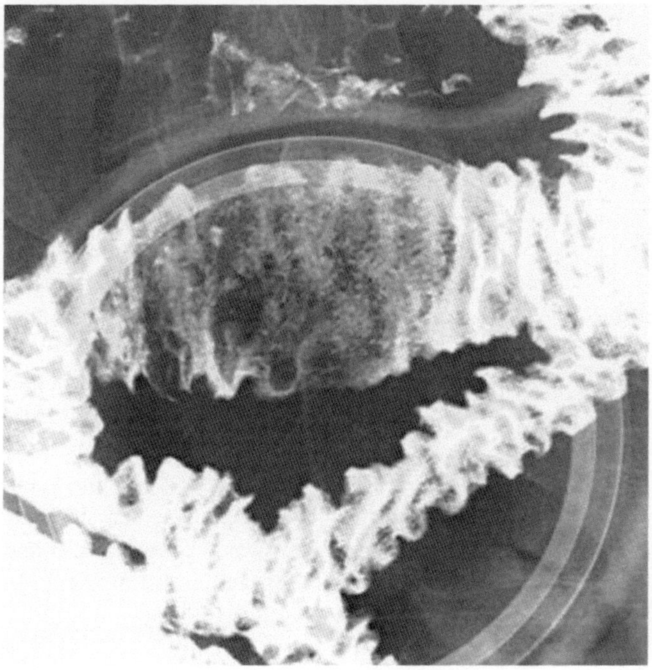

Fig. 23.32 Radiography. Under compression, enlargement of the folds and tiny barium flecks were evident

23.12.2 Lupus Enteritis (Figs. 23.32 and 23.33)

- Systemic lupus erythematosus is a chronic, intractable autoimmune disease that causes inflammatory lesions in multiple organs around the body. Although it may cause lesions throughout the gastrointestinal tract, the incidence of gastrointestinal lesions due to SLE itself is 8–27 %, with small intestinal lesions appearing at a frequency of around 5 %.
- Gastrointestinal lesions in SLE are broadly divided into lupus enteritis caused by vasculitis and protein-losing enteropathy. Lupus enteritis caused by the latter is rarely reported.
- Characteristic endoscopic findings of protein-losing enteropathy are considered to comprise enlarged villi, lymphangiectasia, and villous defects.

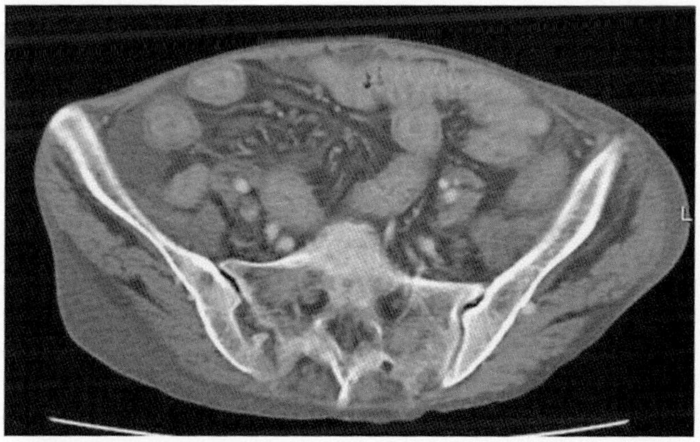

Fig. 23.33 Abdominal contrast-enhanced CT. A ring-shaped, enlarged intestinal loop within the pelvis and the accumulation of ascites were evident

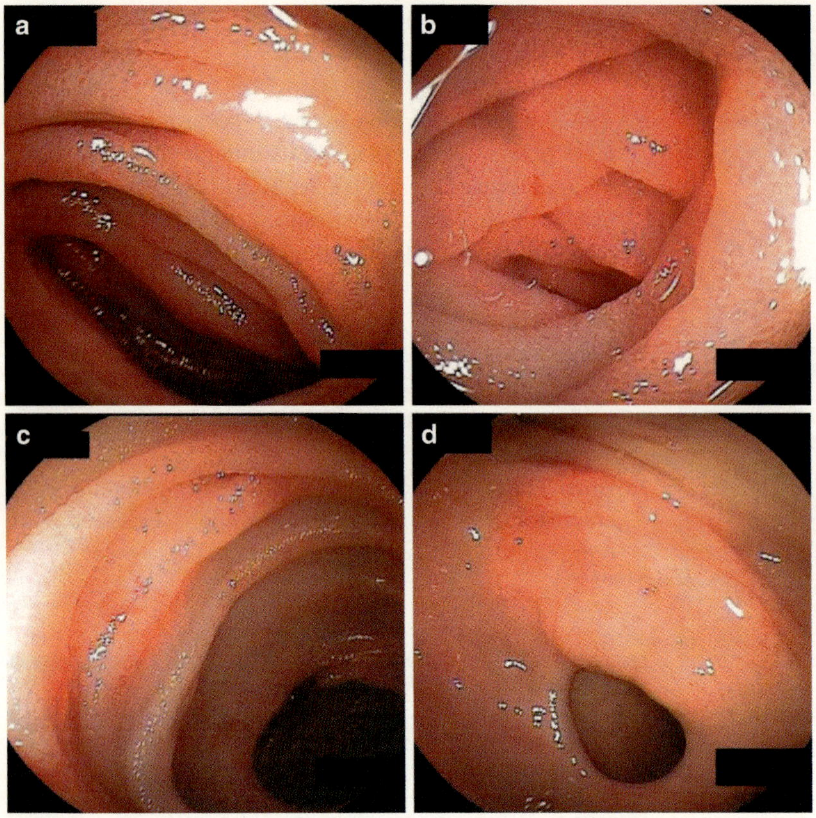

Fig. 23.34

23.13 Case 17 [10]

23.13.1 Female, 50s (Fig. 23.34a–d)

- The patient had undergone radiotherapy (50 Gy in 25 fractions) following surgical resection and chemotherapy for hepatocellular carcinoma. Black stool and anemia appeared 4 months later.
- The mucosa displayed a markedly edematous appearance, with scattered redness and small erosions (a, b).
- The mucosa was reddened and engorged, with somewhat irregular small erosions (c).
- The mucosa was edematous, and Kerckring's folds were indistinct (d).

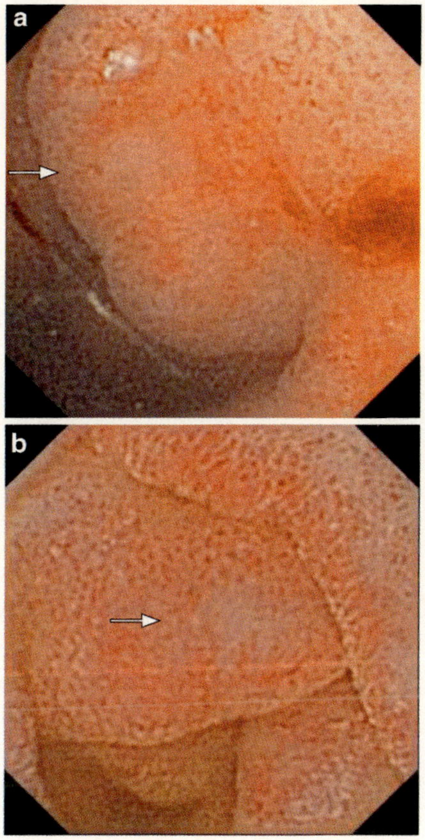

Fig. 23.35 CE showed edematous reddened mucosa and somewhat irregular, shallow ulceration (*arrow*)

23.13.2 Radiation Enteritis (Fig. 23.35a, b)

- Occurs mainly as a complication of radiotherapy applied for the treatment of malignant tumors.
- Complaints during early-stage damage include diarrhea, abdominal pain, and bleeding, and those during late-stage damage appear as symptoms such as disturbances of bowel movement.
- The small intestine is highly sensitive to radiation, and symptoms such as ulceration, stenosis, and perforation are common following exposure to 60 Gy.
- Endoscopically, redness, engorgement, edema, erosions, and bleeding are seen in early-stage damage.

Findings of late-stage damage include vascular ectasia, congestion, edema, and fibrotic stenosis.

- Radiographically, early-stage damage comprises poor barium adhesion, multiple erosions, and shallow ulceration. In late-stage damage, luminal narrowing or stenosis may be evident.

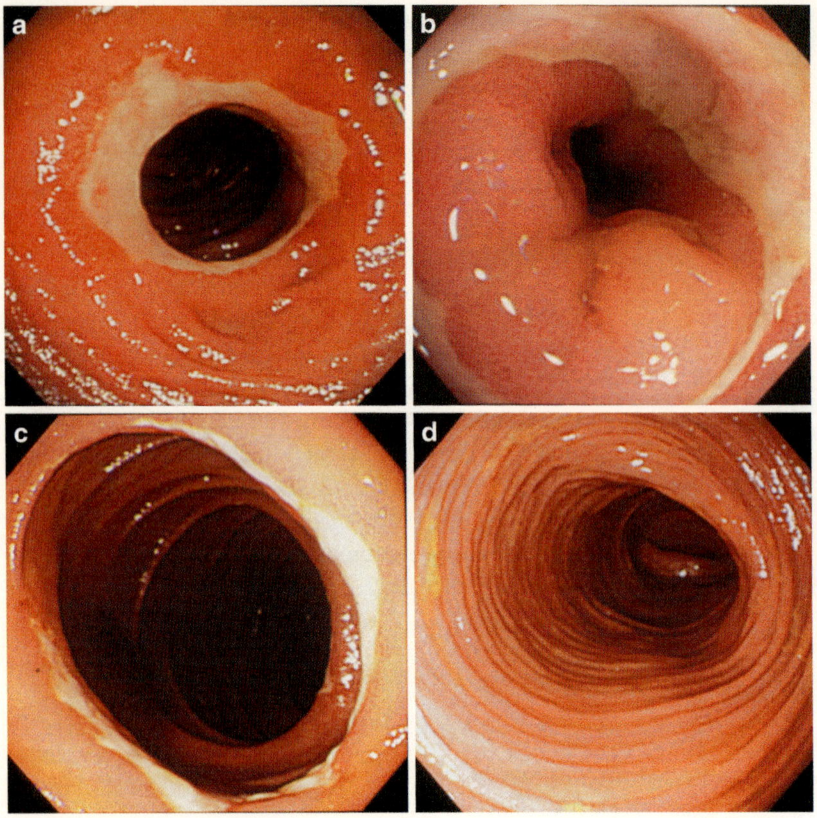

Fig. 23.36

23.14 Case 18 [11]

23.14.1 Male, 20s (Fig. 23.36a–d)

- Since 4 years old, the patient had suffered from persistent abdominal rugitus and distension, as well as symptoms due to anemia. He was admitted with severe anemia (Hb 3.9 g/dL). All endoscopic images represent intraoperative endoscopic images acquired during laparotomy.
- A circumferential ulcer and mild narrowing were evident in the ileum. The ulcer margins were mildly irregular. Very mild enteric edema was also present. There were no obvious inflammatory changes of the surrounding mucosa (a, b).
- Shallow ulcer extending four-fifths of the way around the circumference. The part of the intestinal tract that contained the ulcer was generally dilated, and multiple comparative luminal narrowings were evident at the site of ulcer formation (c).
- There were no obvious inflammatory changes in the non-ulcerated area in the dilated intestine (d).

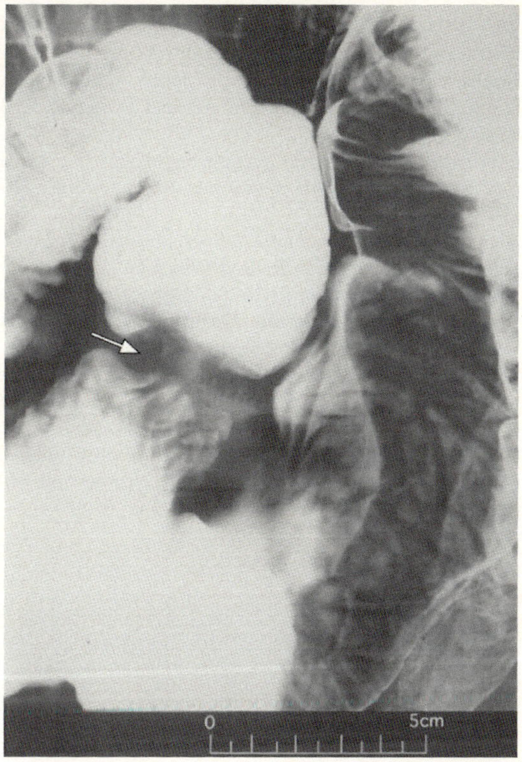

Fig. 23.37 Radiography revealed pronounced dilation of the intestinal tract, relative narrowing of the lumen (*arrow*) and barium flecks suggesting ulceration at the same site, and aberrant Kerckring's folds

23.14.2 Hypoganglionosis (Figs. 23.37 and 23.38)

- This congenital condition occurs in newborns and children, and adult small intestinal cases are extremely rare.
- Radiographically, it is characterized by pronounced intestinal dilation, relative narrowing of the lumen (arrow), and barium flecks suggesting ulceration at the same site. Other findings include ulcer scarring and aberrant Kerckring's folds. This ulceration is a secondary symptom due to congestion of intestinal fluid or residue.
- Pathological characteristics comprise atrophy of Auerbach's plexus in the proximal side of the dilated intestine and a decreased number of neurons.

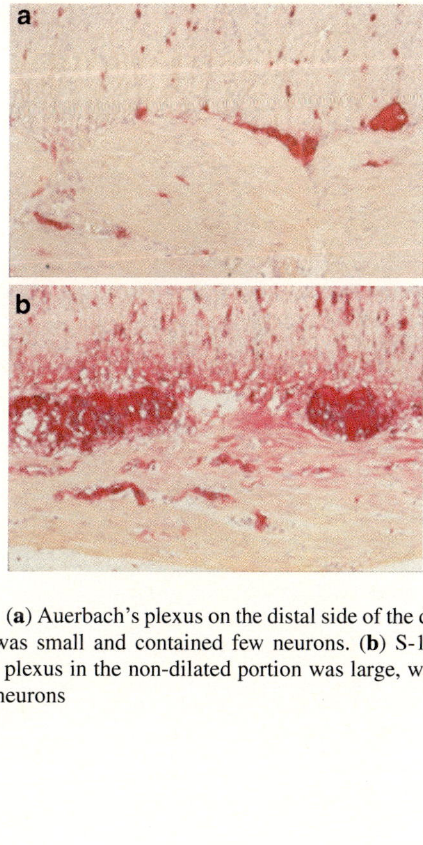

Fig. 23.38 (**a**) Auerbach's plexus on the distal side of the dilated intestinal tract was small and contained few neurons. (**b**) S-100 staining. Auerbach's plexus in the non-dilated portion was large, with a normal number of neurons

References

1. Matsui T et al. Intestinal anisakiasis. Clinical and radiologic features. Radiology. 1985;157:299–302.
2. Arakawa D et al. Outcome after enteroscopy for patients with obscure GI bleeding: diagnostic comparison between double-balloon endoscopy and videocapsule endoscopy. Gastrointest Endosc. 2009;69:866–74.
3. Hayashi Y et al. Non-steroidal anti-inflammatory drug-induced small-bowel lesions identified by double-balloon endoscopy: endoscopic features of the lesions and endoscopic treatments for diaphragm disease. J Gastroenterol. 2009;44:57–63.
4. Mok CC. Investigations and management of gastrointestinal and hepatic manifestations of systemic lupus erythematosus. Best Pract Res Clin Rheumatol. 2006;19:741–66.
5. Chung SY, Ha HK, Kim FH, et al. Radiological findings of behçet syndrome involving the gastro-intestinal tract. Radiographics. 2001;21:911–26.
6. Sharma BC et al. Diagnostic value of push-type enteroscopy: a report from India. Am J Gastroenterol. 2000;95:137–40.
7. Nakamura N et al. Diagnostic yield of double-balloon enteroscopy with intestinal juice analysis for intestinal strongyloidiasis. Dig Endosc. 2010;22:370–2.
8. Hamdulay SS et al. Wireless capsule endoscopy in the investigation of intestinal Behçet's syndrome. Rheumatology. 2008;47: 1231–4.
9. Hizawa K et al. Double-contrast radiographic assessment of lupus-associated enteropathy. Clin Radiol. 1998;53:825–9.
10. Kuroki F et al. Intraoperative endoscopy for small intestinal damage in radiation enteritis. Gastrointest Endosc. 1992;38: 196–7.
11. Taguchi T et al. New classification of hypoganglionosis: congenital and acquired hypoganglionosis. J Pediatr Surg. 2006;41: 2046–51.
12. Hisabe T et al. Small bowel lesions detected with wireless capsule endoscopy in patients with active ulcerative colitis and with post-proctocolectomy. Dig Endosc. 2011;23:302–9.

Case Presentations: Erosive Lesions

24

Issei Egashira, Shin Fujioka, Yoichiro Ono, Takashi Hisabe, and Motohiro Esaki

24.1 Case 1 [1]

24.1.1 Female, 70s (Fig. 24.1a–d)

- The patient was examined for the principal complaint of watery diarrhea persisting for over 6 months. She had a previous history of pulmonary tuberculosis.
- An area of atrophic scarring, erosions, and multiple inflammatory polyps were evident in the ileocecal area (a, b).
- Mild crimping (or convergence) in the neighborhood of the ileocecal valve was evident due to the effect of the area of atrophic scarring (a, b).
- Erosion and redness were present on the ileocecal valve, which was expanded as a result of ulcer scarring.
- Multiple erosions and shallow circular ulcers with irregular margins were present in the terminal ileum (c, d).
- The mucosa surrounding the ulcers was edematous and reddened (c, d).
- The white coat on the ulcer bed was thin, with prominent bumps.
- Although mild narrowing of the lumen due to the circular ulcers was seen, the endoscope was able to pass through to the proximal side.

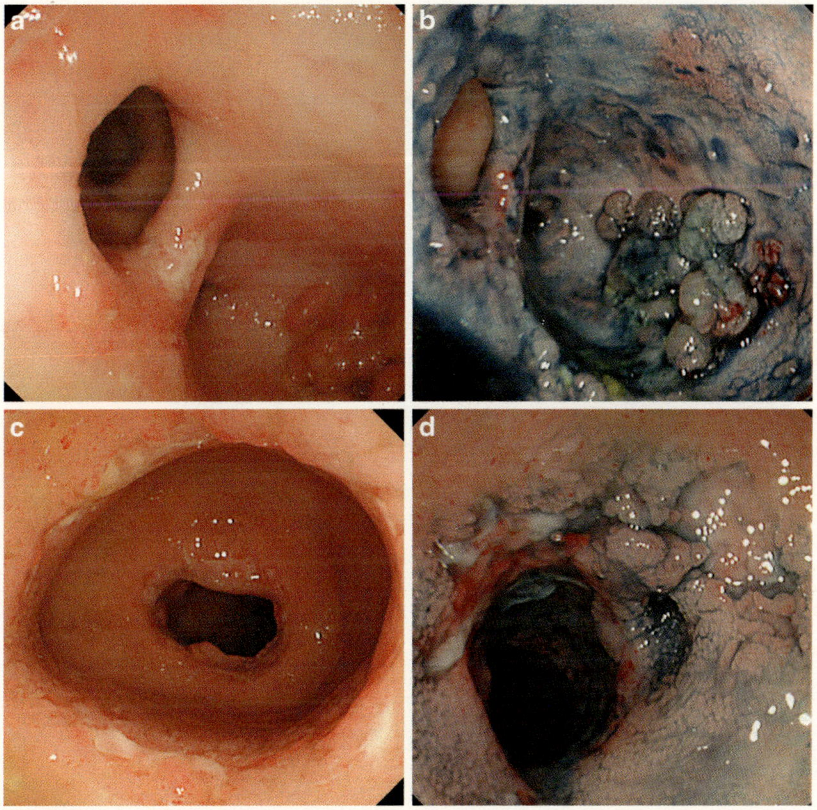

Fig. 24.1

I. Egashira (✉) • S. Fujioka • M. Esaki
Department of Medicine and Clinical Science, Graduate School of Medical Sciences, Kyushu University, 3-1-1, Maidashi, Higashi-ku, Fukuoka City 812-8582, Japan
e-mail: iega@intmed2.med.kyushu-u.ac.jp

Y. Ono • T. Hisabe
Department of Gastroenterology, Fukuoka University Chikushi Hospital, 1-1-1 Zokumyoin, Chikushino 818-8502, Japan

T. Matsui et al. (eds.), *Endoscopy in the Diagnosis of Small Intestine Diseases*, DOI 10.1007/978-4-431-54352-7_24, © Springer Japan 2014

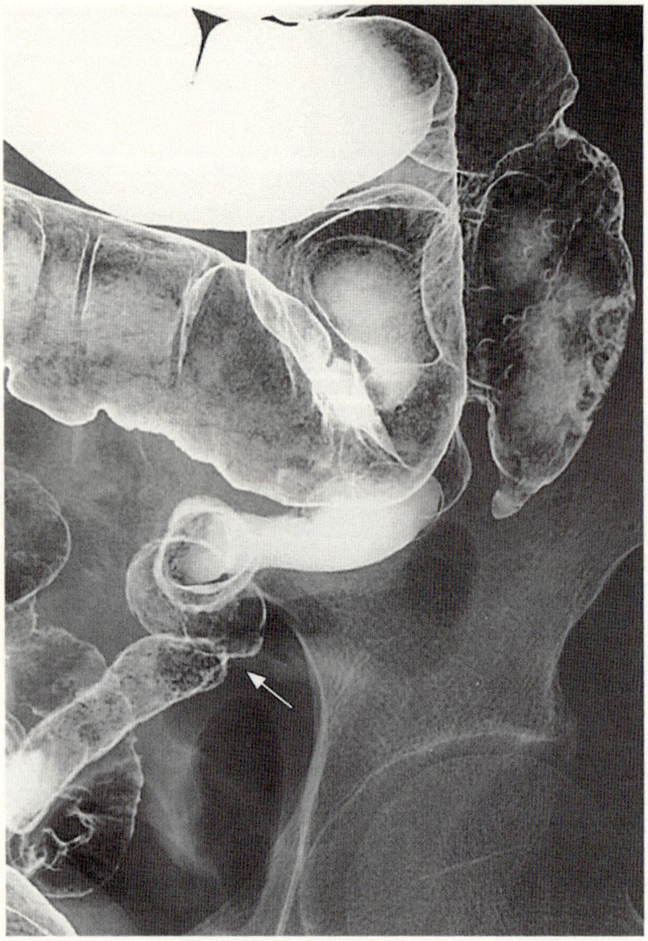

Fig. 24.2 The ileocecal valve was dilated, and multiple circular ulcers (*arrow*) and erosions were present in the terminal ileum

24.1.2 Intestinal Tuberculosis (Figs. 24.2 and 24.3)

- This commonly occurs in people aged in their 50s. Although the great majority of cases are asymptomatic, patients with extensive lesions and open ulcers may experience symptoms including fever, diarrhea, and abdominal pain.
- Intestinal tuberculosis is characterized by a wide variety of ulcer morphologies, including circular, girdle-like, round, irregular, and small ulcers. Ulcer margins resemble the marginal appearance of type IIC early gastric cancer.
- Most ulcers are around U1-II-III in severity, but serosal granulomas may also be present in patients with extensive ulcers.
- Individual ulcers have a strong tendency to heal, with fibrosis of the submucosal layer and regeneration of mucosal epithelium occurring easily. Ulcers in a variety of different stages will thus coexist in the same patient.

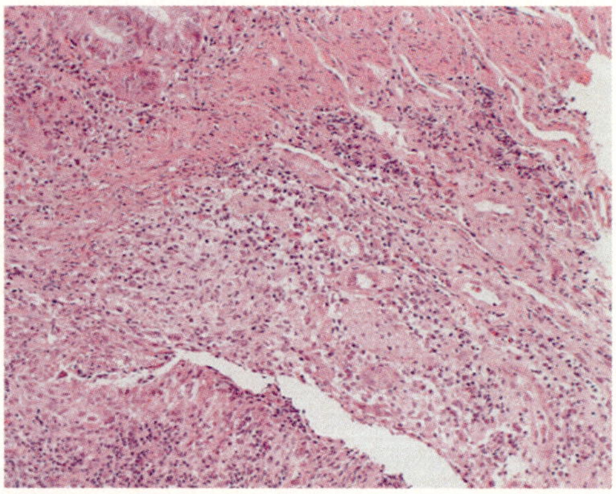

Fig. 24.3 Biopsy specimen from an erosion on the ileocecal valve. Epithelioid cell granuloma was evident immediately below the muscularis mucosa

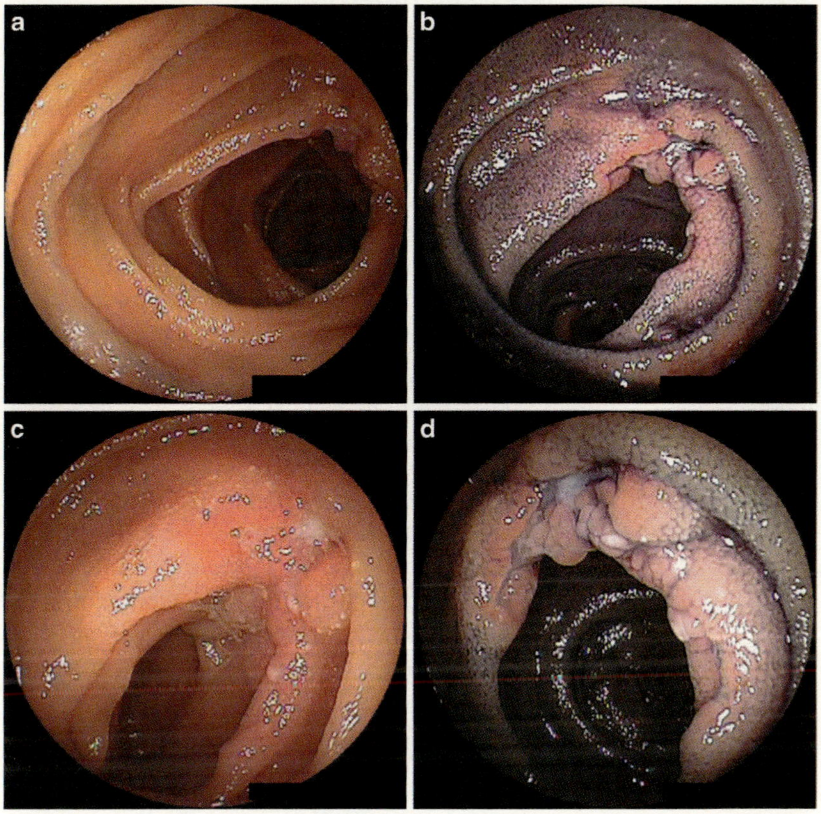

Fig. 24.4

24.2 Case 2 [2]

24.2.1 Female, 50s (Fig. 24.4a–d)

- The patient underwent contrast-enhanced small intestinal radiography at a local clinic because of abdominal pain, and an abnormality of the middle small intestine was identified. Her husband had a previous history of pulmonary tuberculosis.
- A circular ulcer extending one-quarter of the way around the circumference of the intestine was evident on Kerckring's folds in the middle small intestine.
- The surroundings of the ulcer were reddened and edematous. A white protrusion believed to represent lymphangiectasia was present in the neighborhood of the ulcer.
- Epithelium comprising enlarged villi was present within the ulcer, which was regarded as partly healed. A white coat adhered to the areas in which this epithelium was lacking.

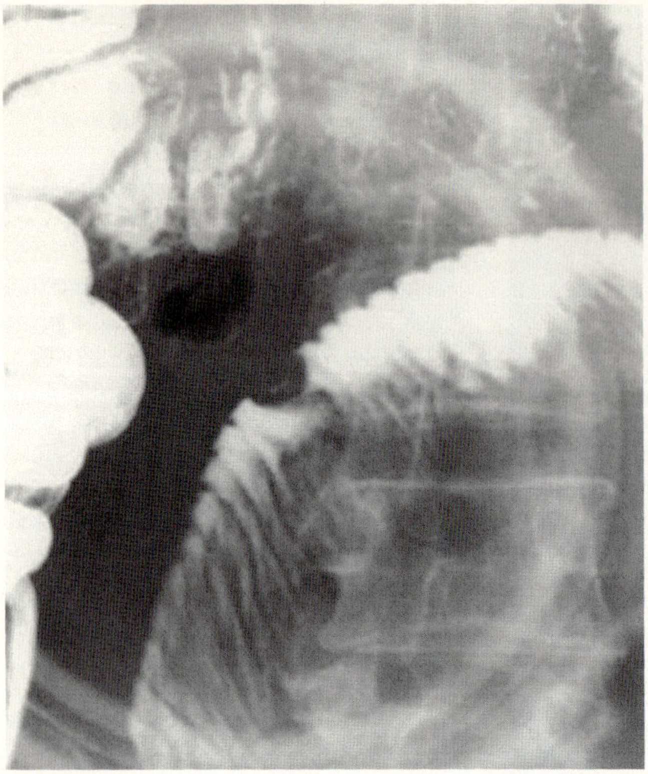

Fig. 24.5 Contrast-enhanced radiography performed by the previous attending physician. A small ulcer with a surrounding protrusion was evident in the middle small intestine

24.2.2 Intestinal Tuberculosis (Figs. 24.5 and 24.6)

- Lesions commonly occur in the ileocecal area or the right colon.
- This condition causes a range of symptoms, including abdominal pain, diarrhea, melena, fever, abdominal distension, and weight loss, although many cases are asymptomatic.
- In the early stages, there may be no symptoms other than aphthous ulcers or irregular small ulceration.
- Small ulcers often develop along the short axis of the intestine, resulting in an annular arrangement or circular ulcers. If a circular ulcer becomes chronic, this can cause stenosis due to fibrosis.
- Diagnosis is made by Mycobacterium tuberculosis culture from feces or biopsy tissue, Ziehl-Neelsen staining, polymerase chain reaction, or histopathological confirmation of caseating granuloma. However, intestinal tuberculosis may be clinically suspected even in unconfirmed cases, and if the characteristic imaging findings are apparent, administration of antituberculosis drugs should be considered.

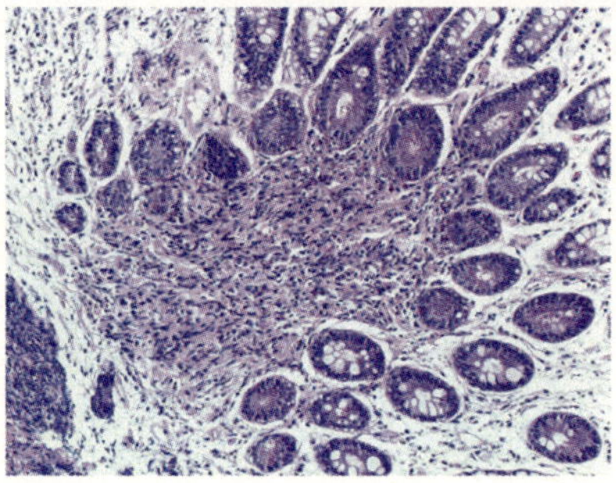

Fig. 24.6 Granuloma-like lesions composed of aggregations of histiocytes were evident in biopsy tissue from a small ulcer. In this case, Mycobacterium tuberculosis culture from biopsy tissue was also positive

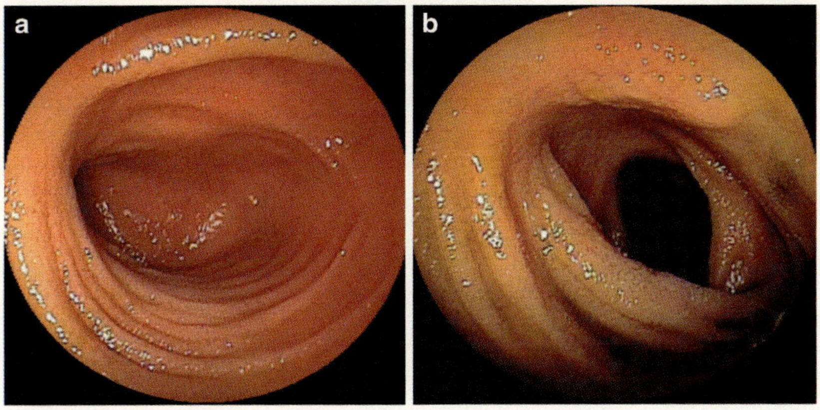

Fig. 24.7

24.3 Case 3, 4 [3]

24.3.1 Male, 30s (Fig. 24.7a, b)

- Treatment: Enteral nutrition and maintenance infliximab administration.
- Longitudinal ulcer scarring with mucosal convergence was evident in the ileum. Each scar caused unilateral deformity, with some luminal stenosis.

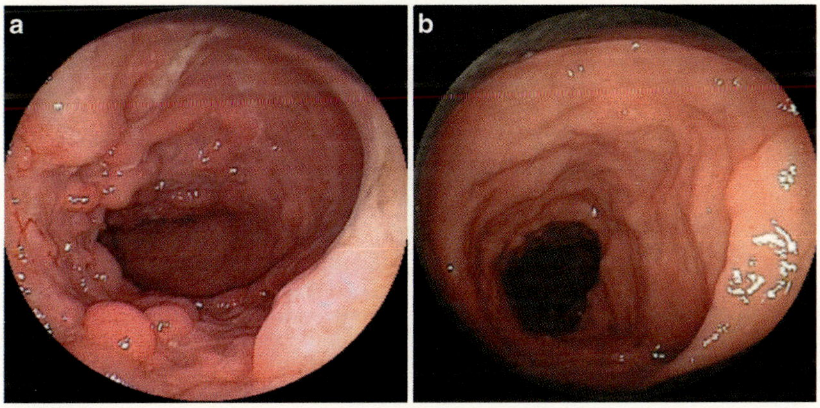

Fig. 24.8

24.3.2 Male, Teens (Fig. 24.8a, b)

- Treatment: Maintenance administration of infliximab
- Before treatment (a)
- There were multiple irregularly shaped and longitudinal ulcers in the terminal part of the ileum, and the surrounding tissue showed a cobblestone appearance. These were typical active-phase small intestinal lesions.
- After three administrations of infliximab (b)
- Ulcers in this area of the terminal part of the ileum had scarred, causing some narrowing, and multiple inflammatory polyps were present. These were findings of mucosal healing (b).

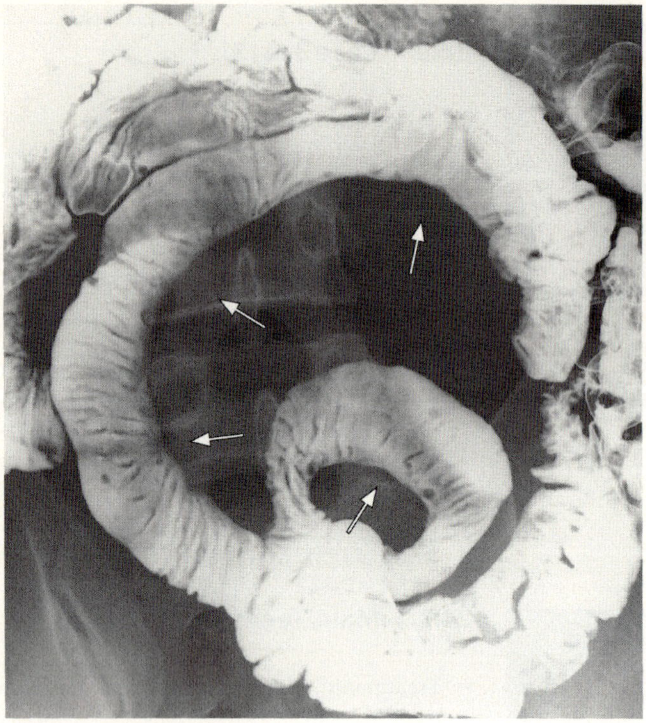

Fig. 24.9

24.3.3 Crohn's Disease (Fig. 24.9)

- Longitudinal ulcers, the active lesions in this condition, scar when they enter the healing phase. They are frequently surrounded by inflammatory polyps, but these may be difficult to distinguish from the cobblestone appearance seen during the active phase if the latter is mild.
- Open, irregularly shaped, or longitudinal ulcers cause unilateral deformity due to scarring when they heal, and this may result in luminal narrowing or stenosis.
- In recent years, the use of mucosal evaluation via small intestinal endoscopy and the emergence of biologic drugs to bring about mucosal healing have gained attention.

Case 3: Radiography. Scarring of a longitudinal ulcer with a unilateral deformity of the intestinal tract and pronounced mucosal convergence was evident.

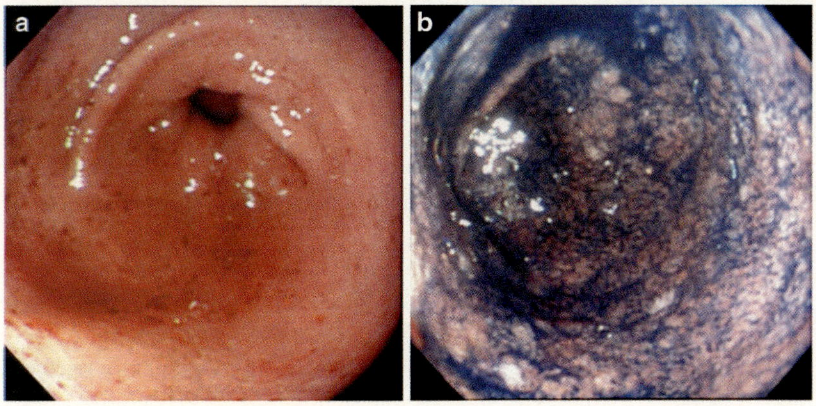

Fig. 24.10

24.4 Case 5, 6 [4]

24.4.1 Female, 20s (Fig. 24.10a, b)

- The patient had suffered from inflammatory ulcerative colitis of the entire colon since 2001.
- Diffuse redness and erosions were evident in the gastric antrum.
- Diffuse erosions and coarse, fragile mucosa were evident in the jejunum, and Kerckring's folds had disappeared.

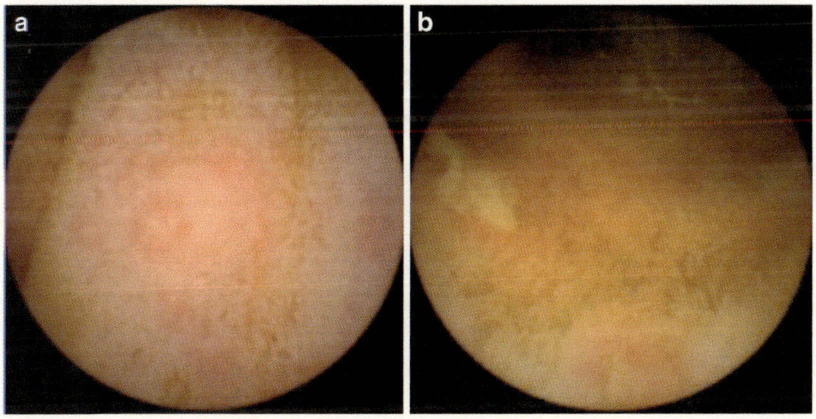

Fig. 24.11

24.4.2 Female, Teens (Fig. 24.11a, b)

- The patient had suffered from inflammatory ulcerative colitis of the entire colon since 2008.
- CE revealed diffuse redness and aphthae in the upper small intestine.
- Diffuse reddened, edematous mucosa and small ulcers were evident in the lower small intestine.

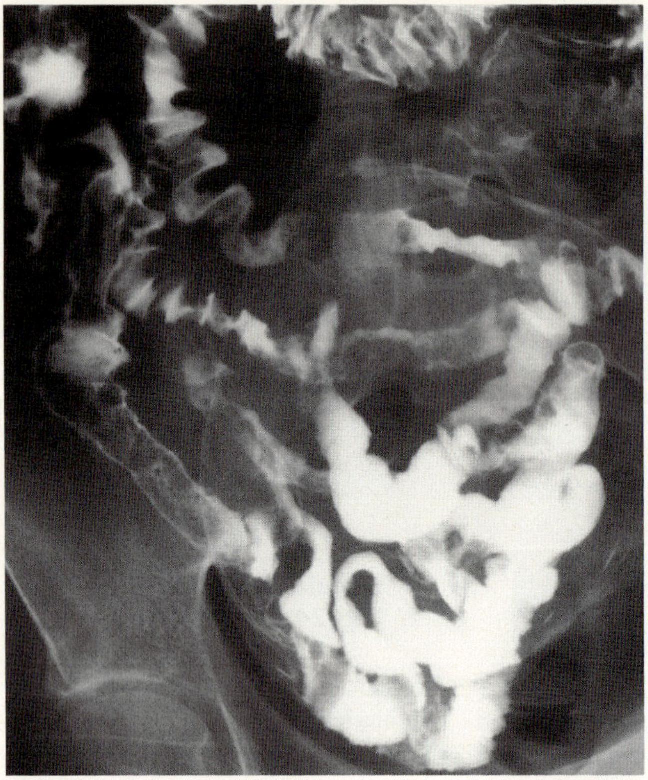

Fig. 24.12 Case 5: Radiography. Coarse mucosa and diffuse findings with a fluffy appearance at the margins were evident throughout the small intestine, with the middle small intestine having a particularly pronounced edematous appearance

24.4.3 Ulcerative Colitis-Associated Intestinal Lesions (Fig. 24.12)

- Ulcerative colitis is a condition localized in the large intestine that causes diffuse inflammation of the mucosa, and which may also cause diffuse or continuous inflammation of the upper gastrointestinal tract or small intestine.
- Endoscopic findings take a variety of forms, including edematous mucosa, redness, aphthae, erosions, and irregularly shaped ulcers.
- Diffuse lesions of the small intestine frequently occur in patients with active-phase inflammatory ulcerative colitis of the entire intestine or pouchitis.

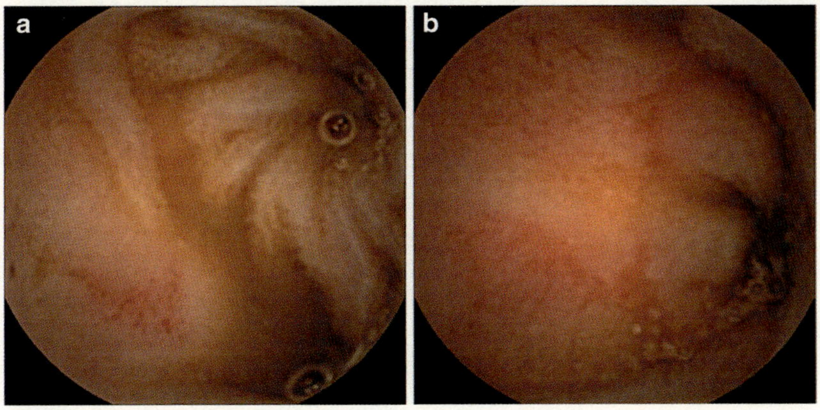

Fig. 24.13

24.5 Case 7, 8 [5]

24.5.1 Male, 70s (Fig. 24.13a, b)

- The patient was referred to our department for detailed testing to investigate lower abdominal discomfort and anemia. He was taking aspirin due to stenosis of bilateral carotid arteries and old cerebral infarction.
- CE revealed mucosal redness and multiple aphthae/erosive lesions from the middle to the lower small intestine.
- Some of the mucosal lesions were linear or irregularly shaped.

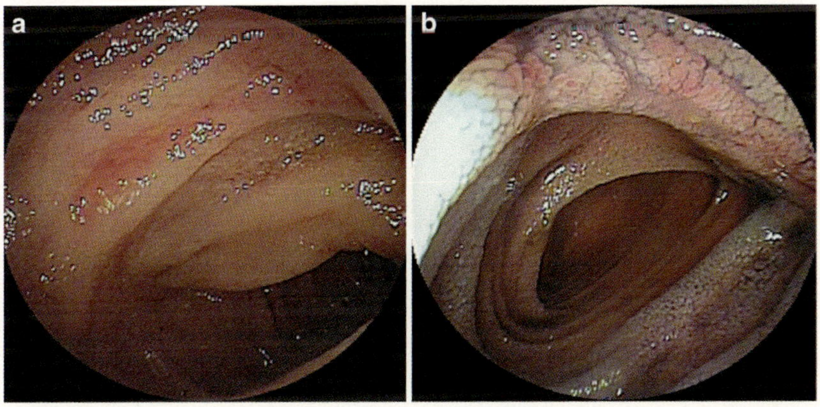

Fig. 24.14

24.5.2 Female, 30s (Fig. 24.14a, b)

- The patient was undergoing chemotherapy for acute lymphocytic leukemia. When she took oral loxoprofen for fever, large quantities of tarry stool and anemia (Hb 6.7 g/dl) appeared.
- CE carried out 1 week after loxoprofen was discontinued revealed an open ulcer in the jejunum.
- DBE carried out 3 weeks after loxoprofen was discontinued showed that the ulcer had almost healed.

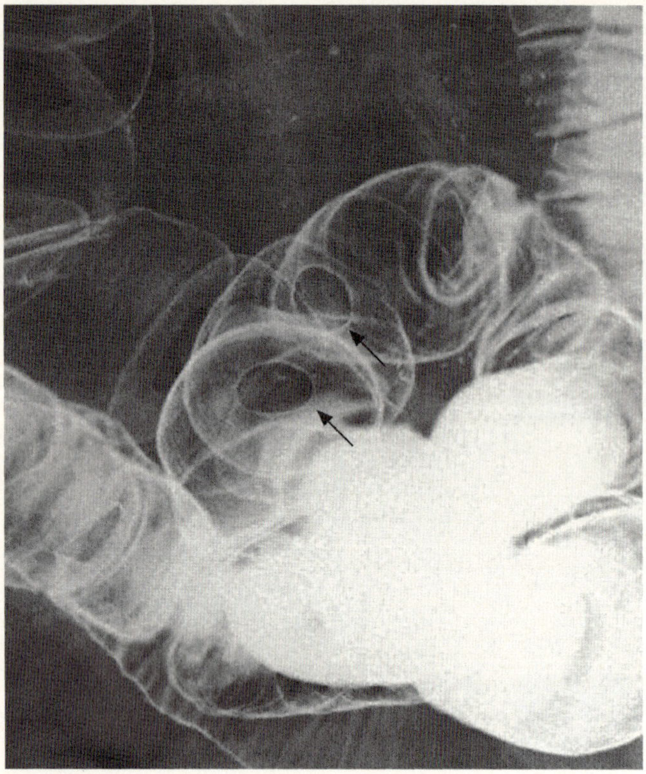

Fig. 24.15

24.5.3 NSAID-Induced Enteropathy (Fig. 24.15)

- The main mechanisms whereby intestinal damage is caused by NSAIDs are abnormal mitochondrial metabolism within small intestinal epithelial cells and increased mucosal permeability as a result of drug exposure.
- Although the frequency of appearance and severity of small intestinal lesions depend on the type of NSAID and duration of use, CE of long-term NSAID users has found that erosions and small ulcers are present in 30–40 % of cases.
- Endoscopy is better than radiography for visualizing erosions and ulcer scarring. Circular ulcer scarring can be visualized radiographically.
- Discontinuation of NSAID use is the basic principal of treatment, but if discontinuation is difficult owing to the underlying disease, the patient should be switched to a different medication. Mucosal lesions improve quickly when NSAID use is discontinued.

References

1. Lee YJ et al. Analysis of colonoscopic findings in the differential diagnosis between intestinal tuberculosis and Crohn's disease. Endoscopy. 2006;38:592–7.
2. Sato S et al. Colonoscopy in the diagnosis of intestinal tuberculosis in asymptomatic patients. Gastrointest Endosc. 2004;59:362–8.
3. Buchman AL et al. Videocapsule endoscopy versus barium contrast studies for the diagnosis of Crohn's disease recurrence involving the small intestine. Am J Gastroenterol. 2004;99:2171–7.
4. Hisabe H et al. Small bowel lesions detected with wireless capsule endoscopy in patients with active ulcerative colitis and with post-proctocolectomy. Dig Endosc. 2011;23:302–9.
5. Goldstein JL et al. Video capsule endoscopy to prospectively assess small bowel injury with celecoxib, naproxen plus omeprazole, an placebo. Clin Gastroenterol Hepatol. 2005;3:133–41.

Case Presentations: Diffuse Granular or Diffuse Coarse Mucosal Lesions

25

Shotaro Nakamura, Shunichi Yanai, Tomohiko Moriyama, Minako Hirahashi, Naoki Ohmiya, Masahiro Kishi, and Takashi Nagahama

25.1 Case 1

25.1.1 Female, 60s (Fig. 25.1a–d)

- The patient was admitted to hospital with principal complaints of abdominal pain, diarrhea, and weight loss.
- Upper gastrointestinal endoscopy revealed numerous small protrusions in the second part of the duodenum (a, b).
- Retrograde DBE showed fine granular mucosa consisting of enlarged villi together with diffuse small protrusions (c, d).

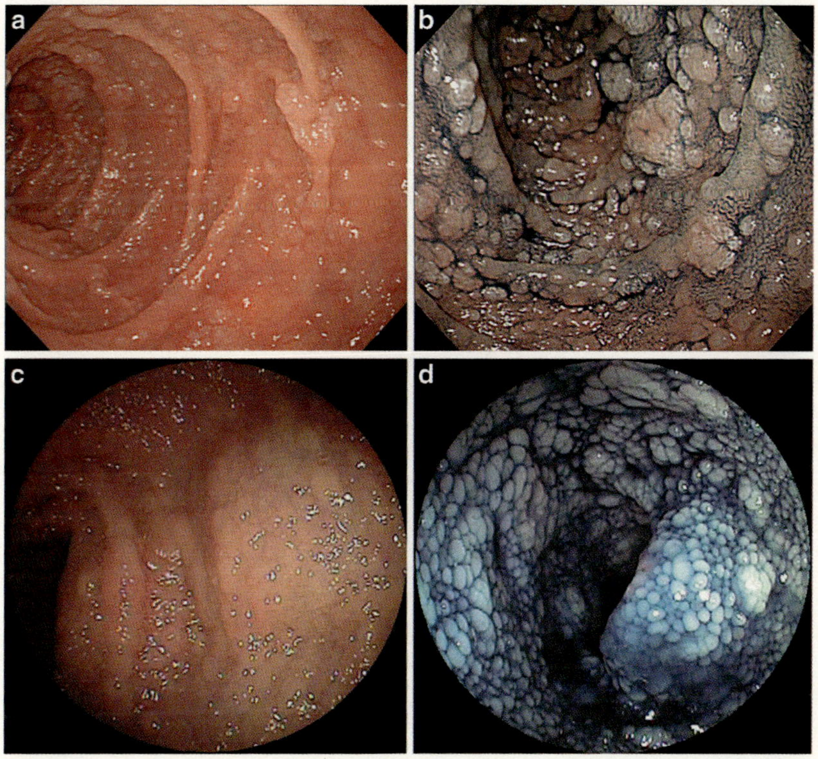

Fig. 25.1

S. Nakamura (✉) • T. Moriyama • M. Hirahashi
Department of Medicine and Clinical Science, Graduate School of Medical Sciences, Kyushu University, 3-1-1, Maidashi, Higashi-ku, Fukuoka City 812-8582, Japan
e-mail: shonaka@intmed2.med.kyushu-u.ac.jp

S. Yanai
Japan Seamen's Relief Association Moji Hospital, 1-3-1 Kiyotaki, Moji-ku, Kitakyushu 801-8550, Japan

N. Ohmiya
Department of Gastroenterology, Nagoya University Graduate School of Medicine, 65 Tsurumai-cho, Showa-ku, Nagoya 466-8550, Japan

M. Kishi • T. Nagahama
Department of Gastroenterology, Fukuoka University Chikushi Hospital, 1-1-1 Zokumyoin, Chikushino 818-8502, Japan

T. Matsui et al. (eds.), *Endoscopy in the Diagnosis of Small Intestine Diseases*,
DOI 10.1007/978-4-431-54352-7_25, © Springer Japan 2014

25.1.2 Immunoproliferative Small Intestinal Disease (Figs. 25.2 and 25.3)

- Immunoproliferative small intestinal disease (IPSID) is a condition classified histologically as a specific type of MALT lymphoma. This pathology causes diarrhea, weight loss, malabsorption, and protein-losing gastroenteropathy and is also known as α-chain disease or Mediterranean lymphoma.
- Radiography and endoscopy show diffuse, fine granular small protrusions across a wide area of the small intestine, mainly in the duodenum and jejunum.
- Monoclonal proliferation of IgA-positive lymphoplasmacytes is evident.
- This condition is more common in countries bordering the Mediterranean and Middle East, and is rare in Japan.
- *Campylobacter jejuni* infection has been implicated in its etiology, and treatment with tetracycline antibiotics may be effective.

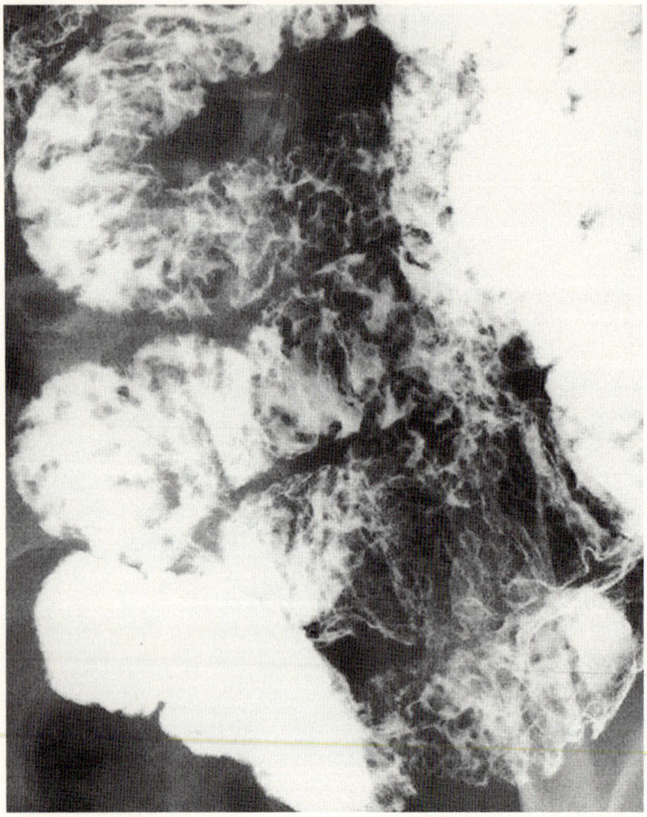

Fig. 25.2 Radiography showed diffuse, fine granular small protrusions were evident across a wide area of the small intestine

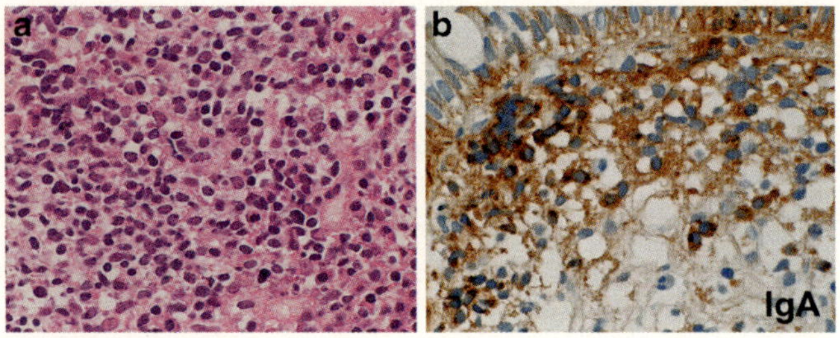

Fig. 25.3 Histology showed monoclonal proliferation of IgA-positive lymphoplasmacytes

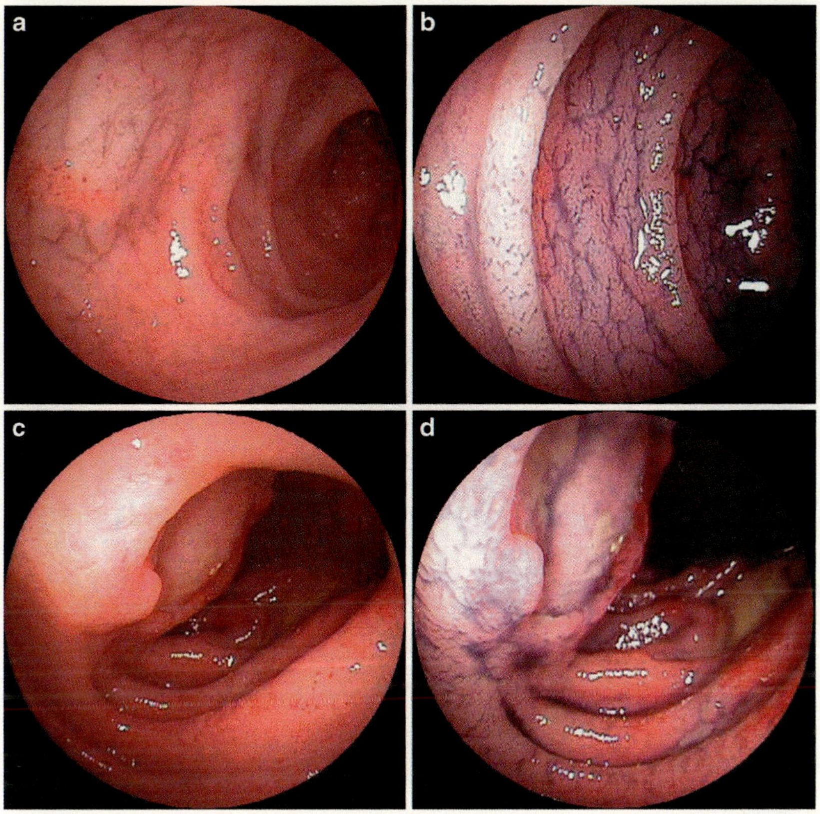

Fig. 25.4

25.2 Case 2 [2]

25.2.1 Male, 70s (Fig. 25.4a–d)

- The patient was admitted to hospital with loss of appetite, diarrhea, and weight loss as principal complaints.
- Antegrade DBE showed enlarged, indistinct Kerckring's folds in the upper jejunum (a).
- Dye spraying revealed coarse changes with a crack-like appearance in the jejunal mucosa (b).
- When the endoscope was advanced further to the distal side, a clearly demarcated ulcerative lesion with gradual marginal rising appearance was observed (c, d).

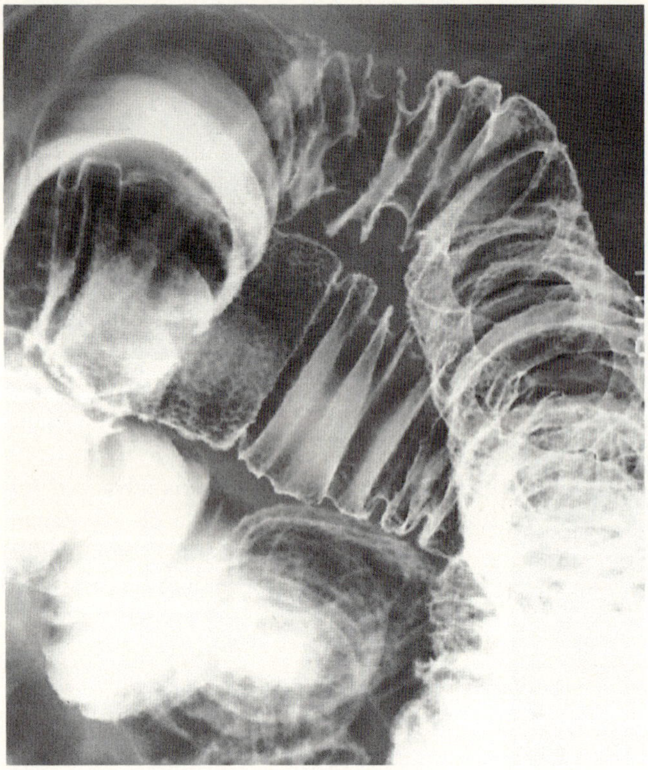

Fig. 25.5 Diffuse enlargement of the folds was evident from the upper jejunum to the ileum, and the mucosal surface had a fine granular appearance

25.2.2 Enteropathy-Associated T-Cell Lymphoma (ETL) (Fig. 25.4)

- This intraepithelial T-lymphocyte-derived lymphoproliferative disease causes chronic diarrhea and malabsorption, usually resulting in intestinal perforation. The prognosis is poor.
- The condition is broadly divided into types 1 and 2, depending on whether or not celiac disease is also present, but this distinction is not always exact.
- The case illustrated here was positive for anti-tissue transglutaminase antibodies, suggesting the presence of celiac disease.
- In addition to swelling of Kerckring's folds from the duodenum to the jejunum and diffuse fine granular mucosa, ulcerative tumor formation is also seen.
- It is important to distinguish this condition from amyloidosis, parasitosis, and immunoproliferative small intestinal disease (IPSID), a specific type of MALT lymphoma.

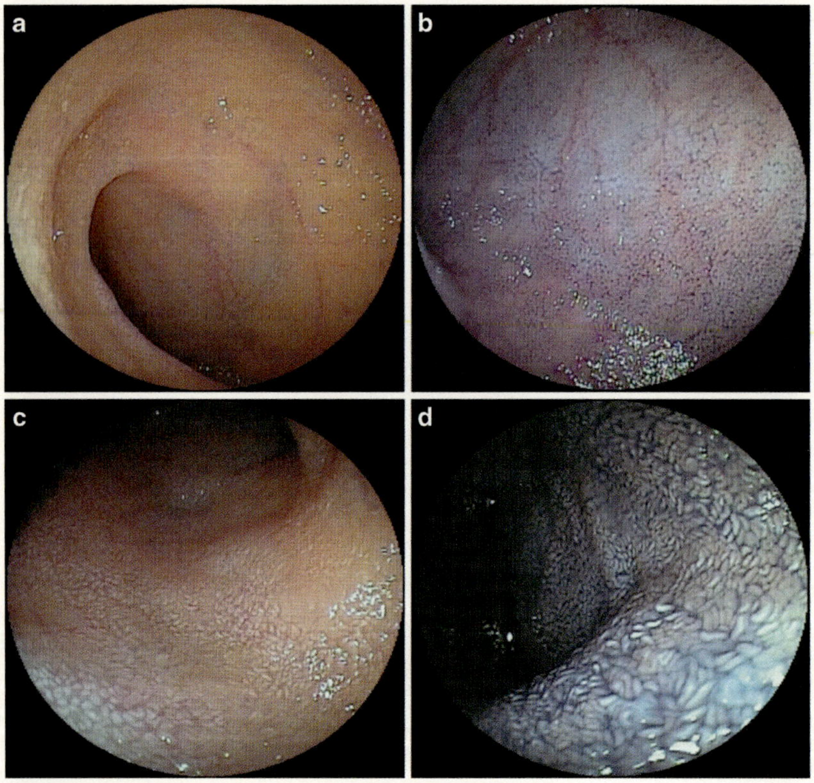

Fig. 25.6

25.3 Case 3 [3]

25.3.1 Female, 60s (Fig. 25.5a–d)

Principal complaints: vomiting, diarrhea

- Underlying disease: rheumatoid arthritis (disease duration 18 years)
- The jejunal mucosa displayed a fine granular appearance (a, b).
- The jejunal villi were somewhat enlarged, and the mucosa was coarse (c, d).
- Whitish changes considered to be due to lymphangiectasia were also evident in part of the mucosa (c, d).

25.3.2 Type AA Intestinal Amyloidosis (Fig. 25.6a–c)

- In this condition, serum amyloid A protein is deposited mainly in the lamina propria and submucosal vascular walls.
- It is often complicated by chronic infections such as tuberculosis, or chronic inflammatory diseases such as rheumatoid arthritis or Crohn's disease.
- Refractory diarrhea, malnutrition, and gastrointestinal bleeding are common principal complaints.
- Radiographically, characteristics include coarse or fine granular mucosa, bumpy Kerckring's folds, and luminal narrowing.
- In addition to those listed above, characteristic endoscopic findings also include whitish changes and friability of the mucosa.

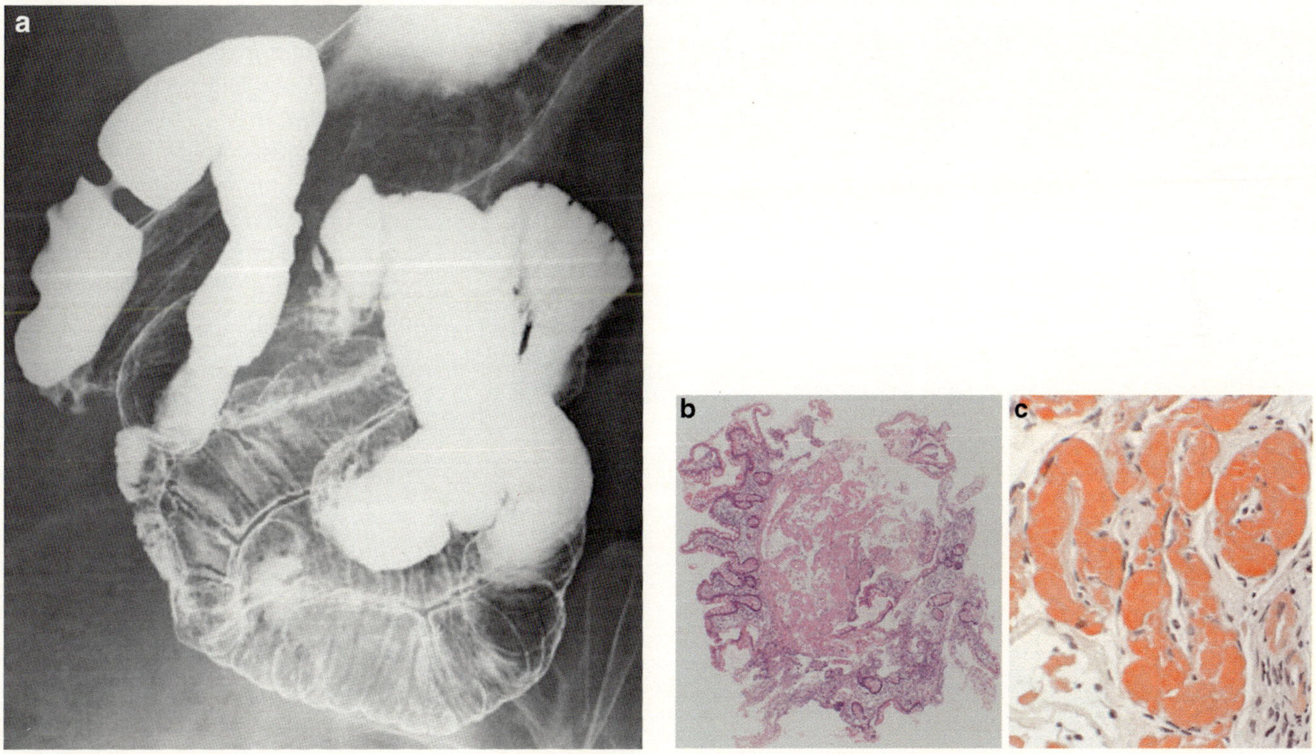

Fig. 25.7 The mucosa had a fine granular or coarse appearance from the second part of the duodenum to the jejunum, with scattered small erosions (**a**). Eosinophilic thickening of vascular walls in the submucosal layer was evident in biopsy tissue (**b**), and immunostaining was positive for anti-amyloid A antibodies (**c**)

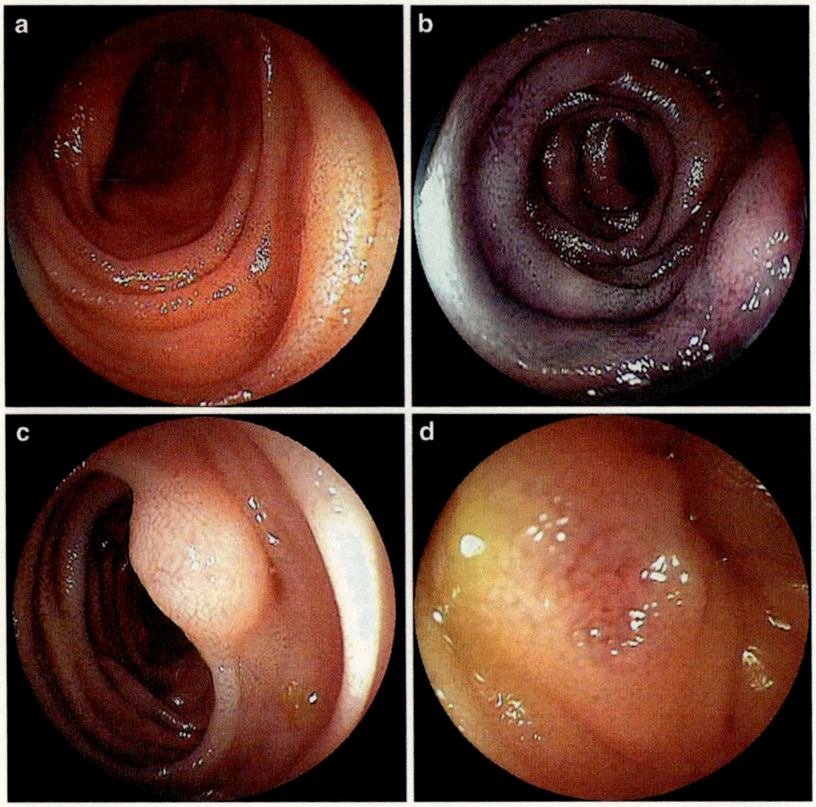

Fig. 25.8

25.4 Case 4 [4]

25.4.1 Male, 50s (Fig. 25.7a–d)

Principal complaints: melena with no abdominal pain

- Underlying disease: none
- Edematous enlargement of Kerckring's folds in the jejunum and scattered yellowish-white submucosal tumor-like small protrusions were evident (a).
- Dye spraying revealed no changes to the villous structure of the mucosa, and the small protrusions had no relationship to Peyer's patches (b).
- A somewhat glossy, yellowish-white submucosal elevation with a smooth surface was present on Kerckring's folds (c).
- The peak of the protrusion was somewhat depressed, with discernable erosion and villous atrophy (d).

25.4.2 AL-Type Intestinal Amyloidosis (Fig. 25.8a–c)

- AL amyloid protein consists of all or part of a variant region of the immunoglobulin L chain, and although this condition may occur as a complication of multiple myeloma or macroglobulinemia, the underlying disease is unknown in many cases.
- Most cases of primary intestinal amyloidosis are the AL type, and it is comparatively rare for this condition to be localized in the gastrointestinal tract.
- Characteristic radiographic and endoscopic findings comprise multiple mild yellowish-white submucosal elevation and swelling of Kerckring's folds.
- Although amyloid deposition is present in all layers of the gastrointestinal wall, the AL type shows a particularly strong tendency for deposition of amyloid in clumps in the muscularis mucosa, submucosal layer, and intrinsic muscle layer; this is not inconsistent with findings supporting multiple submucosal elevation and enlargement of the folds.

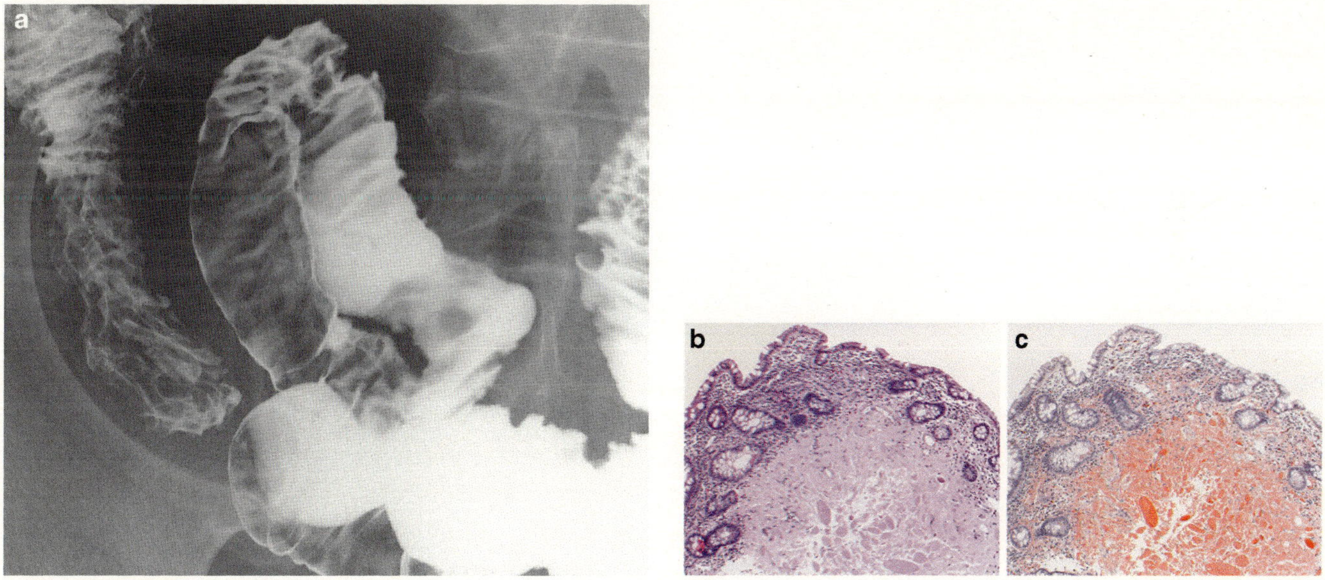

Fig. 25.9 Kerckring's folds were enlarged, and scattered submucosal tumors and bumpy mucosal irregularities were evident (**a**). Eosinophilic unstructured amyloid protein was deposited in clumps in the muscularis mucosa and lamina propria interstitium, and villi were flattened (HE staining, Dylon staining) (**b**, **c**)

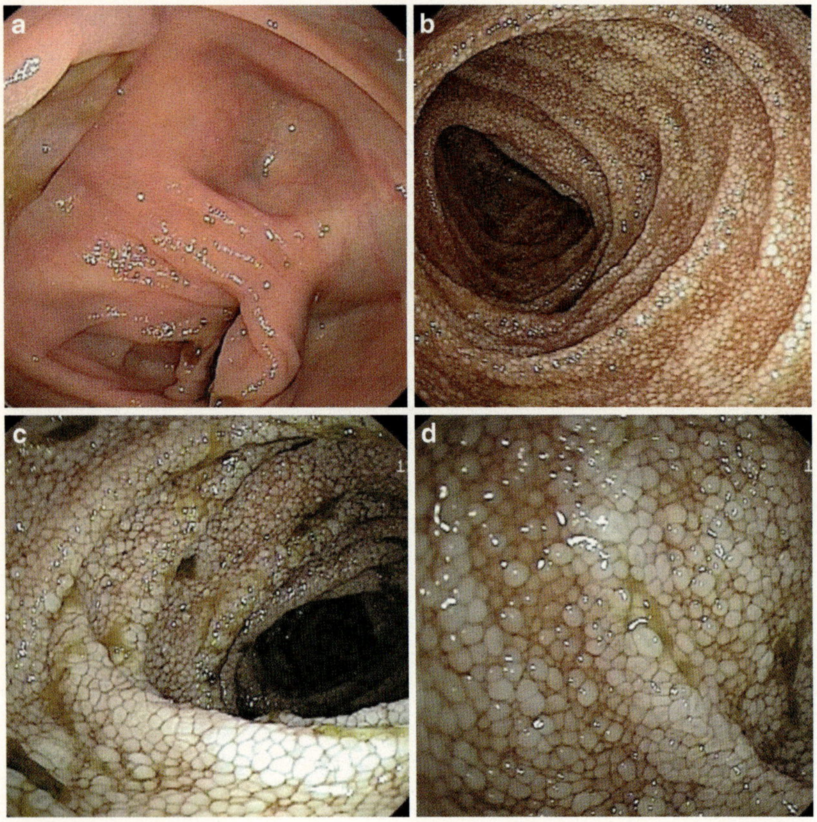

Fig. 25.10

25.5 Case 5 [5]

25.5.1 Male, 40s (Fig. 25.9a–d)

Principal complaints: watery diarrhea, edema of the legs

- Underlying disease: macroglobulinemia
- There was a dense concentration of short, white villi on the ileocecal valve (a). Short white villi were also densely concentrated in the terminal part of the ileum, but scattered normal villi were also present (b).
- Enlarged white villi were densely concentrated in the upper ileum, with no gaps between them (c, d).

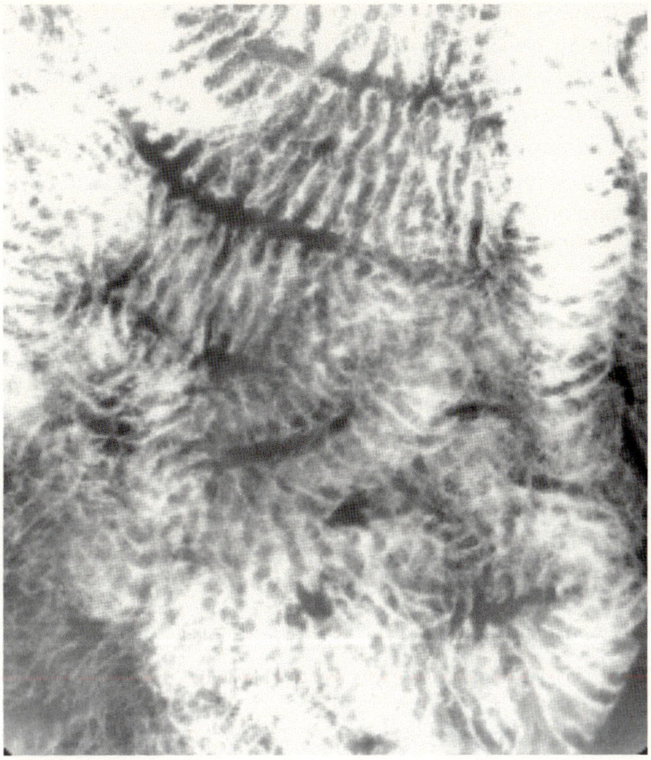

Fig. 25.11 Diffuse thickening of Kerckring's folds, scattered coarse granules, and hazy barium imaging were evident

25.5.2 Intestinal Lymphangiectasia (Fig. 25.10)

- This condition causes pronounced dilation of the intestinal lymph ducts and protein-losing enteropathy due to impaired lymph flow and elevated pressure within the lymph ducts. It is sometimes associated with chylothorax, chylous ascites, and edema of the limbs. Principal complaints include edema, diarrhea, and steatorrhea.
- Radiography reveals thickening of Kerckring's folds throughout the small intestine, multiple granular protrusions, and hazy barium imaging due to excessive lymph secretion.
- Endoscopically, this pathology exhibits the four characteristics of white villi, scattered white spots, small white protrusions, and submucosal elevation, and occurs more commonly in the duodenum and jejunum.

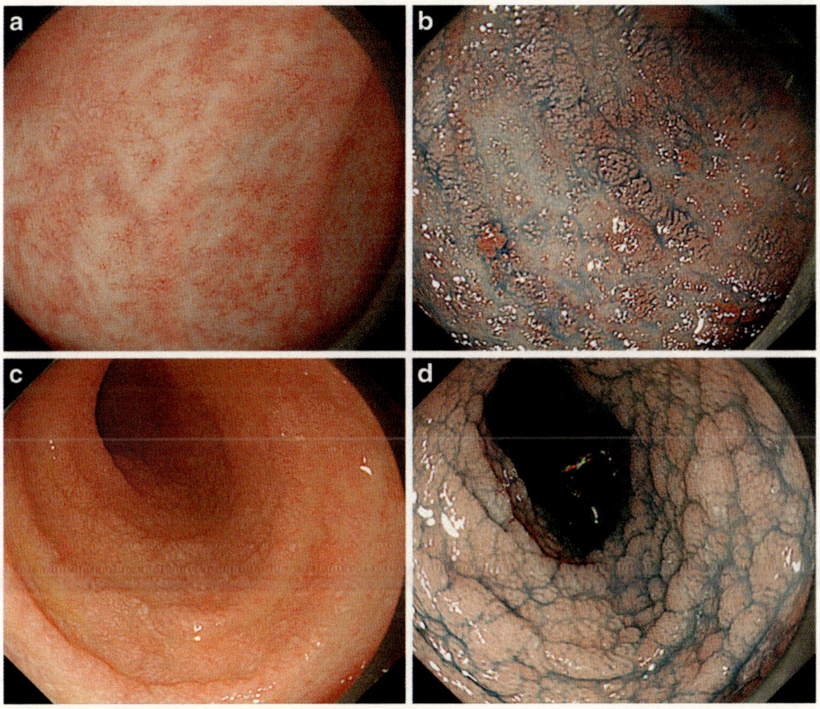

Fig. 25.12

25.6 Case 6 [6]

25.6.1 Female, 60s (Fig. 25.11a–d)

Principal complaints: watery diarrhea, weight loss

- Atrophy and loss of villous structure in the duodenal bulb was evident both in normal observation and after dye spraying (a, b).
- Kerckring's folds in the second part the duodenum were flattened, and scalloping of the mucosa as a result of atrophy of the villous structure was visible (c, d).

25.6.2 Celiac Disease (Fig. 25.12a, b)

- This condition occurs with a frequency of around 1 % in Europe and the US, but is rare in Japan.
- Principal complaints include weight loss and diarrhea.
- Symptoms worsen with a gluten-containing diet, and improve with a gluten-free diet.
- Radiographically, the pathology is characterized by a tendency toward significant disappearance of Kerckring's folds in the proximal intestinal tract and fine granular changes.
- Endoscopically, it is characterized by flattening of Kerckring's folds starting from the duodenum, and atrophy or loss of villous structure.

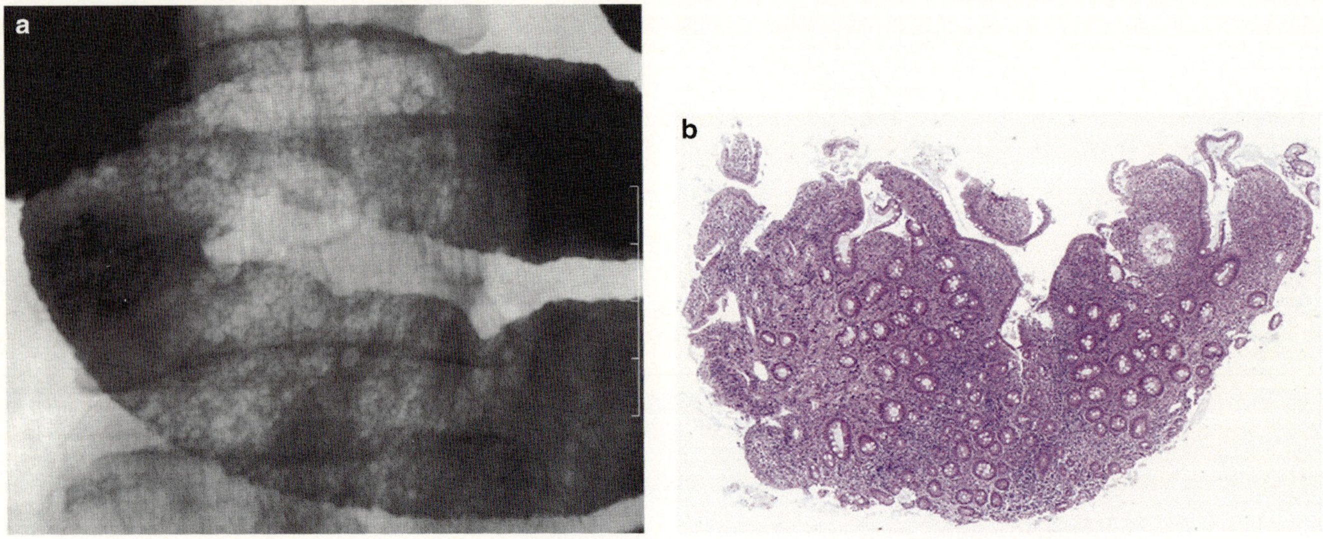

Fig. 25.13 (**a**) Radiography revealed a tendency toward loss of Kerckring's folds and slight granular changes in the jejunum. (**b**) Histopathology of a biopsy specimen from the duodenum revealed flattening of the villous structure and lymphocyte infiltration of the mucosa

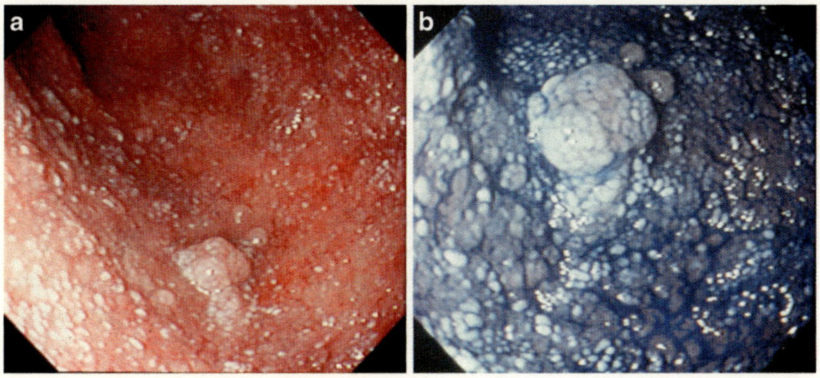

Fig. 25.14

25.7 Case 7, 8 [7]

25.7.1 Female, 30s (Fig. 25.13a, b)

- Generalized alopecia and amenorrhea had appeared at 17 years old, severe diarrhea at 20 years old, and abdominal pain, vomiting, diarrhea, and mild muscle spasms at 36 years old.
- Kerckring's folds had disappeared, the mucosal surface was reddish, and fine granular mucosal changes with scattered white patches were evident, as were polypoid protrusions formed by aggregations of enlarged villi.

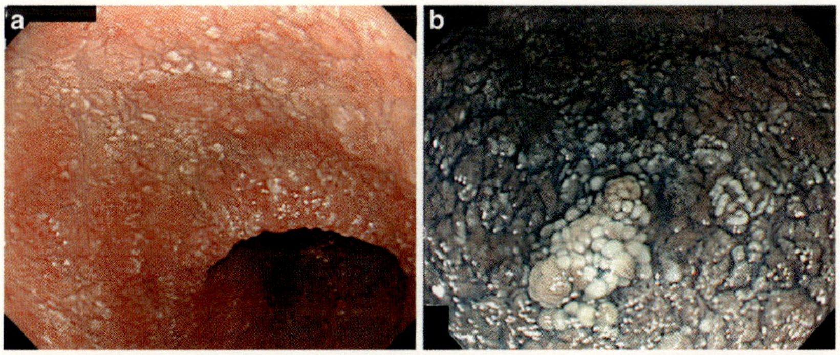

Fig. 25.15

25.7.2 Female, 30s (Fig. 25.14a, b)

- Generalized alopecia, severe diarrhea, and occasional muscle spasms had appeared at 16 years old, and amenorrhea at 30 years old. Muscle spasms and diarrhea worsened at 36 years old.
- Findings were similar to those in Case 1.

25.7.3 Satoyoshi Syndrome (Fig. 25.15a, b)

- This condition of unknown origin has three main characteristics: progressive muscle spasms (cramps); generalized alopecia; and diarrhea. Onset commonly occurs in women in their teens.
- Organic abnormalities of the digestive tract may be present in patients with severe diarrhea, causing malabsorption syndrome.
- Endoscopic findings comprise mottled redness of the mucosal surface, fine granular mucosal changes with scattered white patches, and polypoid protrusions formed by aggregations of enlarged villi.
- Radiographically, a pumiceous appearance is evident (a).
- Histopathologically, atrophy of the glands and epithelial detachment are evident, as are thickening and fibrosis from the lamina propria to the submucosa and cystic dilation of the glandular ducts in the mucosa and submucosa, with the appearance of gastroenterocolitis cystica polyposa (b).

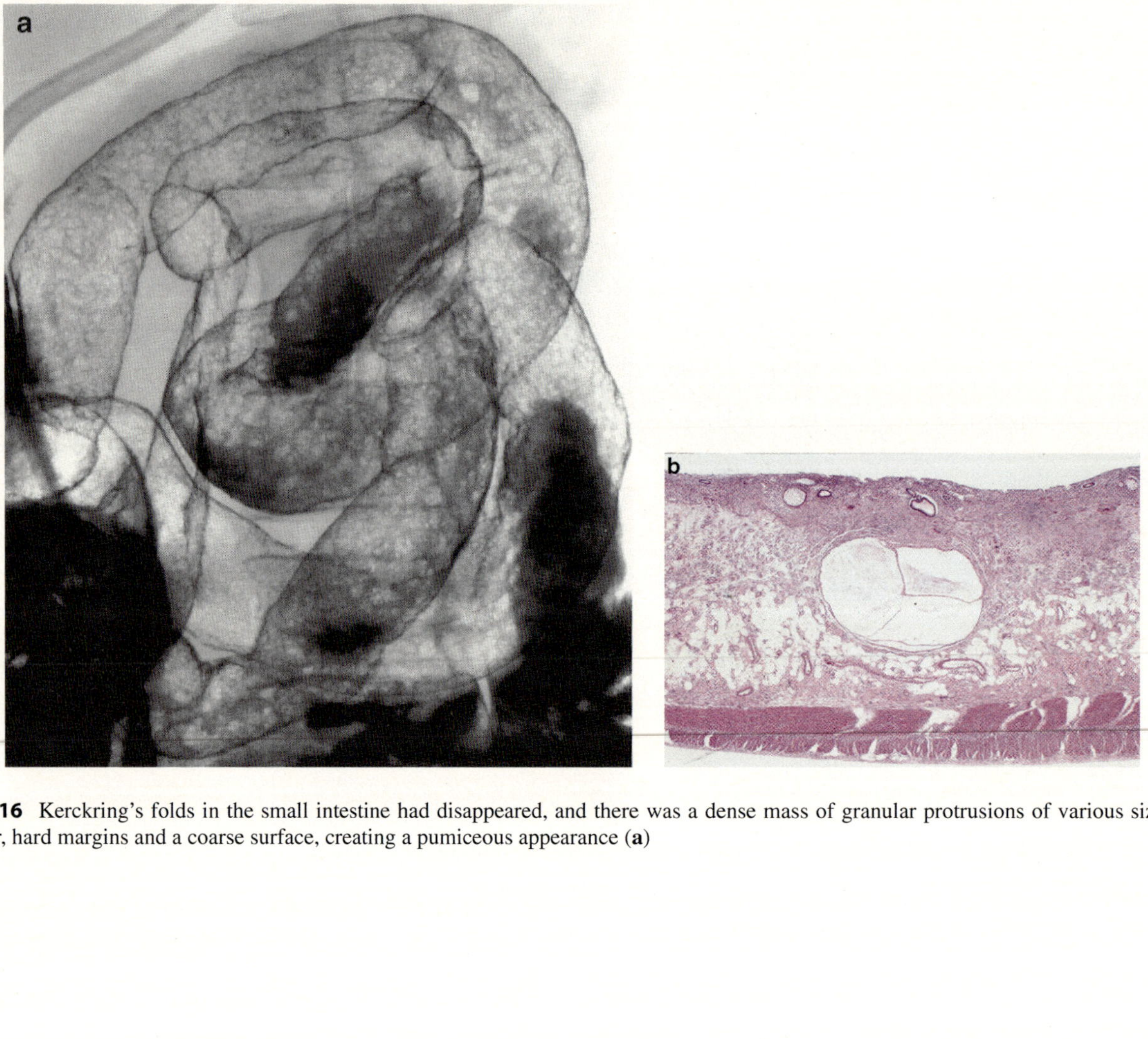

Fig. 25.16 Kerckring's folds in the small intestine had disappeared, and there was a dense mass of granular protrusions of various sizes with irregular, hard margins and a coarse surface, creating a pumiceous appearance (**a**)

References

1. Nakamura S et al. A clinicopathologic study of primary small intestine lymphoma: prognostic significance of mucosa-associated lymphoid tissue-derived lymphoma. Cancer. 2000;88:286–94.
2. Yanai S et al. Endoscopic findings of enteropathy-type T-cell lymphoma. Endoscopy. 2007;39 Suppl 1:E339–40.
3. Tada S et al. Endoscopic features in amyloidosis of the small intestine: clinical and morphologic differences between chemical types of amyloid protein. Gastrointest Endosc. 1994;40:45–50.
4. Tada S et al. Endoscopic features in amyloidosis of the small intestine: clinical and morphologic differences between chemical types of amyloid protein. Gastrointest Endosc. 1994;40:45–50.
5. Takenaka H et al. Endoscopic and imaging findings in protein-losing enteropathy. J Clin Gastroenterol. 2012;46:575–80.
6. Yao K et al. Comprehensive atlas of HRE and NBI. In: Cohen J, editor. Comprehensive atlas of high resolution endoscopy and narrow-band imaging. New York: Blackwell; 2007. p. 83–103.
7. Nagahama T et al. GI manifestations of Satoyoshi's syndrome. Gastrointest Endosc. 2006;64:143–5.

Case Presentaions: Whitish Multi-nodular Lesions

26

Koichi Eguchi and Kunihiko Aoyagi

26.1 Case 1 [1]

26.1.1 Male, 40s (Fig. 26.1a–d)

- No symptoms.
- Abnormality of the ileum was identified during endoscopy while the patient was undergoing treatment for ulcerative colitis.
- Small nodules and submucosal elevations, some of which were fused, were scattered in the ileum.
- The marginal rising appearance was shallow compared with that of epithelial neoplasm (a, b).
- Closer to the lower small intestine, the protrusions became clearer.
- Submucosal elevations of varying sizes that were the same color as the surrounding normal mucosa were aggregated in the terminal part of the ileum (c, d).

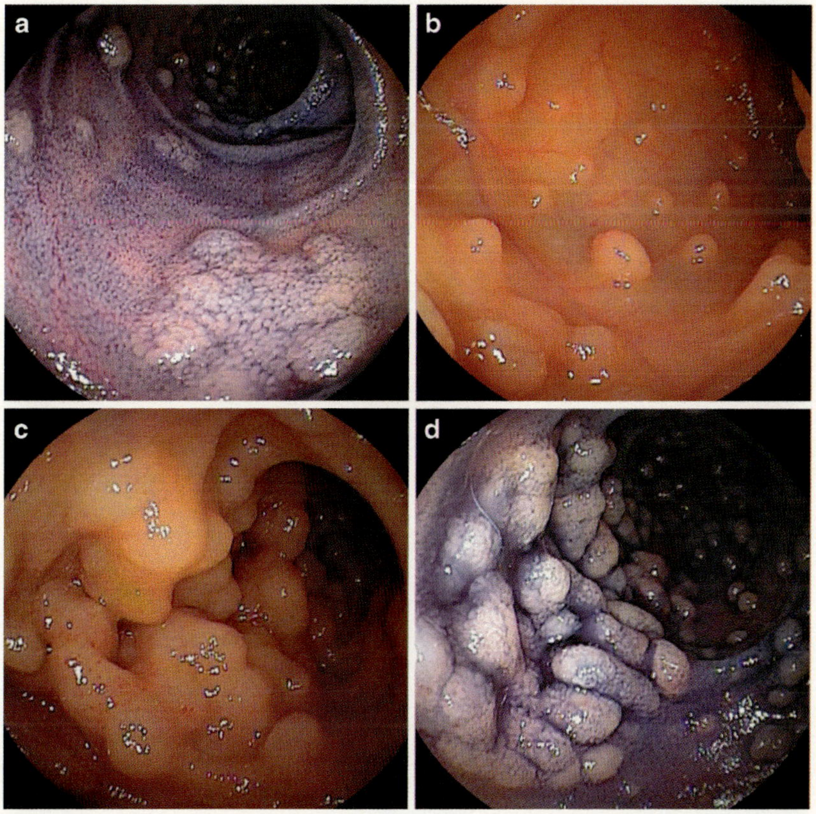

Fig. 26.1

K. Eguchi (✉) • K. Aoyagi
Department of Gastroenterology and Medicine, Fukuoka University Faculty of Medicine, 7-45-1 Nanakuma, Jonan-ku, Fukuoka 814-0180, Japan
e-mail: keguchi@minf.med.fukuoka-u.ac.jp

T. Matsui et al. (eds.), *Endoscopy in the Diagnosis of Small Intestine Diseases*, DOI 10.1007/978-4-431-54352-7_26, © Springer Japan 2014

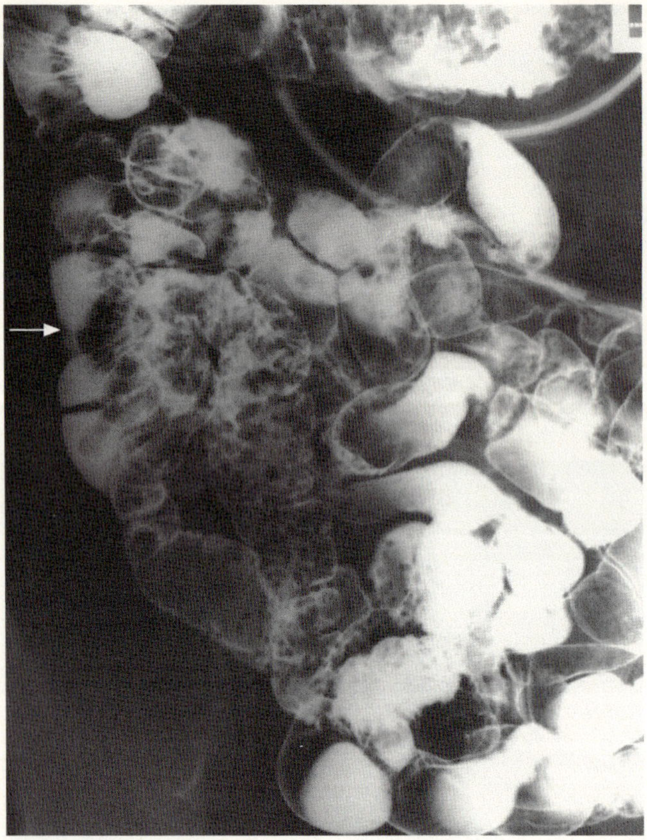

Fig. 26.2 Multiple small protrusions of varying sizes were evident, mainly in the terminal ileum. The ileocecal valve (*arrow*) was also enlarged

26.1.2 Follicular Lymphoma (Fig. 26.2)

- The multiple lymphomatous polyposis-like (MLP) type is a macroscopic type of follicular lymphoma or mantle cell lymphoma that takes the form of countless protruding lesions across a wide area of the gastrointestinal tract.
- Follicular lymphoma commonly occurs in middle to old age, with no sex difference. It is frequently asymptomatic. This tumor progresses slowly and has low malignant potential, with lesions occurring in the duodenum in many cases.
- Characteristic endoscopic findings are white granular mucosa in the small intestine and MLP-type macroscopic findings.
- If ileal lesions are present, they may have the appearance of multiple small nodules or submucosal elevations of the same color as the surrounding normal mucosa.
- Radiological characteristics of the MLP type are that it is frequently evident throughout the small intestine, with protrusions becoming clearer toward the lower small intestine.

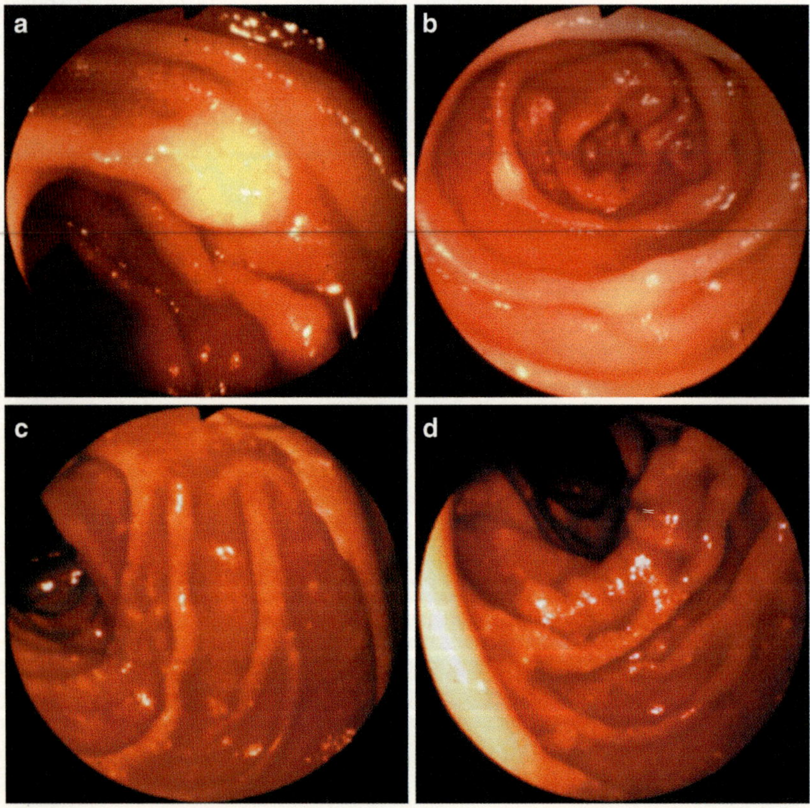

Fig. 26.3

26.2 Case 2 [2]

26.2.1 Female, 70s (Fig. 26.3a–d)

Principal complaints: diarrhea, edema of the legs

- A white protruding lesion was present in the jejunum. The surrounding folds were slightly enlarged (a, b).
- Scattered white spots were also visible in the jejunum (c, d).

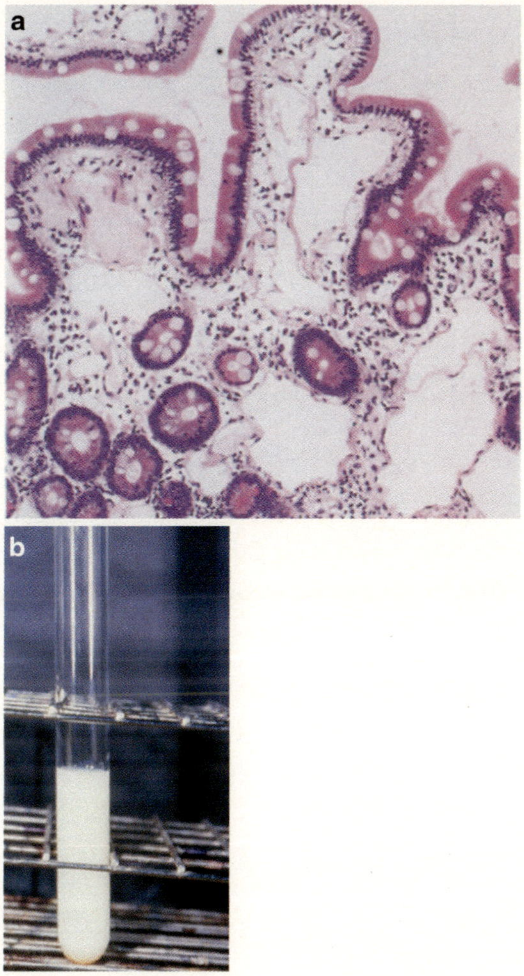

Fig. 26.4 (**a**) Lymphangiectasia was evident within the mucosa. (**b**) Chylous ascites

26.2.2 Intestinal Lymphangiectasia (Fig. 26.4a, b)

- This condition causes pronounced dilation of the intestinal lymph ducts and protein-losing enteropathy due to impaired lymph flow and elevated pressure within the lymph ducts.
- Principal complaints are diarrhea, edema and steatorrhea, and chylous ascites and pleural effusion may also be present.
- Radiographically, it is characterized by filling defects and uneven enlargement of the mucosal folds, with hazy imaging due to leakage of lymph. There is no erosion or ulceration.
- Endoscopically, it is characterized by small white protrusions from the duodenum to the upper small intestine, faint white mucosa with white villi, scattered white spots formed by aggregations of small white spots, and submucosal tumor-like protrusions formed by enlargement of the folds (with no white changes).

References

1. Nakamura S et al. Endoscopic features of intestinal follicular lymphoma: the value of double-balloon enteroscopy. Endoscopy. 2007;39 Suppl 1:E26–7.
2. Aoyagi K et al. Characteristic endoscopic features of intestinal lymphangiectasia: correlation with histological findings. Hepatogastroenterology. 1997;44:133–8.

27 Case Presentations: Intraluminal Growth

Koichi Abe

27.1 Case 1 [1]

27.1.1 Male, 50s (Fig. 27.1a–d)

Principal complaint: Black stool

- Upper and lower gastrointestinal endoscopy revealed no findings that might indicate the cause of bleeding.
- Separately from the lumen (A), the proximal jejunum also contained a diverticulum (B) (a, b).
- Another diverticulum could also be seen further to the distal side of the lesion above (c, d).

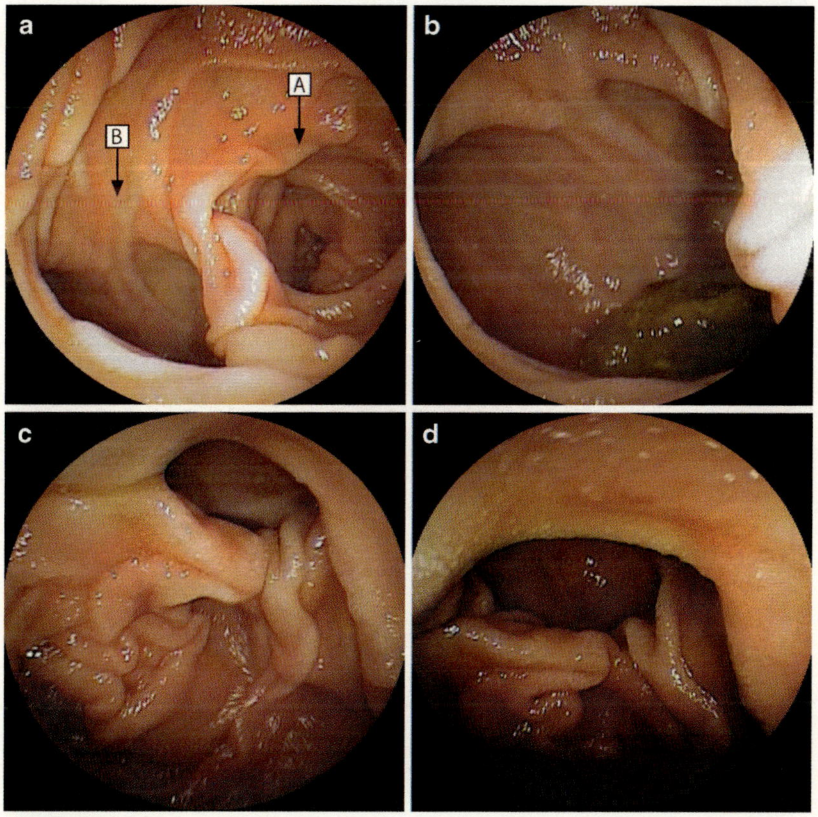

Fig. 27.1

K. Abe (✉)
Department of Gastroenterology and Medicine, Fukuoka University Faculty of Medicine, 7-45-1 Nanakuma, Jonan-ku, Fukuoka 814-0180, Japan
e-mail: k.abe@minf.med.fukuoka-u.ac.jp

T. Matsui et al. (eds.), *Endoscopy in the Diagnosis of Small Intestine Diseases*, DOI 10.1007/978-4-431-54352-7_27, © Springer Japan 2014

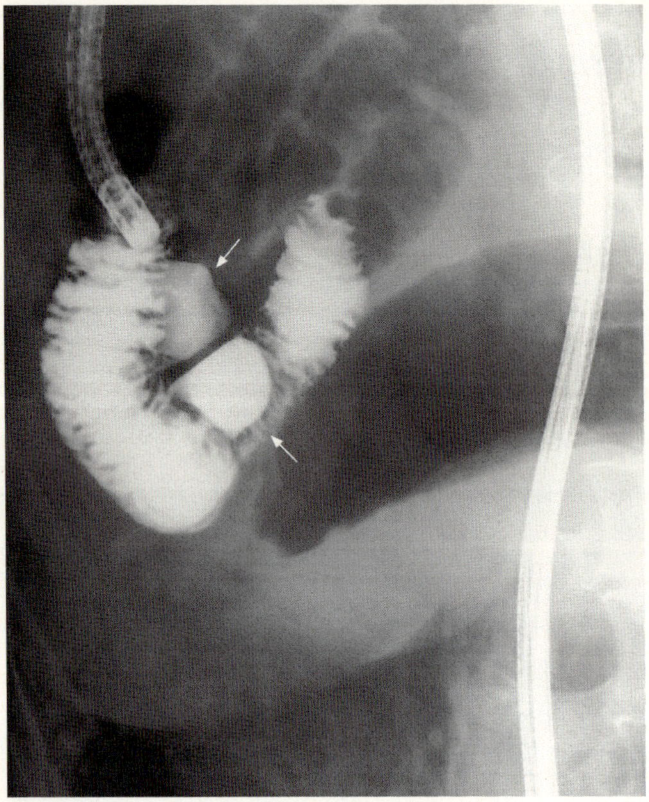

Fig. 27.2 Two contrast-enhanced cystic diverticula were visible in the proximal jejunum

27.1.2 Diverticulum of the Small Intestine (Fig. 27.2)

- In this condition, part of the small intestinal wall protrudes in a cystic manner on the serosal side.
- Diverticula of the small intestine may be true diverticula, in which all the layers of the intestinal tract (mucosa, muscle layer, and serosa) protrude, or pseudodiverticula, which lack the muscle layer. Other than Meckel's diverticulum, all diverticula of the small intestine are pseudodiverticula.
- This condition is common in older people, and occurs more frequently in the proximal jejunum.
- Although many cases are asymptomatic, bleeding, diverticulitis, perforation, intestinal obstruction, and nutritional impairment may occur.
- In small intestinal contrast enhancement, diverticula are enhanced as round, half-round, or cystic protrusions.

Reference

1. Ohmiya N et al. Diagnosis and treatment of obscure GI bleeding at double balloon endoscopy. Gastrointest Endosc. 2007;66(3 Suppl):S72–7.

Part III

Basic Knowledge and Classification

28 On Tumors

Shotaro Nakamura

This is the general classification used in Japan (Table 28.1) [1].

This is the most recent international classification of gastrointestinal tumors (Table 28.2) [2].

S. Nakamura (✉)
Department of Medicine and Clinical Science, Graduate School of Medical Sciences, Kyushu University, 3-1-1 Maidashi, Higashi-ku, Fukuoka 812-8582, Japan
e-mail: shonaka@intmed2.med.kyushu-u.ac.jp

T. Matsui et al. (eds.), *Endoscopy in the Diagnosis of Small Intestine Diseases*, DOI 10.1007/978-4-431-54352-7_28,

Table 28.1 Histological classification of small intestinal tumors [1]

A. Epithelial neoplasms	
1. Benign	1. Adenoma
	2. Adenomatosis
2. Malignant	1. Adenocarcinoma
	2. Mucinous cancer
	3. Signet-ring cell carcinoma
	4. Undifferentiated cancer
B. Endocrine neoplasms	Carcinoid tumor
C. Non-epithelial neoplasms	
1. Benign	1. Lipoma
	2. Lymphangioma
	3. Hemangioma
	4. Leiomyoma
	5. Neurogenic tumors
2. Malignant	1. GIST
	2. Leiomyosarcoma
	3. Neurogenic tumors
	4. Kaposi's sarcoma
D. Lymphatic neoplasms	Malignant lymphomas
	1. MALT lymphoma
	2. Follicular lymphoma
	3. Mantle cell lymphoma
	4. Diffuse large B-cell lymphoma
	5. Burkitt lymphoma
	6. T-cell lymphoma
E. Secondary neoplasms	Metastatic tumors
F. Tumorous lesions	1. Hamartoma
	2. Brunner's gland hyperplasia
	3. Inflammatory fibroid polyp (IFP)
	4. Benign lymphatic polyp
	5. Intestinal endometriosis

Quoted from reference [1] under the permission of the publisher

Table 28.2 WHO classification of tumors of the small intestine [2]

Epithelial tumors
Premalignant lesions
Adenoma
Tubular
Villous
Tubulovillous
Dysplasia (intraepithelial neoplasm), low-grade
Dysplasia (intraepithelial neoplasm), high-grade
Hamartomas
Juvenile polyp
Peutz-Jeghers polyp
Carcinoma
Adenocarcinoma
Mucinous adenocarcinoma
Signet-ring cell carcinoma
Adenosquamous carcinoma
Medullary carcinoma
Squamous cell carcinoma
Undifferentiated carcinoma
Neuroendocrine neoplasms
Neuroendocrine tumor (NET)
NET G1 (carcinoid)
NET G2
Neuroendocrine carcinoma (NEC)
Large-cell NEC
Small-cell NEC
Mixed adenoneuroendocrine carcinoma
Enterochromaffin (EC) cell, serotonin-producing NET
Gangliocytic paraganglioma
Gastrinoma
L-cell, Glucagon-like peptide-producing or PP/PYY-producing NET
Somatostatin-producing NET
Mesenchymal tumors
Leiomyoma
Lipoma
Angiosarcoma
Gastrointestinal stromal tumor (GIST)
Kaposi sarcoma
Leiomyosarcoma
Lymphomas
Secondary tumors

Quoted from reference [2] under the permission of the publisher

This is the most recent international classification of malignant lymphomas (Table 28.3) [3].

This is a modified version of the Ann Arbor classification generally used for malignant lymphomas, and use of this classification is recommended for gastrointestinal lymphomas (Table 28.4 and Fig. 28.1) [4, 5].

Table 28.3 WHO classification of tumors of lymphoid tissues (seen in the small intestine) [3]

Precursor lymphoid neoplasms
B lymphoblastic leukemia/lymphoma
T lymphoblastic leukemia/lymphoma
Mature B-cell neoplasms
Chronic lymphocytic leukemia/small lymphocytic lymphoma
B-cell prolymphocytic leukemia
Lymphoplasmacytic lymphoma (Waldenström macroglobulinemia)
Heavy-chain disease
α-Heavy chain disease (immunoproliferative small intestinal disease, IPSID)
γ-Heavy chain disease
μ-Heavy chain disease
Plasma cell myeloma
Extraosseous plasmacytoma
Extranodal marginal zone lymphoma of mucosa-associated lymphoid tissue (MALT lymphoma)
Follicular lymphoma
Mantle cell lymphoma
Diffuse large B-cell lymphoma
Burkitt lymphoma
B-cell lymphoma, unclassifiable
Mature T-cell or NK-cell neoplasms
T-cell prolymphocytic leukemia
Aggressive NK-cell leukemia/lymphoma
Systemic EBV-positive T-cell lymphoproliferative disease of childhood
Adult T-cell leukemia/lymphoma
Extranodal NK/T-cell lymphoma, nasal type
Enteropathy-associated T-cell lymphoma
Hepatosplenic T-cell lymphoma
Peripheral T-cell lymphoma, NOS (not other specified)
Angioimmunoblastic T-cell lymphoma
Anaplastic large cell lymphoma, ALK positive or negative

Neoplasms that commonly occur in the gastrointestinal tract are underlined

Quoted from reference [3] under the permission of the publisher

Table 28.4 Clinical staging of gastrointestinal lymphomas: the Lugano International Conference classification [4]

	Localized to the gastrointestinal tract with no serosal infiltration
	1 Single
Stage I	2. Multiple (non-secondary)
Stage II	Invasion of the peritoneum from the primary site, lymph node infiltration
	1. II1 Infiltration of regional lymph nodes (gastric or intestinal regional lymph nodes)
	2. II2 Infiltration of distant lymph nodes (para-aortic, para-inferior vena cava, pelvic cavity, and mesenteric lymph nodes)
Stage II E[a]	Infiltration of adjacent organs with serosal infiltration
	1. Penetration, direct infiltration
	2. Perforation, peritonitis
Stage IV	Widespread dissemination into extranodular organs or infiltration of lymph nodes beyond the diaphragm

[a]Stage III is not defined, with "E" standing for "Extending"

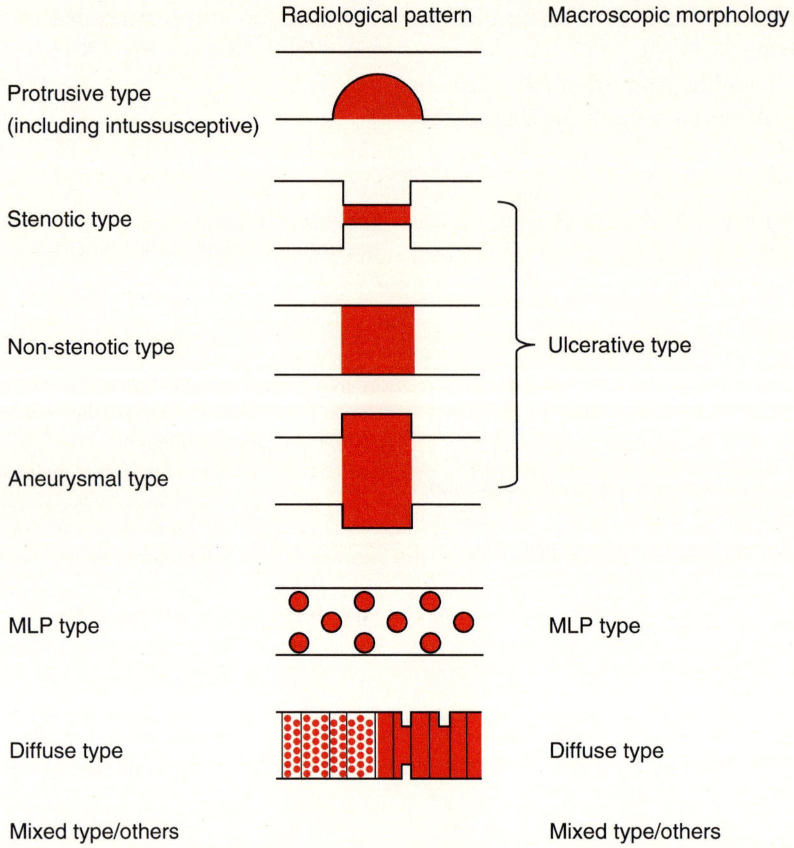

Fig. 28.1 Radiological patterns and macroscopic classifications of small intestinal malignant lymphomas [5]

Table 28.5 GIST risk classification

	Tumor size	Mitotic count*
Very low risk	<2 cm	<5/50 HPF
Low risk	2–5 cm	<5/50 HPF
Intermediate risk	<5 cm	6–10/50 HPF
	5–10 cm	<5/50 HPF
High risk	>5 cm	>5/50 HPF
	>10 cm	Any mitotic rate
	Any size	>10/50 HPF

*The number of tumor cells exhibiting mitosis per 50 high-power fields (HPF) [6]

In the absence of an internationally accepted classification, this classification is used comparatively frequently in Japan.

This is the standard internationally used classification (Table 28.5 and Fig 28.2) [6, 7].

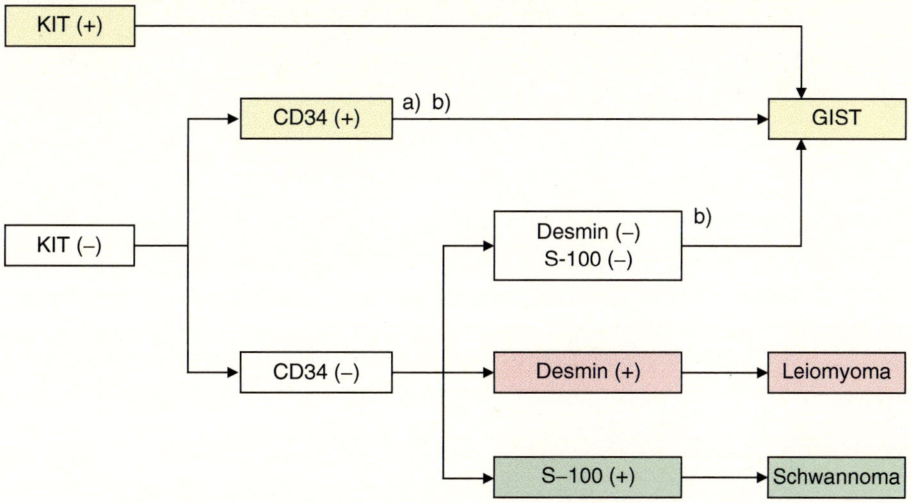

Fig. 28.2 Differentiation of major gastrointestinal mesenchymal cell tumors by immunohistochemical staining. (**a**) Must be distinguished from solitary fibrous tumor. (**b**) In this case, C-kit and PDGFRA point mutation screening is useful for diagnosis [7]

References

1. Jass JR, Sobin LH. WHO International histological classification of tumours. In: Histological Typing of Intestinal Tumours, 2nd edn. Springer-Verlag; 1989. p. 5–6.
2. Shepherd NA et al. Chapter 6, Tumours of the small intestisne. In: Bosman FT, Carneiro F, HrubanRH, et al. editors. WHO Classification of Tumours of the Digestive System, 4th edn. IARC: Lyon; 2010. p. 95–118.
3. Swerdlow SH et al., editors. WHO Classification of Tumours of Haematopoietic and Lymphoid Tissues. 4th ed. IARC: Lyon; 2008.
4. Rohatiner A et al. Report on a workshop convened to discuss the pathological and staging classifications of gastrointestinal tract lymphoma. Ann Oncol. 1994;5:397–400.
5. Yao T et al., editors. Shocho Shikkan no Rinsho. Igaku Shoin: Tokyo; 2004. p. 340 (in Japanese).
6. Fletcher CD et al. Diagnosis of gastrointestinal stromal tumors: a consensus approach. Hum Pathol. 2002;33:459–65.
7. JSCO, JGCA, Japanese Study Group on GIST, editors. In: GIST Shinryo Guideline, 2nd edn. Kanehara Shuppan: Tokyo; 2010. p. 7 (in Japanese).

29 On Inflammation

Takashi Hisabe

Inflammatory diseases of the small intestine are diagnosed overall by taking into account clinical symptoms, general test results, and imaging findings (Table 29.1).

Chronic non-specific multiple ulcers of the small intestine display specific findings in terms of the distribution of lesions and macroscopic morphology (Table 29.2).

A detailed medical history, including types of food eaten and the incubation period, is required when diagnosing infectious diseases of the small intestine (Table 29.3).

Radiographic images of the small intestine enable an objective evaluation of the sites and distribution of lesions, deformity of the intestinal tract, and changes over time (Tables 29.4 and 29.5).

A severity classification in line with the classification of the European Crohn's and Colitis Organization (ECCO) was added when the diagnostic guidelines were revised (Table 29.6).

The CDAI is the most widely used activity index based on clinical symptoms (Table 29.7).

CDEIS is an activity index based on endoscopic findings mainly of large intestinal lesions (Table 29.8 and 29.9).

Rutgeerts score is an activity index based on endoscopic findings of postoperative recurrence in the terminal part of the ileum (Table 29.10).

The Fukuoka index is an activity index based on imaging findings of lesions in the small and large intestine (Tables 29.11).

The Kuromaru classification is a widely known classification indicating the patterns of development of intestinal tuberculosis (Table 29.13 and Fig. 29.1).

All three of the criteria listed in Table 29.14 must be met.

Although many diseases cause protein-losing gastroenteropathy, they can be classified according to the three main causes in Table 29.15.

T. Hisabe (✉)
Department of Gastroenterology, Fukuoka University Chikushi Hospital, 1-1-1 Zokumyoin, Chikushino 818-8502, Japan
e-mail: hisabe@cis.fukuoka-u.ac.jp

T. Matsui et al. (eds.), *Endoscopy in the Diagnosis of Small Intestine Diseases*, DOI 10.1007/978-4-431-54352-7_29, © Springer Japan 2014

Table 29.1 Inflammatory diseases of the small intestine

Non-specific		Crohn's disease, ulcerative colitis, intestinal Behçet disease, simple ulcer, chronic non-specific multiple ulcers of the small intestine, eosinophilic gastroenteritis, etc.
Infectious		
	Bacterial	Yersinia enteritis, Campylobacter enteritis, Salmonella enteritis, intestinal typhoid fever, intestinal tuberculosis, etc.
	Protozoan	Giardiasis, isosporiasis
	Parasitic	Strongyloidiasis, anisakiasis, etc.
Vascular		Ischemic enteropathy, etc.
Iatrogenic		Antibiotic-induced enteritis, NSAID-induced enteritis, radiation enteritis, etc.
Others, inflammation due to systemic disease		Amyloidosis, Schönlein-Henoch purpura, systemic lupus erythematosus, systemic sclerosis, etc.

Table 29.2 Clinical findings of typical non-specific small intestinal inflammatory diseases

Disease	Common site	Distribution of lesions	Macroscopic morphology
Crohn's disease	Ileum, terminal part of the ileum (mesenteric side)	Discontinuous, segmental	Longitudinal ulcers, cobblestone appearance, irregular to oval or round-shaped ulcers, multiple aphthae, unilateral stenosis
Ulcerative colitis		Continuous	Diffuse redness, erosions, small ulcers
Intestinal Behçet disease	Terminal part of the ileum (antimesenteric side)	Segmental	Typical lesions are punched-out ulcers, atypical lesions may be oval or round-shaped ulcers or aphthous ulcers
Chronic non-specific multiple ulcers of the small intestine	Ileum	Segmental	Unilateral circular or oblique clearly demarcated ulcers, multiple asymmetric lesions
Eosinophilic gastroenteritis		Segmental	Mucosal edema, redness, erosions

Table 29.3 Clinical findings of typical small intestinal infectious diseases

Disease	Pathogen	Incubation period	Common site	Macroscopic morphology
Campylobacter enteritis	Campylobacter jejuni/coli	2–7 days	Ileum	Shallow ulceration on the ileocecal valve, ileal redness and erosions
Intestinal typhoid or paratyphoid fever	Salmonella typhi/paratyphi	7–14 days	Terminal part of the ileum (antimesenteric side)	Erosions, oval or round-shaped ulcers
Salmonella enteritis	Salmonella enteriditis/typhimurium	8–48 h	Terminal part of the ileum	Edema, erosions
Yersinia enteritis	Yersinia enterocolitica/pseudotuberculosis	1–10 days	Terminal part of the ileum	Enlarged Peyer's patches, erosions, small ulcers
Strongyloidiasis	Strongyloides stercoralis		Upper jejunum	Diffuse mucosal edema, coarse mucosa, erosions
Giardiasis	Giardia lamblia	10–14 days	Upper jejunum	Redness, granular mucosa
Anisakiasis	Anisakis simplex	8–48 h		Mucosal edema
Intestinal tuberculosis	Mycobacterium tuberculosis		Ileum (antimesenteric side)	Circular/girdle-like ulcers

Table 29.4 Radiographic characteristics of small intestinal inflammatory and non-neoplastic diseases

Disease	Distribution	Marginal appearance	Appearance of folds	Mucosal appearance
Acute infectious diseases				
Vibrio enteritis	Segmental, continuous	Segmental edema	Edematous thickening	Normal
Salmonella, Campylobacter enteritis	Segmental, continuous	Segmental edema	Edematous thickening	Mostly normal (multiple protrusions)
Yersinia enteritis, Intestinal typhoid fever	Segmental	Segmental edema	Edematous thickening	Multiple protrusions, barium flecks
Anisakiasis	Regional	Edematous stenosis	Irregular, severe thickening	Normal, parasites visualized
Chronic infections				
Intestinal tuberculosis	Segmental, multiple	Concentric stenosis	Thickening, convergence, loss	Areas of atrophic scarring, barium flecks
Giardiasis	Diffuse	Diffuse edema	Thickening, loss	Mostly normal (mildly granular)
Strongyloidiasis, Isosporiosis	Diffuse	Diffuse edema	Thickening, loss	Granular mucosa, fine barium flecks
Acute inflammatory diseases				
Eosinophilic enteritis	Segmental	Segmental edema	Irregular thickening	Multiple mucosal barium flecks
Ischemic enteritis	Segmental	Thumbprinting sign, tubular stenosis	Edematous thickening	Granular shadows at site of ulcerative stenosis
Allergic purpura	Segmental	Segmental edema	Moderate to severe thickening	Multiple barium flecks
Chronic inflammatory diseases				
Radiation enteritis	Segmental	Tubular stenosis	Moderate thickening	Atrophic mucosa, barium flecks
NSAID-induced small intestinal ulceration	Segmental	Concentric stenosis	Convergence of folds	Normal

Table 29.5 Crohn's disease diagnostic criteria in Japan [1]

1. Major findings	A. Longitudinal ulcer[a] B. Cobblestone appearance C. Non-caseating epithelioid cell granuloma[b]
2. Secondary findings	a. Irregular to oval or round-shaped ulcers or aphthae across a wide area of gastrointestinal tract[c] b. Characteristic anal lesions[d] c. Characteristic gastric/duodenal lesions[e]
Confirmed cases	
1. Patients with major findings A or B[f]	
2. Patients with major finding C and secondary findings a or b	
3. Patients with all of secondary findings a, b, and c	
Suspected cases	
1. Patients with major finding C and secondary finding	
2. Patients with major findings A or B, but who cannot be differentiated from ischemic intestinal lesions or ulcerative colitis	
3. Patients with major finding C only[g]	
4. Patients with one or two secondary findings	

Quoted from reference [1]

[a]In the small intestine, lesions tend to occur on the mesenteric side

[b]Production of a series of continuous sections improves the diagnostic rate. If possible, the determination should be made by a pathologist familiar with the gastrointestinal tract

[c]Lesions are typically longitudinal, but this is not always the case. They must also persist for at least 3 months. Intestinal tuberculosis, intestinal Behçet disease, simple ulcer, NSAID ulceration, and infectious enterocolitis must also be excluded

[d]Anal fissure, cavitating ulcer, anal fistula, perianal abscess, edematous skin tags, etc. Refer to an atlas of macroscopic findings of anal lesions in Crohn's disease, and if possible the diagnosis should be made by a specialist proctologist familiar with Crohn's disease

[e]Bamboo-joint sign, notched depressions, etc. If possible, the diagnosis should be made by a specialist familiar with Crohn's disease

[f]If only longitudinal ulcers are present, ischemic intestinal lesions and ulcerative colitis must be excluded. If only a cobblestone appearance is present, ischemic intestinal lesions must be excluded

[g]Intestinal tuberculosis and other inflammatory diseases that cause granuloma must be excluded

Table 29.6 Crohn's disease severity classification [1]

	CDAI[a]	Complications	Inflammation (CRP level)	Response to treatment
Mild	150–220	None	Slightly elevated	
Moderate	220–450	No obvious intestinal obstruction, etc.	Obviously elevated	No response to treatment for mild cases
Severe	450<	Intestinal obstruction, abscess, etc.	Highly elevated	Poor response to treatment

[a]CDAI: Crohn's disease activity index
Quoted from reference [1]

Table 29.7 Crohn's disease activity index (CDAI) [2]

1. Number of liquid or soft stools over the past 7 days
2. Total score for abdominal pain over the past 7 days
0 = none, 1 = mild, 2 = moderate, 3 = severe
3. Total score for general wellbeing over the past 7 days
0 = well, 1 = not very well, 2 = poor, 3 = bad, 4 = terrible
4. Findings and symptoms attributable to Crohn's disease
One point added to the total for each of items 1–6
(a) Arthritis or joint pain
(b) Cutaneous or oral lesions (pyoderma gangrenosum, erythema nodosum, etc.)
(c) Iritis or uveitis
(d) Anal fissure, anal fistula, or perianal abscess
(e) Other fistula (e.g., intestinovesical fistula)
(f) Fever exceeding 37.8°C during the past 7 days
5. Use of lopemin or opiates for diarrhea
0 = no, 1 = yes
6. Abdominal tumor
0 = no, 1 = yes
7. Hematocrit
Males = 47–hematocrit level, females = 42–hematocrit level
8. Percentage deviation from standard weight
100 × (1–(weight/standard weight)

Quoted from reference [2]

Table 29.8 Crohn's disease endoscopic index of severity (CDEIS) [3]

1. ISRCF (Individual segmental rectocolonic frequency of deep ulceration)[a]
X1 = (number of segments[b] with deep ulceration)/(number of segments observed)
2. ISRCF (Individual segmental rectocolonic frequency of superficial ulceration)
X2 = (number of segments with superficial ulceration)/(number of segments observed)
3. ASSD (Average segmental surfaces involved by the disease (cm2), including ulcerative lesions)[c]
X3 = (sum of surface area of lesions on segmental surface (cm2))/(segmental surface area observed)
4. ASSU (Average segmental surfaces involved by ulcerations only (cm2)[d])
X4 = (sum of surface area of ulceration on segmental surface (cm2))/(segmental surface area observed)
5. PRES (presence or absence of non-ulcerated stenosis)
X5 = presence or absence of non-ulcerated stenosis in the segments observed
0 = no, 1 = yes
6. PRES (presence or absence of ulcerated stenosis)
X6 = presence or absence of ulcerated stenosis in the segments observed
0 = no, 1 = yes

Quoted from reference [3]
[a]ISRCF is calculated by dividing the number of segments that contain lesions by the number of segments observed. ISRCF values range between 0 (no lesions in any segment observed) and 1 (lesions in all segments observed)
[b]Segments comprise the rectum, sigmoid colon and left large intestine, transverse colon, right colon, and ileum
[c]A 10-cm linear analog scale is used to evaluate the percentages of the segmental surface area occupied by the nine lesions included in the list of mucosal lesions below and by ulcerative lesions alone
0: No lesion or ulcerative lesions present
10: Lesions or ulcerative lesions occupying the entire segmental surface
[d]Ulcerative lesions comprise aphthous ulceration, superficial ulceration, deep ulceration, and ulcerated stenosis

Table 29.9 Crohn's disease endoscopic index of severity (CDEIS) [3]

List of nine mucosal lesions	
1. Pseudopolyp	
2. Healed ulceration	Whitish area with a "ground glass" appearance
3. Frank erythema (plaques, bands, or diffuse)	Slight or moderate erythema should be neglected
4. Frankly swollen mucosa	Slight or moderate mucosal swelling should be neglected
5. Aphthoid ulceration	Defined as a tiny (2–3 mm) raised or flat red lesion with a white center
6. Superficial or shallow ulceration	Defined as any ulceration that is neither aphthoid nor deep
7. Deep ulceration	Only frankly deep ulceration should be recorded under this heading
8. Non-ulcerated stenosis	Should be impossible or difficult to pass with an adult endoscope
9. Ulcerated stenosis	Should be impossible or difficult to pass with an adult endoscope

Quoted from reference [3]

Table 29.10 Rutgeerts score [4]

	Score
No lesions in the distal ileum	0
Less than five aphthous lesions	1
Five or more aphthous lesions with normal mucosa between lesions, or skip lesions or lesions confined to ileocolonic anastomosis (<1 cm in length)	2
Diffuse aphthous ileitis with diffusely inflamed mucosa	3
Diffuse inflammation with already larger ulcers, nodules, and/or narrowing	4

Quoted from reference [4]

Table 29.11 Fukuoka index

Protruding lesions (cobblestone appearance or inflammatory polyps)	
0	None
1	Sparse inflammatory polyps only
2	Scattered lesions
3	Lesions intermediate between sparse and dense or densely packed in a narrow area (length <4 cm)
4	Densely packed across a comparatively wide area
Ulcerative lesions (longitudinal ulcers, irregularly shaped ulcers, or scarring)[a]	
0	None
1	Scarring
2	Unknown whether open ulcer or scarring has occurred
3	Active longitudinal ulcer with transverse diameter <5 mm or shallow, broad, irregularly shaped ulcer
4	Active longitudinal ulcer with transverse diameter ≥5 mm or clearly demarcated, deep, broad, irregularly shaped ulcer
Stenosis[b]	
0	None
1	No dilation on the proximal side of the stenosis, with the width of the lumen in the stenotic area at least half that of the adjacent normal intestine
2	No dilation on the proximal side, with lumen width in the stenotic area being less than half
3	Pronounced narrowing of the lumen, with dilation of the intestine on the proximal side

Quoted from reference [5]

The small intestine is divided into four segments comprising the upper, middle, and lower small intestine and the terminal ileum (around 30 cm from the ileocecal valve), and the severities of protruding lesions, ulcerative lesions, and stenosis are scored for each segment

[a]Ulcers ≥5 cm in length are regarded as longitudinal ulcers, and those <5 cm in length are regarded as irregularly shaped ulcers

[b]Stenosis is determined on double-contrast images with an adequate amount of insufflation

Table 29.12 Pouchitis disease activity index (PDAI) [6]

Clinical findings	Endoscopic findings	Histological findings
Stool frequency	Edema 1	Multinuclear leukocyte infiltration
Usual stool frequency 0	Coarse granular mucosa 1	Mild 1
1–2 stools/day > usual frequency 1	Friability 1	Moderate + crypt abscess 2
3 or more stools/day > usual frequency 2	Loss of vascular pattern 1	Severe + crypt abscess 3
Anal bleeding	Mucus exudates 1	Ulceration (low-power field)
None or rare 0	Ulceration 1	<25 % 1
Present daily 1		25–50 % 2
Frequent bowel movements or abdominal pain		>50 % 3
None 0		
Occasional 1		
Usual 2		
Fever (≥37.8°C)		
Absent 0		
Present 1		

Quoted from reference [6]
Pouchitis is diagnosed for total score ≥7

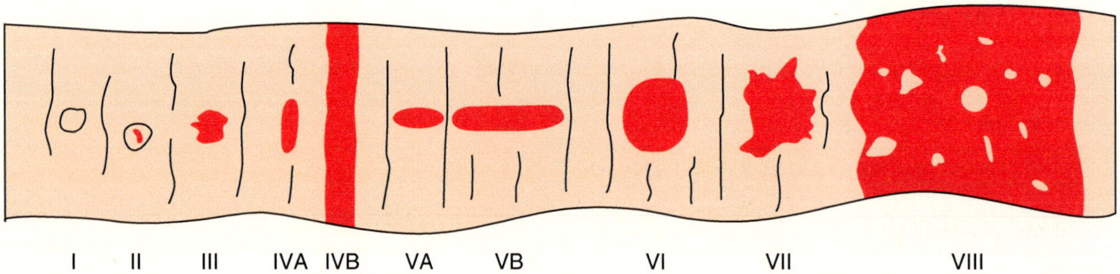

Fig. 29.1

Table 29.13 Macroscopic classification of intestinal tuberculosis [7]

Type I	Early lesions, tuberculous nodules the size of grains of millet or hemp seeds
Type II	Tuberculous nodules become necrotic; necrotic substances break down the mucosa and are released into the lumen, forming small ulcers
Type III	Type II small ulcers enlarge to the size of azuki beans or almonds
Type IV	Ulcers elongate along the transverse axis of the intestinal canal, progressing to form circular or girdle-like ulcers.
	(A: longest diameter ≤2 cm; B: longest diameter ≥2 cm)
Type V	Ulcers elongated along the longitudinal axis of the intestinal canal
	(A: longest diameter ≤2 cm; B: longest diameter ≥2 cm)
Type VI	Round or oval ulcers larger than the size of an almond
Type VII	Irregularly shaped ulcers larger than the size of an almond
Type VIII	Ulcers have fused together to form widespread ulceration

Quoted from reference [7]

Table 29.14 Eosinophilic gastroenteritis diagnostic criteria [8]

1. Presence of gastrointestinal symptoms
2. Biopsy demonstrating eosinophil infiltration of at least one site in the gastrointestinal tract, or eosinophilia of peripheral blood together with characteristic radiological findings
3. Exclusion of parasitic infection and other conditions that exhibit eosinophilia

Quoted from reference [8]

Table 29.15 Diseases causing protein-losing gastroenteropathy

1. Lymphostasis	Primary intestinal lymphangiectasia, retroperitoneal fibrosis, Whipple's disease
2. Gastrointestinal mucosal damage	Crohn's disease, non-specific multiple ulcers of the small intestine, amyloidosis, celiac disease, drug-induced enteritis, radiation enteritis, infectious enteritis, parasitic enteritis
3. Unknown mechanism, enhanced capillary permeability	Rheumatoid arthritis, systemic scleroderma, systemic lupus erythematosus, Sjögren's syndrome, eosinophilic gastroenteritis

References

1. Ueno F et al. Evidence-based clinical practice guidelines for Crohn's disease, integrated with formal consensus of experts in Japan. J Gastroenterol. 2013; 48:31–72.
2. Best WR, Becktel JM, Singleton JW, Kern F. Development of a Crohn's disease activity index. Gastroenterology. 1976;70:439–44.
3. Mary JY et al. Development and validation of an endoscopic index of the severity for Crohn's disease: a prospective multicentre study. Group d'Etudes Thepapeutiques des Affections Inflammatoires du Tube Digestif (GETAID). Gut. 1989;30:983–9.
4. Rutgeerts P et al. Predictability of the postoperative course of Crohn's disease. Gastroenterology. 1990;99:956–63.
5. Sou S et al. Clinical and endoscopic healing after infliximab treatment in patients with Crohn's disease. Dig Endosc. 2006;18: 29–33.
6. Sanborn WJ et al. Pouchitis after ileal pouch-anal anastomosis: a Pouchitis Disease Activity Index. Mayo Clin Proc. 1994;69:409–15.
7. Kuromaru G. Pathology of the intestinal tuberculosis. Tokyo: Igakushoin; 1952. p.28 (in Japanese).
8. Tally NJ et al. Eosinophilic gastroenteritis: A clinicopathological study of patients with disease of the mucosa, muscle layer, and subserosal tissue. Gut. 1990;31:54–8.

Index

T. Matsui et al. (eds.), *Endoscopy in the Diagnosis of Small Intestine Diseases*,
DOI 10.1007/978-4-431-54352-7, © Springer Japan 2014

Printed by Printforce, the Netherlands